FIGHTING FOR
HEALTH

The *History of Medicine in Southeast Asia* Series promotes academic research in all aspects of the history of medicine and health in Southeast Asia from the ancient to modern times. In order to foster closer fellowship among medical historians and greater cooperation among scholars and students, especially those practicing in the region, it provides a forum for the international exchange of research on various topics from the history of traditional medicine to the postcolonial fate of biomedicine in the region. Both monographs and edited volumes will be considered.

Series Editor: Laurence Monnais

FIGHTING FOR HEALTH

Medicine in Cold War Southeast Asia

Edited by

C. Michele Thompson,
Kathryn Sweet & Michitake Aso

NUS PRESS
SINGAPORE

© 2024 C. Michele Thompson, Kathryn Sweet & Michitake Aso

Published by:

NUS Press
National University of Singapore
AS3-01-02, 3 Arts Link
Singapore 117569
Fax: (65) 6774-0652
E-mail: nusbooks@nus.edu.sg
Website: http://nuspress.nus.edu.sg

ISBN: 978-981-325-256-1 (paper)
ePDF ISBN: 978-981-325-257-8
ePub: 978-981-325-276-9

National Library Board, Singapore Cataloguing in Publication Data
Name(s): Thompson, Claudia Michele, editor. | Sweet, Kathryn, editor. |
    Aso, Michitake, editor.
Title: Fighting for health : medicine in Cold War Southeast Asia / edited by
    C. Michele Thompson, Kathryn Sweet & Michitake Aso.
Other Title(s): History of medicine in Southeast Asia series.
Description: Singapore : NUS Press, [2024]
Identifier(s): ISBN 978-981-325-256-1 (paperback) |
    ISBN 978-981-325-257-8 (PDF) | 978-981-325-276-9 (ePub)
Subject(s): LCSH: Public health—Southeast Asia—History—20th century. |
    Medical care—Southeast Asia—History—20th century. | Medical policy—
    Southeast Asia—History—20th century. | Cold War.
Classification: DDC 362.10959—dc23

Cover image: The photo depicts a young, ethnic woman (possibly Khmu, based on her clothing) in the uplands of northern Laos in the mid-1970s. She is carrying a medical first aid kit on her front, and a pack loaded with rocket-propelled grenades (RPGs) on her back. Source: Lao News Agency/KPL archives, Vientiane.

Typeset by: Westchester Publishing Services UK
Printed by: Integrated Books International

Contents

List of Illustrations

Figures

Maps

Tables

Acknowledgments

The inspiration for this volume came from John Harley Warner, who noted on several occasions that the history of health and medicine during the Cold War in Southeast Asia would make a fascinating book. This book began to take shape during subsequent meetings of the History of Medicine in Southeast Asia (HOMSEA) group in Vientiane and Jakarta. The editors of this volume would like to thank the organizers of both of those conferences and the officers and editorial board of HOMSEA for their encouragement and support. We would also like to thank C. Michele Thompson's graduate assistant Elias Papadimitriou for his work on the bibliography, glossary and index for this volume. The outside readers of this volume offered valuable insights to all of our contributors and the staff of the NUS Press has been uniformly informative and encouraging.

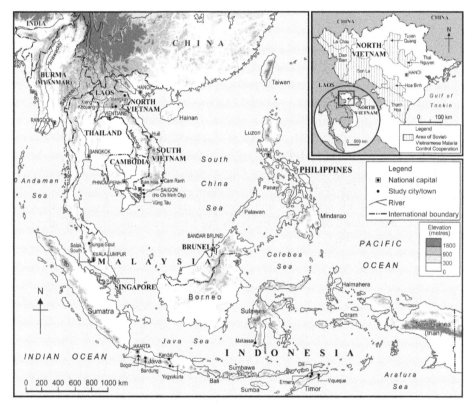

Frontispiece Map 1 Cold War Southeast Asia c. 1965 with places mentioned in the text.

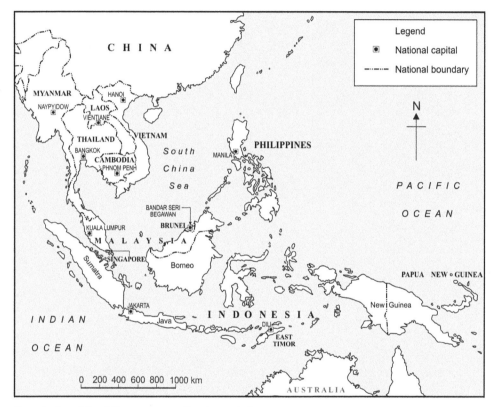

Frontispiece Map 2 Contemporary Southeast Asia.

INTRODUCTION

History of Medicine Inflected by COVID-19

As with all scholarship, this book is a product of its time. More than that, it is an argument for the need to understand medicine in its global context and to bring a historical perspective to bear on contemporary problems. As of November 2022, over 600 million people have been infected with SARS-CoV-2, the coronavirus that causes COVID-19. Of these people, around 6.6 million have died from the disease. These numbers are surely minimums as many cases have passed unconfirmed, or unnoticed, and there are many incentives to undercount cases and deaths. In addition, several vaccines have been rapidly developed and brought to market, and close to 13 billion doses given. Yet, 30 long months into the pandemic, new variants of SARS-CoV-2 most likely mean that the virus will pose a threat into the future.[1]

The effects of the COVID-19 pandemic extend beyond the biological to the economic, political, cultural and social. A moment early in 2020 foreshadowed some of these effects. The cruise ship MS *Westerdam* was turned away from multiple ports because of fears that its passengers were infected with SARS-CoV-2 after having docked at Hong Kong. When Cambodian leader Hun Sen ordered Sihanoukville to accept the cruise ship, his act was celebrated by the World Health Organization (WHO) and Cambodians were proud that their country had carried out such a humane act. Yet, Hun Sen was also criticized for prioritizing his relationship with China over the health of the Cambodians and others around the world. Moreover, Hun Sen's refusal to wear a mask signaled his denial of the seriousness of the disease and foreshadowed later debates about the need for preventive equipment, resources and protocols. Finally, the pandemic put a temporary halt to the mass tourism represented by the cruise ship and the jet travel that enabled its passengers to make their ways home.[2] The subsequent, though ephemeral, celebrations in the national media in Southeast Asia of zero or low death rates also suggested trends in the politics of the pandemic that would develop more fully later on.[3]

From the beginning of this pandemic, people have searched for explanations of the progress of the virus and the relative success or failure of countries in dealing with it. These explanations have been based on several factors: differences in medical precautions, such as quarantines and lockdowns; comparative politics, including an analysis of the competence of government response and the politics of mask wearing; and more abstract categories such as communal versus individualistic societies and other sterile dichotomies. Some commentators have worried about, or even argued for in the case of China, the necessity of a medical authoritarianism, a question historians of medicine have long examined.

More fruitful questions grounded in the past have been posed about how understandings of previous outbreaks have framed individual and social responses. The most common analogy made has been with the 2003–04 severe acute respiratory syndrome (SARS) outbreak. There are good reasons for this comparison. While SARS-CoV-1 infected and killed relatively few people, it restricted travel and made a big impact on the awareness of individuals and governments in Asia.[4] Others have gone further back in time to the influenza pandemic that began in 1918, which killed an estimated minimum of 30 million people. Indeed, there are many similarities, from the images of masked populations to widespread fear, while the diagnostic technologies, vaccine development capacities, international organizations, speed of travel and wartime context are just a few of the important differences.[5]

The co-editors of this volume originally conceived of it as an invitation to explore medicine and health in Southeast Asia during the Cold War (1945–91). We had four objectives for the book. First, we saw this edited volume as a chance to reframe how histories of medicine of Southeast Asia are taught in Euro-American universities. For far too long, Southeast Asia has been treated as a static backdrop for the exploits and discoveries of Western biomedical doctors. Yet, Southeast Asians have been vital to the significant developments in the prevention and treatment of diseases that have taken place in the region. Moreover, Southeast Asia is home to a rich diversity of medical traditions that have long held lessons for global health. Second, new perspectives and methods have emerged from research presented at regional conferences, including the History of Medicine in Southeast Asia (HOMSEA) series. We hoped to use these insights to challenge dominant models of the medical humanities. Third, we wanted to foster greater inter-Asia dialogue about shared methodologies and subjects by including specialists on South Korea and China, thus moving our study of Southeast Asia beyond national and regional boundaries and past the restrictions of the area studies model.[6] Fourth, we sought to examine the intersection of the histories of development and of medicine in Southeast

Asia, as health has been one of the most powerful engines, and symbolic vessels, of development.[7]

These goals remain. However, recent circumstances have added to them a related set of questions inflected, or infected, by COVID-19. How can an exploration of the Cold War context of medicine and health in Southeast Asia shed light on the region's (and the world's) experience with COVID-19? What structures were set in place after 1945 that may have guided individual and social responses across the region? What lessons have been learned, and forgotten?[8]

We argue that looking to previous outbreaks and pandemics is not the only useful exploration of the past. Doing so encourages teleological narratives of progress. Instead, we argue that eras need to be understood on their own terms. Our volume adopts a period-focused approach to examine a period from which many of the institutions and people that have shaped the responses to COVID-19 emerged. In other words, many current trends were framed in deeper, less visible ways by the Cold War.

We also argue that the diversity of approaches to health in Cold War Southeast Asia reminds us of the possibilities, and limits, of medical intervention in the face of political, social, economic and microbial realities. More than just a source of emerging infectious diseases, the people and places of Southeast Asia have provided a clinical trial for different health regimes.

For example, while Cambodia has remained open for business during COVID-19, the Vietnamese government, like China to the north and Australia and New Zealand to the south, initially attempted a zero-COVID policy. Or take the variety of approaches to vaccines. While many Southeast Asian countries have accepted vaccines developed in China, Russia, Japan, Europe and the United States, Indonesia, Thailand and Vietnam have worked to develop their own vaccines. In other words, Southeast Asian histories of medicine and health continue to have profound implications for the contemporary moment.[9]

The chapters in our volume are organized around these arguments to throw into relief the complexities that always threaten to make a mess of neat intellectual categories. Now, let us turn to the specific Cold War contexts of these histories.

Military Medicine for Wars of Decolonization

The process of decolonization, or the proliferation of nation-states after World War II, shaped, and was shaped by, the fighting of the Cold War in Southeast Asia. More than any other world region, Southeast Asians were affected by "hot" wars. And as the cover image of our edited volume suggests, medicine played a key role in this violent process. The sprawling Indochina Wars (first, second and third), along with numerous smaller police actions and emergencies, had profound effects on medicine and health in the region. Not surprisingly, much medical effort was put into the service of the military. For example, of the 1,000 medical doctors in South Vietnam in 1966, 700 were on active duty. In 1969, 1,000 out of 1,400 physicians were in the military. This percentage increased to 90 percent by the end of the war.[10]

Government archives show the importance of war in procuring medical supplies as well. A 1954 report from the Democratic Republic of Vietnam (DRV) evaluating material received from the People's Republic of China (PRC) categorized such aid in its relationship to the First Indochina War and anticipated peace. As the DRV produced very few medical goods of its own, it needed to import them from the PRC. When negotiating the terms of this aid, the Ministry of Commerce (Bo Mau Dich) placed items into four categories: (1) things needed now, and subsequently for peacetime; (2) things needed now but not later; (3) things not needed yet but that would be needed immediately during peacetime; and (4) things needed only well into the future.[11]

While the military claimed the lion's share of medical attention, medicine could benefit as well from the resources dedicated to fighting. As Por Heong Hong notes in her chapter on the Malayan Emergency, "while medicine benefits from war, the military too seem to gain from medicine in return."[12] In a direct way, soldiers were the targets of medical advances meant to keep them fit enough to fight. In an era of "limited" war, governments and guerillas both saw the necessity of fighting diseases and improving medical techniques that affected production and war-making ability.

Civilian populations, too, could benefit medically from the efforts to win "hearts and minds." These benefits could range from new health clinics to haircuts, as John P. DiMoia notes in his chapter on the South Korean military in the Republic of Vietnam (RVN).[13] Yet just as often, resources were drained away from civilian medicine. Moreover, the violence of war created conditions conducive to the spread of disease. Migrant populations, domestic and foreign soldiers, and changed ecological conditions often led to an increase in diseases such as malaria, plague and typhus. Loose government control over villages meant that preventative measures were difficult to put in place.

Even medicine and health in countries not directly at war were affected by the violence in Mainland Southeast Asia. US soldiers stationed in Thailand and the Philippines, or on rest and relaxation (R&R) in Singapore, could bring with them venereal diseases.[14] As Por Heong Hong points out, soldiers from throughout the British Empire were brought into Malaya, a movement that threatened to spread bancroftian filariasis.[15] As several authors also note, medical personnel from allied countries traveled to war zones. People in ostensibly neutral Laos were sprayed with herbicides, including Agent Orange.[16] Diseases such as cholera and malaria that were exacerbated by war conditions threatened to spill over borders into other Southeast Asian countries. From the socialist side, communists throughout the region also drew on international medical aid.

Thus, while medicine and health in post-1945 Southeast Asia cannot be reduced to wars, they cannot be discussed without reference to this violence. As is evident in all of the chapters of this edited volume, especially those by Por Heong Hong, Kathryn Sweet and John P. DiMoia, the language of warfare became the language of healing.

State Medicine in International Relations

The Korean War, the First Indochina War, the Berlin Crisis, the Cuban Missile Crisis, the Vietnam War, the Third Indochina War—these touchstones for the Cold War in Southeast Asia roll off the tongue like the Billy Joel song.[17] While these names and dates are useful for familiar political and military framings of the Cold War, a history of health and medicine calls for a focus on different actors, frameworks and timelines.

Following work over the past decade that has shifted the sole focus off the US and the USSR in Cold War histories, our volume seeks to decenter the two superpowers while still analyzing the parts they played in Southeast Asia.[18] Thus Annick Guénel's chapter examines how Soviet experts worked with their counterparts in the Democratic Republic of Vietnam (North Vietnam) to combat malaria. As Guénel shows, Soviet aid "was not a mere material assistance, but included training, research and participation in health activities."[19] Like exchanges elsewhere in the socialist world, medical transfers in Southeast Asia were ideological, material and organizational. But Soviet aid was uneven throughout the region and our volume's chapters evaluate its effects in specific places. Likewise, even though more hegemonic, US aid, as Kathryn Sweet shows in the case of Laos, could be quite thick in some places and thin in others. Further, as Vivek Neelakantan reminds us, leaders such as Indonesia's President Soekarno often understood their best option as playing one superpower off the other.

One aspect that distinguished Southeast Asia from most other regions was the importance of China as a regional actor.[20] Many chapters in our volume show this importance. After 1949, for example, Chinese aid to the Viet Minh helped them win their war against the French. China could also provide moral support, as Por shows for the guerillas in Malaya. But the People's Republic of China was going through upheavals of its own and, as a regional power, its guidance waxed and waned and was felt (for better and for worse) most directly in countries that shared a land border with it. China did not exert the kind of medical sway over Southeast Asia that the United States exerted over Latin America in the 20th century.[21]

Another point that comes through clearly in this volume is the interaction among smaller political and military powers on both sides of the Cold War. On the capitalist side, DiMoia shows how South Koreans thought they could import a medical modernity to their anti-communist allies in South Vietnam through civic actions and construction. On the socialist side, Sweet shows how the first DRV and then the Socialist Republic of Vietnam played a key role in forming Laos' medical system, both before and after 1975. Often one individual such as Phạm Ngọc Thạch could play both the role of instructor, as Por shows in the case of a communist nurse from Malaya trained in the DRV, and of collaborator and junior partner, as Guénel shows in the case of interactions with Soviet malaria experts.[22]

The importance of South–South exchanges contributes to the burgeoning studies of the so-called Second World that compliments the previous emphasis on the internationalism of the US/West/North. Scholars have paid some attention to the political and cultural exchanges associated with socialist internationalism, the Non-Aligned Movement, Afro-Asian solidarity and the Bandung Conference.[23] Tracing the contours of medical exchange among such groups can yield rich insights, as Neelakantan's analysis of Soedjono Djoened Poesponegoro's international cooperation in pediatrics shows.[24]

The Cold War was a time when the institutions of socialist internationalism were being created and travel was an important aspect of this internationalism and the Second World.[25] Such travel included a small number of elites engaged in medical tourism and health trips. Experts also engaged in friendship projects, as analyzed by Applebaum for Czechoslovakia.[26] Similarly, Friendship hospitals were common throughout Southeast Asia, in the DRV, Cambodia and Laos.[27] Although relatively small in number, experts associated with such projects had an outsized influence, as Guénel's and Sweet's chapters show.

Medical exchanges followed, served and promoted commercial relations in both the communist and capitalist blocs as well.[28] As Fang's chapter shows, this was true of the overseas Chinese, who were viewed by the Chinese Communist Party (CCP) as both a source of danger and of valuable foreign exchange. Given this dual role, internal party documents marked returning Chinese as the source of cholera outbreaks (based on rather weak circumstantial evidence);

public pronouncements, however, attempted to avoid stigmatizing these returnees.[29] DiMoia's chapter shows how medical exchanges served South Korea's interests in expanding both its military and commercial reach. As the South Korean government set up offices of the Korea Overseas Trade Agency (KOTRA) around the world, in the RVN, it sought to apply the "lessons" it had learned on the Korean peninsula regarding health.[30] After the end of the Vietnam War, the South Korean government was quick to establish ties with its erstwhile enemy. Now the Socialist Republic of Vietnam is the fourth largest trading partner of the Republic of Korea, behind only China, the US and Japan. In return, many Vietnamese scientists, including those in the field of medicine, now receive their training and start their careers in the ROK.[31]

At the same time, there continued seemingly atavistic forms of international political organization. For example, the Marshall Plan for reconstructing Europe had repercussions in Southeast Asia through its effects on the efforts of Britain, France, Portugal and the Netherlands to hold on to their colonies, which in the case of Timor-Leste continued until 1975.[32] In addition to high politics, there were the experiences of ordinary people.[33] There were people-to-people, direct medical interactions, without the mediation of governments.

Moreover, the end of World War II triggered mass migrations which had an impact on global health. For example, large numbers of soldiers distributed throughout the Japanese Empire, including Timor-Leste and elsewhere in Southeast Asia, returned to Japan, where some compatriots feared that these survivors would bring diseases with them. The beginning of the Cold War also witnessed the migration of another kind of soldier, those working for the kingdom of God. As Por shows, after the CCP victory in 1949, British missionaries were expelled from China. There was less fear that these missionaries would bring diseases with them, but they were important for healthcare in Southeast Asia, as many of them had at least some medical training and were called upon to care for those injured and sick.[34]

During the Cold War, even as certain borders were hardening and walls were being constructed (for example the 17th and 38th parallels and the Berlin Wall), international mobility expanded in the post-1945 world. Travelers included soldiers (men), experts, entrepreneurs (mostly men) and growing numbers of tourists (including medical and sex tourists). Take soldiers for instance. As Por shows, soldiers of the British Empire brought, or were feared to have brought, diseases with them. Because of this, their bodies were viewed with suspicion, but they also received special attention and care. US soldiers, too, migrated throughout Southeast Asia during their R&R breaks, including Thailand and Singapore, bringing diseases, especially venereal diseases, with them.[35] Since the Cold War, Singapore has shed its reputation as a seedy playground for foreigners and is now considered by many scholars to be an Asian center for research and development in biomedical sciences.

It was not just American soldiers that were on the move. Chinese advisors and troops saw extensive activity in the DRV and Laos during the Vietnam War. While we know less about their experience with disease, they suffered no doubt from malaria and other diseases in an unfamiliar land.[36] On a much smaller scale, in both the socialist and capitalist arenas there were individual medical experts and in some cases whole teams of medical personnel on the move.[37] There was also elite travel for medical treatment in centers such as Beijing and Moscow.

Finally, alongside states and people, institutions operated at the international level. The Rockefeller Foundation was meaningful in its absence as its influence was largely superseded in communist-controlled areas.[38] Newer organizations such as the WHO also had to navigate ideologically tricky waters. Phạm Ngọc Thạch, considering whether or not to participate in WHO efforts, evaded the issue in 1960 by arguing that the DRV was not in a position to join.[39] Later, the WHO officially recognized the importance of socialist approaches to medicine at the Alma Ata conference on Primary Health Care in 1978.

Preventative Medicine as Nationalist Politics

The struggle for control over a nation that occurred as part of decolonization also had profound effects on medicine and health. Different factions within the boundaries of a nation, supported by either socialist or capitalist internationalism, or both, battled for the hearts and minds of people through medicine. The politics of health were complex. At times, all sides saw the benefits of a healthier population. As Por shows, Malaya's medical care providers were almost never attacked by communist forces during the emergency. At other times, health was viewed as a zero-sum game, and if one side was perceived as bringing healthcare services to the population, the other side was seen as losing, at least ideologically. Sweet shows, for example, how in Laos the provision of healthcare buttressed claims to legitimacy.[40]

Non-communist nationalists were one of these groups. These non-revolutionary reformers were often determined to create a post-colonial nation, yet they did not view communism as the proper economic system to do so. The physician often embodied the nationalist project and suffered from its tensions. Por's chapter shows how such nationalists had to navigate between imperial powers and communist revolutionaries. Many military medical doctors in the Republic of Vietnam felt similar tensions. Tran Xuan Dung received training from French and American instructors and fought against communist forces. He and Nguyen Manh Tien, medical doctors in the army of the Republic of Vietnam, both faced moments of great danger.[41]

Even physicians far behind the front lines had to position themselves with respect to the nation. Neelakantan's chapter offers a close look at three such medical doctors-cum-politicians: M. Sardjito, Sarwono Prawirohardjo and Soedjono Djoened Poesponegoro. As Neelakantan notes, one distinctive aspect of the growth of science in Indonesia "was the niche occupied by physicians."[42] Neelakantan argues that these medical doctors urged the state to address the health problems of its citizens, such as malnutrition. A productivist logic, such as articulated by M. Sardjito, was used to argue for the importance of dealing with such problems.[43] Meanwhile, in the Philippines, medical doctors and nurses had to position themselves vis-à-vis anti-communist authoritarian regimes.

With the exception of elites in Thailand, which retained its government through the upheavals of the Pacific War years, nationalists across the region had to build, or rebuild, institutions to bring their politics to fruition. In terms of medicine, this could mean embedding medical doctors in other organizations such as the military. It could also mean creating the educational and research centers of medicine. Birth control and maternal and child healthcare were both key issues.[44] Family planning was emphasized by medical doctors such as Sarwono Prawirohardjo, professor of obstetrics and gynecology at Universitas Indonesia.[45] More successfully, Soedjono Djoened Poesponegoro promoted pediatrics and nutritional research, a less controversial program that was more palatable to religious groups.[46] Such campaigns touched on the reproduction of the nation and treated the household as a site of medical exchange.

Within medical establishments, questions of language, race and ethnicity were raised. As Por shows, moderate nationalists in Malaya viewed Malayanization of the medical services as an important step in the decolonization of society.[47] This undertaking also aimed to ensure the status of Malayans in a society where Chinese and Indian people had come to occupy important roles in professional fields. In Indonesia, as Neelakantan's chapter shows, the "Nationalization Decree (1946)" designated Bahasa Indonesia as the language of higher education. Particular ethnic communities, such as the overseas Chinese communities spread throughout Southeast Asia, both contributed to the health of broader society and existed in tension with it. Medical doctors from these communities also earned global fame, including Wu Lien-Teh, who initiated the widespread use of facemasks during the 1910–11 plague outbreak in China.[48]

Finally, as in Latin America, the question of indigeneity was important for health in Southeast Asia. Groups such as the Orang Asli, which had received little medical care during the colonial era, became viewed as quite important during the Cold War as potential allies. In the DRV, so-called ethnic minorities, for example Thái Mèo, became the target of malaria reduction efforts.[49]

Local Health beyond the Battlefield

Scholars have recently explored the ways in which Cold War experiences were structured by local contexts. For example, the mass killings in 1965 in Indonesia, and those perpetrated by the Khmer Rouge in Cambodia, played out at the village level. Such violence had an immediate impact on health—the death of many—as well as longer-term implications for mental health and community trust.[50]

There were echoes as well of the past, both the recent colonial past and more distant times, in the fact that urban–rural relations and inter-ethnic relations, domestic, regional and more widely international, were mediated in part through medicine and healthcare. For example, the hunting and gathering aspects of the trade, both domestic and international, in spices and medicaments from Southeast Asia to the rest of the world have been dominated by minority peoples such as the Tai of Mainland Southeast Asia or the Dayak of Borneo, rather than by the governing ethnic groups of any polity in Southeast Asia for at least 2,000 years.[51] This is a pattern that has characterized the trade in *materia medica* throughout Southeast Asia down to the present time.[52]

Even today Southeast Asia is ethnically, linguistically and ecologically diverse.[53] Each and every country in the region is multi-ethnic and multilingual, and this has been so throughout recorded history.[54] For at least two millennia this mixture of ethnicities has included groups indigenous to each and every Southeast Asian polity, groups indigenous to several polities, and groups exogenous to the entire region.[55] Each and every group has had, and most still have, their own traditional healers and medical beliefs that reflect the influence of every religion and outside cultures that they have had sustained contact with. The colonial era encouraged the in-migration of exogenous groups, contact with biomedical beliefs and practices, and the codification of those "traditions" that were "recognized" by colonial governments.

During the wars of decolonization, combatants and civilians, both Southeast Asian and foreign, interacted with, and experienced many, ecological and ethnological zones. The essays in this volume reflect this. So does the photograph on our cover, which features a young female medic in upland Laos who in terms of nationality was Lao, in terms of ethnicity was likely Khmu (based on her clothing), and who carried a medical pack (first aid kit) with the

Red Cross popularized by the Swiss as a symbol of medicine, along with weapons quite possibly manufactured in the Soviet Union, China or Vietnam.[56]

Just as the overarching Cold War was structured through a series of binaries—capitalism/communism, West/East, North/South, urban/rural, lowland/upland, modern/traditional, good/evil—so too was local experience. As in Latin America, urban–rural relations were mediated in part through specialized medicine and healthcare.[57] Indeed, the term "rice roots," which frequently appeared in developmentalist literature, was often a reference to a backward, non-state space with a sparse population, as Por's chapter in this book illustrates. These places were sometimes simply *assumed* to have specific diseases such as malaria. There were also assumed to be solutions appropriate to each term of the binary, though these solutions could be modified in practice. Christopher Shepherd's chapter shows how the state adopted either religion or medicine to address what it saw as a problem, animism, depending on a cost-benefit analysis of the economics and politics of the situation. As Shepherd writes, "in the mountainous swidden realm it was cheaper to have the clergy save souls than for the state to cure ailing bodies."[58]

Much recent work has looked beyond these dichotomies to examine how they have obfuscated lived experience as much as they have clarified it. The young woman on the cover of our volume was someone who traversed intellectual constructs of upland and lowland as well as modern and traditional. Likewise, Nara Oda's practitioners of Eastern Medicine in RVN sought to modernize, use science and blend categories. Such figures, and those trained in biomedicine, moved between city and country. They created both new models and tensions as existing ways were challenged.[59]

Diseases of Specific Environments

In addition to trade and travel, Southeast Asia has been linked to the world through its microbes and environments. It continues to be treated as a "sentinel" for pandemics.[60] This volume adopts a critical approach to the understandings of the relationships that exist between environments and human diseases developed by the scientific discipline called disease ecology.[61] During World War II, malaria was a major concern of both the Japanese and the American militaries in Southeast Asia and it affected both of these militaries differently at different times. Malaria continued to be a key disease during the Cold War, and it shows up in several of this volume's chapters. It defied generalizations and could primarily affect lowlands, midlands and/or uplands, depending on the specific configurations of mosquitoes and people. In

Timor-Leste, as Shepherd shows, malaria struck people living in the lowlands and meant those areas remained sparsely populated despite the presence of arable land. Moreover, Shepherd's chapter reminds us that animism's "cold body" and malaria were not the same disease. The language of sacred land, *lulik*, and that of barriers to development projects called for different responses.

As Guénel's chapter shows, the disease ecology of malaria in Vietnam was different, where falciparum had higher incidence in the uplands. Yet, Soviet and DRV experts spoke a similar developmentalist language of barriers to agricultural development and human welfare. Throughout Southeast Asia the use of dichloro-diphenyl-trichloroethane (DDT) was a common method of malaria control, suggesting a shared material history in the region and indeed the globe.[62]

Other familiar diseases remained important killers as well. Xiaoping Fang's chapter examines cholera, but tuberculosis, smallpox and plague were all spread by wartime conditions. Much like those diseases that have more recently been in the news, such as SARS, bird flu and Zika, public health officials and medical doctors were concerned that these diseases might lead to outbreaks and large-scale epidemics (pandemics were not commonly evoked). These diseases also remind us of the importance of human–animal interaction, just as bats (and civets, tanuki and now American deer) have served as hosts of SARS-CoV-2 virus.[63]

Cold War processes were linked to specific diseases in other ways as well. Much of the region, largely rural at the time, experienced rapid urbanization; population increase and urban migration, however, were not intrinsic to decolonization and instead were the results of Cold War strategies. Modernization theorists such as Walt Rostow viewed urban growth as a necessary precondition for capitalist development; but rapidly expanding urban populations in Saigon, Manila, Bangkok, Jakarta and elsewhere experienced air and water pollution, as well as the growth of chronic diseases such as diabetes. Heavy use of chemicals in industrial production led to health problems as well.[64]

Finally, the weapons used to fight the Cold War contributed to a range of health problems. Herbicides, including Agent Orange, which were sprayed throughout the region, had long-terms effects. In Vietnam, dioxin, a contaminant found in the herbicides used by the US and RVN militaries, has had devastating consequences.[65] In addition, suspicions of the United States' use of biological warfare, or weaponized medicine, were a staple of Cold War rhetoric. During the COVID-19 pandemic, there has been a recurrent discussion of the possibility of a laboratory leak in Wuhan. While the situation may echo earlier times, this research was at least partially funded by the US, a decidedly post-Cold War process.

Though inextricably intertwined, the epistemology of medicine and the geopolitical, social, and other contextual factors that affect medical ideas and practices can be separated for analytical purposes. For COVID-19, more robust understandings of human and non-human virus exchanges, or the rapid development of gene sequencing techniques over the past decade, have played key roles in understanding the origin and spread of the SARS-CoV-2 virus while mRNA knowledge has led to the most effective vaccines for COVID-19.[66] This introduction focuses more on external factors, not because the co-editors privilege those above internalist medical developments in response to disease, but for the very practical reason that there is not enough space to do justice to changes over time in all of the branches of medicine and public health covered in this volume. The co-editors have left it to individual authors to examine the intellectual histories of medicine necessary for their specific cases.

Origins and Organization of This Volume

This volume's most immediate lineage can be traced back over 30 years to a book edited by Norman G. Owen, *Death and Disease in Southeast Asia*, published in 1987.[67] Recent HOMSEA volumes have continued that tradition with a focus on Southeast Asia, medicine and health in the world. All of the editors have been involved in that revival as authors, and one of us (C. Michele Thompson) was co-editor of an earlier volume in this series. One difference to note between the Owen volume and more recent publications in the HOMSEA series is that Owen's volume called on economic, social and political historians to write about health, while the HOMSEA series has drawn from the expertise of History of Medicine scholars, especially those living in Southeast Asia.[68]

It also struck the editors that a focus on medicine and health during the Cold War would push the field forward. For one, it was next in line after the colonial era, which has been the subject of more scholarship. There are other reasons as well. While Michitake Aso has argued for profound continuities in malaria prevention and control in 20th-century Vietnam, the Cold War era did have discontinuities, at least deformations of previous forms into something unrecognizable. As Shepherd makes clear, the Cold War and its imperatives changed the trajectory of medicine. Development imperatives pressured the Portuguese to change the nature of their interventions. This was not business as usual.

The placement of medicine and health at the center of the political struggles of the Cold War, both global and local, is observable in other regions. In addition to the literature on Eastern Europe and China, there is also a recent, and important, work on Latin America by Anne-Emanuelle Birn and Raúl

Necochea López.[69] Our volume brings Southeast Asia into this conversation in a focused way and explores Third World connections in the region that hosted the Asian–African Bandung Conference of 1955.

This volume organically emerged out of presentations at HOMSEA conferences over a number of years. Ironically our volume has been shaped by governmental actions, including lockdowns, border closures and other limits on movement that recall the travel restrictions of an earlier era.

The volume's eight chapters address Cold War effects on health and/or medicine in six countries, including nations such as Timor-Leste and Laos that are rarely represented in collections on Southeast Asia, as well as the Chinese diaspora and South Korea's medical outreach in the region. The editors approached scholars who research other Southeast Asian nations, but they were unable to participate in this project for various reasons. The volume does not attempt to cover all countries in the region, and we are therefore very cognizant that our coverage of Cold War and health is not exhaustive. There are certainly other, sometimes related, stories that remain to be researched, and which have the potential to bring new appreciation and perspectives to the themes explored in this volume.

The difficulties of editing a book about the entwinement of medicine and politics were brought home to us in terms of theoretical considerations and also in practical ways. Some of our original authors had to drop out; others had to delay when they could not legally access their research materials within their own cities; one of the editors got COVID-19; and another was stranded while attempting to relocate internationally through the quirks and restrictions of multiple international laws and regulations!

Notwithstanding the above, we are pleased that our authors were able to continue with this project. They include a healthy mix of younger and more established scholars, including those from within and those from outside Southeast Asia itself, and those based in East Asia, Southeast Asia, South Asia, Europe, North America and Australia. It is a diverse mix of authors for a diverse region.

There is a risk in addressing head-on an ongoing pandemic: the pace of events will always outrun any analysis that scholars can bring to it. Yet this ongoing pandemic provides continuing insights, and changing urgencies—when to stop writing and hit "Send"? This volume has been so seriously shaped in both intellectual and practical ways by the pandemic that not to note this fact would seem odd. Drawing on a potent animal native to Southeast Asia, it would be avoiding the elephant in the room.

The chapters in our volume are organized in a roughly chronological and broadly thematic way. They range from 1945 to the 1970s, but they address the prehistory of Cold War in the region, including colonialism, languages, traditional medicine in modern form, environments and trade. They also bring in the context of the long durée migration patterns of the Chinese diaspora. The historical approach highlights the importance of context, time and place, and past layers throughout. Our broadly thematic organization also allows our volume to challenge the dichotomies discussed earlier, as well as the siloed disciplines of agriculture and medicine, among others.

Chapter Summaries

Christopher Shepherd's chapter on Timor-Leste leads off the volume for both chronological and thematic reasons. It takes up an apparent anomaly in the Southeast East Asian experience of the Cold War: Timor-Leste was the last place to win independence from a European colonizer, Portugal. After doing so in 1975, East Timor was promptly occupied by another Southeast Asian country, Indonesia. Timor-Leste was also an exception of sorts in that the staple grain during the Cold War was maize, not rice, mirroring a pattern seen elsewhere in the uplands. Shepherd's chapter examines a place and people fascinating in and of themselves and highlights, through an exception, what held elsewhere in the region. His chapter calls into conversation indigenous, anthropological and government views of health. Shepherd emphasizes what he terms "medicalized agricultural development," reflecting a key insight that agriculture, medicine and animism were inextricably linked. Such a holistic approach to being in the world, though previously dominant, has been suppressed in favor of a siloed, disciplinary emphasis of the Cold War's modernizers. By placing animism and agriculture at the heart of health, Shepherd unmasks "the modernization of medicine as well as the impression thereof [that] served as key components of Portugal's attempt to find its way between these conflicting constraints." Finally, Shephard's chapter completes its unexpected trajectory through the Cold War by showing that the Portuguese "used international development to consolidate their imperial ambitions just as that same developmentalist ideology undermined the legitimacy of their presence."[70]

The next two chapters focus on military medicine in two heartlands of the region, Malaya and Laos. Por Heong Hong's chapter charts the impacts of local dynamics and international Cold War on health services during the Malayan Emergency period (1948–60). Facing multiple post-war challenges, the British government attempted to bolster its legitimacy by announcing a shift in its anti-communist strategy from a military oriented one to one that emphasized the government's social responsibility, including provision of healthcare. Contradicting this claim, Por shows that the government budget largely went to anti-communist warfare, leaving health services scant resources. To fill the void, the government encouraged the voluntary and missionary sectors to provide health services in the New Villages and other resettlement areas, which it built to segregate communist influence. The missionaries expelled from communist-controlled China in 1949 were soon deployed as an anti-communist medical brigade. In this way, the government consciously made use of the health services it did provide in the New Villages and the Orang Asli jungle forts to win the "hearts and minds" of the people. Thus, Por argues, health services were an "instrument of war" disguised as "medical benevolence" and were simultaneously exclusive and intrusive during the Malayan Emergency. At the war front, the relationship between medicine and anti-communist forces was characterized by mutual influence and mutual benefit. This relationship was also aided by an international network of medical collaboration and research. By contrast, the communist guerrillas, many ethnically Chinese, suffered from the paucity of drugs and medical facilities. Yet, they were creative enough to make use of local healing knowledge and makeshift "operation huts" made of local materials.[71]

Kathryn Sweet's chapter explores the contestation and fragmentation of the Lao health sector during the period from 1950 to 1975. She describes how several new health services—at least three civilian health services and two military services—emerged in Laos in place of the unitary colonial health service in the early years following independence from France. These various health services, in both the Royal Lao Government controlled zone and in the Liberated Zone of the Lao revolutionaries, were motivated by the different priorities of their respective Cold War donors, and employed different technical languages and standards of training and operation. Her chapter provides much-needed context for the diverse health infrastructure, staffing, and professional and technical standards inherited by the Lao PDR regime and the challenges of uniting these divergent health services into a uniform national healthcare system post-1975.

Next, our volume moves away from active fighting and in three chapters turns its attention to medicine in the processes of nation-building and decolonization in South and North Vietnam and Indonesia.

The first chapter in this trio is by Nara Oda. She examines the development of so-called Eastern medicine, or traditional medicine (EM/TM), in the newly created Republic of Vietnam (South Vietnam). In a fascinating case study, Oda offers a necessary addition to the DRV-dominated story of EM/TM in the territory that is now Vietnam and shows how common understandings of EM/TM in RVN have been wrong. Immediately after 1954, the Diem regime left in place colonial-era regulations and in general took a more hard-line stance towards EM/TM than in the north. Diem did this in part because its practitioners were mostly of Chinese descent, and they became suspect when the PRC was formed in 1949. Rather than an antipathy towards EM/TM itself, or overreliance on American support as the DRV claimed, Diem was concerned about the loyalties of those practicing it. With a nod towards Por's chapter, effects of the Emergency period in Malaya were felt in TM in RVN. Oda shows how in 1964, after the end of the Diem regime, the second RVN somewhat relaxed its stance towards EM/TM and its practitioners. Thus, when a study team was sent in 1976 from Hanoi to study conditions in the south, they found an active EM/TM community. Beyond the Cold War dichotomies, approaches to EM began to converge. They were standardized under the slogan of science and institutionalized by law in both North and South Vietnam. The next chapter, by Annick Guénel, looks at the building of a socialist health system through the lens of malaria control in the Democratic Republic of Vietnam. Providing healthcare was an important component of state-building during the First Indochina War. After it ended in 1954, the DRV could build on the initial wartime efforts. It invited teams of foreign experts, in particular from the USSR, whose team arrived in 1955 and continued to participate in malaria control via experts and material until 1975. One of the initial malaria control studies began in Thái Nguyên province. Its midlands ecology and multi-ethnic society meant that it had year-round malaria and the presence of falciparum. It was also an industrial center, and for these reasons politically and economically important.

Malarial control was also an issue in the South and the use of DDT in RVN started in 1951, with a WHO-supported eradication program beginning in 1958. In fact, the Soviet Union had left the WHO in 1949, and only returned in 1956. As Guénel notes, the programs in the two countries ran in parallel, with similar timing and a similar approach that, as Guénel puts it, consisted of: preparation, attack, consolidation and maintenance. Malaria control was a key site of decolonization and while the political competition between the DRV and RVN has been analyzed, the biomedical competition has been rarely examined historically. Of course, malaria remained a battlefield issue and the leading Vietnamese malariologist, Dang Van Ngu, was killed in 1967 while carrying out studies on malaria.

The final chapter in this trio is by Vivek Neelakantan. He examines how applied medical sciences, particularly nutrition and pediatrics, were mobilized in nation-building in Indonesia during the 1950s. Unlike the leaders of the RVN and the DRV examined in the previous two chapters by Oda and Guénel, President Soekarno envisioned a technologically self-sufficient Indonesia that was dependent on neither the US nor the USSR. The most salient feature of Soekarnoist science, a concept Neelakantan develops in his chapter, was its reflection of the proverbial Bandung Spirit, which emphasized solidarity with post-colonial Asian and African nations. Soekarno understood science functionally and strategically with reference to Indonesia's needs and its Cold War aspirations as leader of the Non-Aligned Bloc. That is, science could help provide for the needs of the people and play a role in international relations. Moreover, a prosopography of three Indonesian physicians, Neelakantan argues, shows that "the legacy of nationalist physicians in shaping the trajectory of scientific thinking continued in terms of symbolically aligning medical research with national exigencies, arising partially in response to the Cold War." Neelakantan concludes by evaluating the outcomes of Soekarnoist science. Soekarno's syncretism in appropriating international ideas contributed to, Neelakantan observes, a variant of post-colonial science with a distinctive Indonesian flavor.[72]

The last two chapters expand out again from Southeast Asia, exploring migration, international relations and development in the region's relationship with the PRC and the Republic of Korea (ROK).

Xiaoping Fang's chapter discusses the transnational politics of the seventh global cholera pandemic (*Vibrio cholerae* El Tor). It focuses on the Chinese diasporic community, disease, and migration between Southeast Asia and China, which, according to Fang, arose from a context of colonialism, trade and political turmoil dating from the beginning of the 19th century. Chinese migrants faced racial and social prejudice often linked to disease. Then, as Por and Oda note in their chapters, Cold War forces reshaped Chinese migration and disease patterns. In particular, Fang follows the so-called overseas Chinese who returned to the PRC during the early 1960s, and the fears about cholera that they might have brought with them. Fang argues that wars of decolonization and the Cold War provided the ecological conditions that turned cholera outbreaks in Indonesia into a global pandemic. He also shows how the PRC simultaneously attempted to entice the overseas Chinese to return and bring their financial resources with them, and to control the potential epidemiological and political fallout of the introduction of cholera to mainland China. Chinese leaders, Fang argues, chose to isolate their country from the international health community and deliberately used "medical humanitarianism" and the media to legitimize their sociopolitical and ideological power both domestically and abroad.

The final chapter returns to an active battlefield through South Korean civic actions in South Vietnam. During its nine-year participation in the Vietnam War (1964–73), South Korea sent an estimated 300,000 troops. John

DiMoia's chapter opens with one exemplary encounter between South Koreans and Vietnamese: the free haircut. DiMoia shows how this campaign had the aim of limiting the spread of disease in Vietnamese villages and keeping the Republic of Korea troops healthy. As DiMoia shows, for South Koreans, "the imagined relationship between the Korean rural village and its Vietnamese counterpart helped to shape the medical relationship." And even if South Korea conducted tropical medicine for its own benefit through agencies such as Korean Preventive Medicine (KOPREM), the haircut represented one of the most fascinating aspects of the public face of their medical presence in RVN. More than a public health measure, DiMoia argues, the haircut was also meant to create a sense of welfare, especially among the young and elderly Vietnamese, and make the Korean presence more palatable. It was an example of how public health intersected with civil affairs. This insight allows DiMoia to pivot to a discussion of civic outreach and formative developmentalism. Thus, in 1964, KOTRA opened an office in Saigon and when the Dove/Pigeon Brigade arrived in early 1965, it combined the tasks of civil affairs with construction. DiMoia's framework also allows him to discuss the larger context of health through the lens of renewed diplomatic relations between the Republic of Korea and its close neighbors in East and Southeast Asia. Scarcely a decade removed from its own war, the Republic of Korea arrived as a sub-imperial actor intervening at the request of the United States, and, equally, an Asian partner seeking to assist, given its own recent experience with division.[73]

DiMoia's chapter is a useful stopping point as it suggests how medicine and development were inextricably intertwined during the Cold War years. As with the volume as a whole, it tells a Cold War history that questions dichotomies and decenters the United States. Not that this hegemon was absent, just that there are many other important stories about health and medicine to tell.

NOTES

1.   See COVID-19 Dashboard by Johns Hopkins University. Available at: https://coronavirus.jhu.edu/map.html [accessed 19 November 2022]. See also WHO Coronavirus (COVID-19) Dashboard. Available at: https://covid19.who.int/ [accessed 19 May 2023].

2.   "How Did Cambodia's Cruise Ship Welcome Go Wrong?" *BBC News*, 20 February 2020, sec. Asia. Available at: https://www.bbc.com/news/world-asia -51542241 [accessed 19 May 2023].

3.   For Laos, see Kathryn Sweet, "Locked-in, Locked-down: COVID-19 in Laos," *CSEAS* [Center for Southeast Asian Studies] *Newsletter* 78, 2020, Available at: https://covid-19chronicles.cseas.kyoto-u.ac.jp/post-015-html/ [accessed 19 May 2023], along with other articles from around Southeast Asia. For an article critical

of such celebration, see Bill Hayton and Tro Ly Ngheo, "Vietnam's Coronavirus Success Is Built on Repression," *Foreign Policy*, 12 May 2020. Available at: https://foreignpolicy.com/2020/05/12/vietnam-coronavirus-pandemic-success-repression/ [accessed 19 May 2023].

4.   Arthur Kleinman and James L. Watson, ed., *SARS in China: Prelude to Pandemic?* (Stanford, CA: Stanford University Press, 2006).

5.   Francis Gealogo, "The Influenza Pandemic of 1918–1919 and COVID-19 Pandemic of 2020 in the Philippines: Some Historical Parallelisms," presented at the *44th Southeast Asia Seminar on The COVID-19 Pandemic in Japanese and Southeast Asian Perspective: Histories, States, Markets, Societies*, Kyoto, 1 March 2021. For more on the 1918–19 pandemic in Southeast Asia, see Kirsty Walker, "The Influenza Pandemic of 1918 in Southeast Asia," in *Histories of Health in Southeast Asia*, ed. Tim Harper and Sunil S. Amrith (Bloomington, IN: Indiana University Press, 2014), pp. 61–71. For a classic work on the 1918–19 pandemic in the United States, and an eerily prescient preface, see Alfred W. Crosby, *America's Forgotten Pandemic: The Influenza of 1918*, 2nd ed. (Cambridge: Cambridge University Press, 2003). This book was originally published in 1976 at a moment of medical triumphalism, when it seemed like infectious diseases were monsters of the past. Estimated global deaths come from Crosby, p. xii.

6.   Vivek Neelakantan, "History of Pandemics in Southeast Asia: A Return of National Anxieties?" The History of Science Society, IsisCB Special Issue on Pandemics, no. CBE101.3a-v.2021.03.12 (2021). Available at: https://perma.cc/2VDW-D23T [accessed 19 May 2023].

7.   For a historiography of development, Stephen J. Macekura and Erez Manela, "Introduction," in *The Development Century: A Global History* (New York: Cambridge University Press, 2018). For histories of development focused on Cold War Southeast Asia, see among others Bradley R. Simpson, *Economists with Guns: Authoritarian Development and U.S.-Indonesian Relations, 1960–1968* (Stanford, CA: Stanford University Press, 2008) and Edward Garvey Miller, *Misalliance Ngo Dinh Diem, the United States, and the Fate of South Vietnam* (Cambridge, MA: Harvard University Press, 2013).

8.   Cf. other volumes on decolonization such as Christopher E. Goscha and Christian F. Ostermann, ed., *Connecting Histories: Decolonization and the Cold War in Southeast Asia* (Washington, DC: Woodrow Wilson Center Press, 2009); John Robert McNeill and Corinna R. Unger, ed., *Environmental Histories of the Cold War* (Washington, DC: Cambridge University Press, 2010); Hiromi Mizuno, Aaron S. Moore and John DiMoia, ed., *Engineering Asia: Technology, Colonial Development, and the Cold War Order* (London, UK: Bloomsbury Academic, 2018); Macekura and Manela, ed., *The Development Century*; and Anne-Emanuelle Birn and Raúl Necochea López, ed., *Peripheral Nerve: Health and Medicine in Cold War Latin America* (Durham, NC: Duke University Press, 2020).

9. For vaccines in Vietnam, see C. Michele Thompson, "Mission to Macau: Smallpox, Vaccinia, and the Nguyen Dynasty," *Portuguese Studies Review* 9 (2001): 194–231; Annick Guénel, "La Lutte Antivariolique En Extreme-Orient: Ruptures et Continuite," in *L'Aventure de La Vaccination*, ed. Anne-Marie Moulin (Geneva: Fayard, 1996), pp. 82–94; and Laurence Monnais, "Preventive Medicine and 'Mission Civilisatrice': Uses of the BCG Vaccine in French Colonial Vietnam between the Two World Wars," *The International Journal of Asia-Pacific Studies* 2, 1 (2006): 40–66. For a recent work on China, see Mary Augusta Brazelton, *Mass Vaccination: Citizens' Bodies and State Power in Modern China* (Ithaca, NY: Cornell University Press, 2019).

10. Nathalie Huynh Chau Nguyen, "Military Doctors in South Vietnam: Wartime and Post-War Lives," *Oral History* 43, 1 (2015): 86. Nguyên Kiên Ngoc, *Public Health in Viet Nam* (Saigon, Republic of Vietnam: Vietnam Council on Foreign Relations, 1969), p. 5.

11. Trung tâm Lưu trữ quốc gia 3 (National Archives of Vietnam No. 3, hereafter TTLT3), Bộ Y Tế [Ministry of Health] 5412 Công văn, bảng thống kê của Thủ tướng Phủ, Bộ Y Tế về viện trợ thuốc và dụng cụ, cho ngành Y tế từ Bungari, Hungari, Trung Quốc, 1954. The first three categories accounted for 85 to 90 percent of items, with category 4 accounting for 10 percent of items.

12. Por Heong Hong, "Tool of Domination and Act of Benevolence: Medicine and Healthcare during the Malayan Emergency, 1948–60," in this volume, p. 53.

13. Kathryn Sweet, "Health Sector Contestation in Cold War Laos, 1950–75" and John P. DiMoia, "Managing Wartime Conditions: South Korean Developmental Ambitions, Public Health and Emerging Forms of Overseas Medical Outreach, 1964–73," both in this volume, pp. 84 and 214.

14. Simeon Man, *Soldiering through Empire: Race and the Making of the Decolonizing Pacific* (Berkeley, CA: University of California Press, 2018) and Richard A. Ruth, *In Buddha's Company: Thai Soldiers in the Vietnam War* (Honolulu, HI: University of Hawai'i Press, 2011).

15. Hong, "Tool of Domination," in this volume, p. 53.

16. George Black, "The Victims of Agent Orange the U.S. Has Never Acknowledged," *The New York Times*, 16 March 2021, sec. Magazine. Available at: https://www.nytimes.com/2021/03/16/magazine/laos-agent-orange-vietnam-war.html [accessed 19 May 2023].

17. Billy Joel, "We Didn't Start the Fire" from the album *Storm Front*, Columbia Records, 1989.

18. Ang Cheng Guan, *Southeast Asia after the Cold War: A Contemporary History* (Singapore: NUS Press, 2019). For monographs that include treatment of health in individual Southeast Asian countries during the Cold War, see Jan Ovesen and Ing-Britt Trankell, *Cambodians and Their Doctors: A Medical Anthropology of Colonial and Postcolonial Cambodia* (Copenhagen: NIAS Press, 2010) and Vivek Neelakantan, *Science, Public Health and Nation-Building in Soekarno-*

Era Indonesia (Newcastle upon Tyne: Cambridge Scholars Publishing, 2017). For an exploration of the links between South Asia and parts of Southeast Asia, see Sunil S. Amrith, *Decolonizing International Health: India and Southeast Asia, 1930–65* (New York: Palgrave Macmillan, 2006). For medicine in Eastern Europe during the Cold War, see Dóra Vargha, *Polio across the Iron Curtain: Hungary's Cold War with an Epidemic* (New York: Cambridge University Press, 2018). For the PRC, see Miriam Gross, *Chairman Mao's Campaign to Deworm China* (Berkeley, CA: University of California Press, 2016).

19.   Annick Guénel, "Building a 'Socialist Health System': Soviet Assistance in Malaria Control in the Democratic Republic of Vietnam during the Cold War," p. 146 in this volume.

20.   Xiaobing Li, *The Dragon in the Jungle* (London: Oxford University Press, 2020).

21.   Birn and López, ed., *Peripheral Nerve*.

22.   Guénel, "Building a 'Socialist Health System'," p. 146 in this volume.

23.   See for example Rachel Applebaum, "The Friendship Project: Socialist Internationalism in the Soviet Union and Czechoslovakia in the 1950s and 1960s," *Slavic Review* 74, 3 (2015): 484–507; Hong Young-sun, *Cold War Germany, the Third World, and the Global Humanitarian Regime* (New York: Cambridge University Press, 2015); and Su Lin Lewis and Carolien Stolte, "Other Bandungs: Afro-Asian Internationalisms in the Early Cold War," *Journal of World History* 30, 1 (2019): 1–19.

24.   Vivek Neelakantan, "Mobilizing Applied Medical Knowledge in Indonesia: Soekarnoist Science and Asian–African Solidarity in the 1950s," p. 167 in this volume.

25.   Patryk Babiracki and Austin Jersild, ed., *Socialist Internationalism in the Cold War: Exploring the Second World* (Cham, Switzerland: Palgrave Macmillan, 2016); Birn and López, ed., *Peripheral Nerve*.

26.   Rachel Applebaum, *Empire of Friends: Soviet Power and Socialist Internationalism in Cold War Czechoslovakia* (Ithaca, NY: Cornell University Press, 2019).

27.   Jenna Grant, "Friends, Partners, and Orphans: Relations That Make and Unmake a Hospital," *Medicine Anthropology Theory* 5, 2 (2018): 56–72; Jenna Grant, "Repair in Translation," *East Asian Science, Technology and Society* 14, 1 (2020): 15–33.

28.   Mark Harrison, *Contagion: How Commerce Has Spread Disease* (New Haven, CT: Yale University Press, 2013).

29.   Xiaoping Fang, "The Cholera Pandemic, the Chinese Diaspora and the Cold War Politics in Southeast Asia and China during the 1960s," p. 194 in this volume.

30.   DiMoia, "Managing Wartime Conditions," p. 214 in this volume.

31.   See, for example, https://wits.worldbank.org/CountrySnapshot/en/KOR [accessed 19 May 2023] and https://www.asianscientist.com/ [accessed 19 May 2023].

32.   Christopher Shepherd, "Health, Agriculture and Animism in the 'Development' of Portuguese Timor, 1945–75," p. 27 in this volume.

33. Hajimu Masuda, "What Was the Cold War? Imagined Reality, Ordinary People's War, and Social Mechanism," *The Asia-Pacific Journal* 15, 4 (2017): 1–25.
34. Hong, "Tool of Domination," p. 53 in this volume.
35. Peter Bogdanovich, *Saint Jack* (New World Pictures, 1979).
36. Li, *The Dragon in the Jungle*.
37. Guénel "Building a 'Socialist Health System'," p. 146 in this volume.
38. This was also the case in Czechoslovakia. See Bradley M. Moore, "For the People's Health: Ideology, Medical Authority and Hygienic Science in Communist Czechoslovakia," *Social History of Medicine: The Journal of the Society for the Social History of Medicine* 27, 1 (2014): 122–43.
39. TTLT3, BYT 5647 Hội nghị Bộ trưởng Y tế các nước XHCN lần thứ 5 tại Mascova—Liên Xô, 1960. Tập 4, Bungari, Hungari, Mông Cổ, Rumani, Tiệp, Triều Tiên.
40. Sweet, "Health Sector Contestation," p. 84 in this volume.
41. Nguyen, "Military Doctors in South Vietnam," pp. 85–96.
42. Neelakantan, "Mobilizing Applied Medical Knowledge," p. 167 in this volume.
43. Neelakantan, "Mobilizing Applied Medical Knowledge," p. 167 in this volume.
44. Bộ Y Tế, "Vietnam," *International Conference on Children and National Development, Saigon, January 14–23, 1975* (Saigon: Pediatrics Committee, Ministry of Health, 1975).
45. Neelakantan, "Mobilizing Applied Medical Knowledge," p. 167 in this volume.
46. Neelakantan, "Mobilizing Applied Medical Knowledge," p. 167 in this volume.
47. Hong, "Tool of Domination," p. 53 in this volume.
48. Neelakantan, "Mobilizing Applied Medical Knowledge," p. 167 in this volume. See also Hans Pols, C. Michele Thompson and John Harley Warner, ed., *Translating the Body: Medical Education in Southeast Asia* (Singapore: NUS Press, 2017). For more on the use of masks during the plague outbreak, see William C. Summers, *The Great Manchurian Plague of 1910–1911: The Geopolitics of an Epidemic Disease* (New Haven, CT: Yale University Press, 2012) and Christos Lynteris, "Plague Masks: The Visual Emergence of Anti-Epidemic Personal Protection Equipment," *Medical Anthropology* 37, 6 (2018): 442–57.
49. Guénel, "Building a 'Socialist Health System'," p. 146 in this volume. See also Christian C. Lentz, *Contested Territory: Điện Biên Phủ and the Making of Northwest Vietnam* (New Haven, CT: Yale University Press, 2019).
50. For Indonesia, see Geoffrey Robinson, *The Killing Season: A History of the Indonesian Massacres, 1965–66* (Princeton, NJ: Princeton University Press, 2018) and Joshua Oppenheimer, *The Act of Killing* (Drafthouse Films, 2013). For Cambodia, see Alexander Laban Hinton, *Why Did They Kill?: Cambodia in the Shadow of Genocide* (Berkeley, CA: University of California Press, 2005).
51. C. Michele Thompson, "Setting the Stage: Ancient Medical History of the Geographic Space that is now Vietnam," in *Southern Medicine for Southern People: Vietnamese Medicine in the Making*, ed. Laurence Monnais, C. Michele

Thompson and Ayo Wahlberg (Newcastle upon Tyne: Cambridge Scholars, 2012), pp. 21–60.

52. Eric Tagliacozzo, "A Sino-Southeast Asian Circuit: Ethnohistories of the Marine Goods Trade," in *Chinese Circulations: Capital, Commodities, and Networks in Southeast Asia*, ed. Eric Tagliacozzo and Wen-Chin Chang (Durham, NC: Duke University Press, 2011), pp. 432–54; Heather Sutherland, "A Sino-Indonesian Commodity Chain: The Trade in Tortoise Shell in the Late Seventeenth and Eighteenth Centuries," in *Chinese Circulations*, ed. Tagliacozzo and Chang (Durham, NC: Duke University Press, 2011), pp. 172–202; Chiang Bien, "Market Price, Labor Input, and Relations of Production in Sarawak's Edible Birds' Nest Trade," in *Chinese Circulations*, ed. Tagliacozzo and Chang (Durham, NC: Duke University Press, 2011), pp. 407–31; Kenneth R. Hall, "Economic History of Early Southeast Asia," in *The Cambridge History of Southeast Asia*, vol. 1, pt. 1, *From Early Times to c. 1500,* ed. Nicholas Tarling (Cambridge: Cambridge University Press, 1992), pp. 257–60.

53. Peter Bellwood, "Southeast Asia before History," in *The Cambridge History of Southeast Asia*, vol. 1, pt. 1 (Cambridge: Cambridge University Press, 1992): see maps on pp. 108 and 111.

54. Patricia Herbert and Anthony Milner, ed., *South-East Asia: Languages and Literatures, a Select Guide* (Honolulu: University of Hawai'i Press, 1989).

55. Anthony Reid, *Southeast Asia in the Age of Commerce*, vol. 1, *The Lands below the Winds* (New Haven, CT: Yale University Press, 1988) and vol. 2, *Expansion and Crisis* (New Haven, CT: Yale University Press, 1993).

56. The Soviet Union manufactured RPG-2 anti-tank missiles. Similar versions were manufactured in China (Type 56 RPG) and Vietnam (B40, B50). Email correspondence with UXO expert, Phil Bean, 13 February 2022.

57. Birn and López, ed., *Peripheral Nerve*.

58. Shepherd, "Health, Agriculture and Animism," p. 27 in this volume.

59. Nara Oda, "More Eastern than Traditional: The Making of *Đông y* in the Republic of Vietnam during the Cold War," p. 120 in this volume.

60. Amos Zeeberg, "A Lab in Cambodia Is on the Lookout for the next Pandemic," *The New York Times*, 16 February 2021, sec. World. Available at: https://www.nytimes.com/2021/02/16/world/a-lab-in-cambodia-is-on-the-lookout-for-the-next-pandemic.html [accessed 19 May 2023].

61. For a global approach developed by a medical doctor who spent an extended time in Southeast Asia, see Jacques M. May, *Studies in Disease Ecology* (New York: Macmillan, 1961).

62. David Kinkela, *DDT and the American Century: Global Health, Environmental Politics, and the Pesticide That Changed the World* (Chapel Hill, NC: University of North Carolina Press, 2011).

63. Natalie Porter, *Viral Economies: Bird Flu Experiments in Vietnam* (Chicago, IL: The University of Chicago Press, 2019).

64. See for example Steve Ferzacca, *Healing the Modern in a Central Javanese City* (Durham, NC: Carolina Academic Press, 2001).

65. Edwin A. Martini, *Agent Orange: History, Science, and the Politics of Uncertainty* (Amherst, MA: University of Massachusetts Press, 2012) and Amy M. Hay, *The Defoliation of America: Agent Orange Chemicals, Citizens, and Protests* (Tuscaloosa, AL: University Alabama Press, 2021).

66. Nathan D. Wolfe, Peter Daszak, A. Marm Kilpatrick and Donald S. Burke, "Bushmeat Hunting, Deforestation, and Prediction of Zoonotic Disease," *Emerging Infectious Diseases* 11, 12 (2005): 1822–7. Available at: https://doi.org/10.3201/eid1112.040789 [accessed 19 May 2023]. Jon Gertner, "A DNA Sequencing Revolution Helped Us Fight Covid. What Else Can It Do?" *The New York Times*, 25 March 2021, sec. Magazine. Available at: https://www.nytimes.com/interactive/2021/03/25/magazine/genome-sequencing-covid-variants.html [accessed 19 May 2023]. For an example of an intellectual history of hygienic science during the Cold War, see Moore, "For the People's Health," pp. 122–43.

67. Norman G. Owen, ed., *Death and Disease in Southeast Asia: Explorations in Social, Medical and Demographic History* (Singapore: Oxford University Press, 1987). See more recently Harper and Amrith, ed., *Histories of Health in Southeast Asia*, which does not have the same focus on the Cold War and decolonization.

68. Laurence Monnais and Harold J. Cook, *Global Movements, Local Concerns: Medicine and Health in Southeast Asia* (Singapore: NUS Press, 2012); Pols, Thompson and Warner, ed., *Translating the Body*.

69. Birn and López, ed., *Peripheral Nerve*; Hong, *Cold War Germany*; Babiracki and Jersild, ed., *Socialist Internationalism in the Cold War*; and Applebaum, *Empire of Friends*.

70. Shepherd, "Health, Agriculture and Animism," p. 27 in this volume.

71. Hong, "Tool of Domination," p. 53 in this volume.

72. Neelakantan, "Mobilizing Applied Medical Knowledge," p. 167 in this volume.

73. DiMoia, "Managing Wartime Conditions," p. 214 in this volume.

CHAPTER 1

Health, Agriculture and Animism in the "Development" of Portuguese Timor, 1945–75

Christopher Shepherd

East Timor (or Timor-Leste) is a spectacular, mountainous half-island country of about 18,000 square kilometers at the southeastern edge of Southeast Asia. The Portuguese began their colonial project in Timor in the 1500s, and they had consolidated their claim over the eastern half of the island by 1859 with the Dutch occupying the Western half.[1] While Dutch Timor had been absorbed into the new nation-state archipelago of Indonesia by 1949, Portugal, after re-possessing "Portuguese Timor" immediately after Japanese occupation of the island in 1945, resisted decolonization for another 30 years. Portugal, therefore, was the last European colonial power in Southeast Asia to relinquish its overseas territory. Concomitantly, East Timor was the last of all Southeast Asian countries to gain independence, albeit only briefly before the Indonesian invasion of December 1975.[2] This means that the first 30 years of the Cold War, 1945 to 1975, which ushered in a new geopolitics of development throughout Southeast Asia, applied to Portuguese Timor under the distinct conditions of recalcitrant Portuguese colonialism.

This chapter investigates that Cold War distinctiveness of Portuguese Timor in relation to the incipient role of modern medicine in an over-whelmingly indigenous-animist society as the colony pursued agricultural development. What ensued was a kind of medicalized agricultural development whose ideological and material elements emerged from the new global order, but which fell in with a colonial system that struggled to shed its traditional

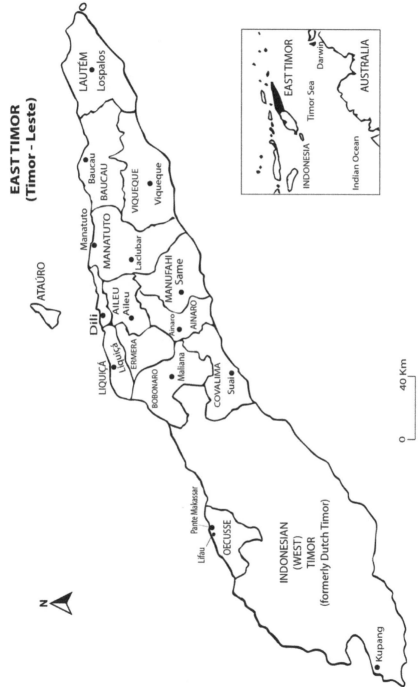

EAST TIMOR (Timor - Leste)

ATAÚRO

LAUTÉM
Lospalos

Baucau
BAUCAU

VIQUEQUE
Viqueque

Manatuto
MANATUTO

Laclubar

MANUFAHI
Same

Dili

AILEU
Aileu

AINARO
Ainaro

LIQUIÇÁ
Liquiçá

ERMERA

BOBONARO
Maliana

COVALIMA
Suai

Lifau
Pante Makassar

OECUSSE

INDONESIAN
(WEST)
TIMOR
(formerly Dutch Timor)

Kupang

N

0   40 Km

EAST TIMOR
Darwin
Timor Sea
INDONESIA
AUSTRALIA
Indian Ocean

Map 1.1. East Timor (or Timor-Leste)

imperialistic methods. I argue that in the post-war period the Portuguese had to find their way between a rock and a hard place: they used international development to consolidate their imperial ambitions just as that same developmentalist ideology undermined the legitimacy of their presence. In effect, I show that the modernization of medicine as well as the impression thereof served as key components of Portugal's attempt to find its way between these conflicting forces. Portugal's paradoxical resistance to Cold War pressures as well as the adoption of its means—including the development of health and agriculture—are precisely those forces which allowed it to hang on to its Southeast Asian "province" (of Portugal) for so long.

To modernize medicine and agriculture involved the suppression of traditional agriculture, traditional medicine and the attendant traditional animist worldview. Timorese traditions were also emergent as they were influenced by the colonial encounter.[3] Either way, the Portuguese continually reinstated the category of "Timorese tradition" in order to devalue tradition against higher civilizing and development goals. This dichotomy propelled interventions, but not uniformly so. Interventions were highly targeted and structured around a value set of interlocking priorities and prejudices that scholars of Southeast Asia are well familiar with.

First, there was the priority accorded to lowlands over highlands as sites more conducive to high-productivity agriculture, the transport of goods, and the governance of people;[4] second was the favor accorded to wet rice as a lowland market crop and the corresponding neglect of maize and dry rice as highland subsistence crops embedded in a shifting or swidden agro-system;[5] third was the relationship between highlands and lowlands, which was no longer one of exchange but a more unidirectional supply and demand whereby highlands provided lowlands with resources (labor, draft animals, water and food);[6] and fourth was the scientific rationality required to sustain these multiple hierarchies, with a correspondingly pejorative view of animist "superstition."[7] To understand the Cold War in post-war Portuguese Timor is to trace a path among this matrix of changing priorities and prejudices, strongly inflected by both old imperialism and new developmentalism.

The Cold War, Post-war Developmentalism and the Defence of Colony

Prior to the Japanese invasion of 1942, the small, remote colony of Portuguese Timor subsisted within a moderately impervious bubble at the margins of the Portuguese Empire. After World War II, that bubble was perforated and finally burst under the pressures of Cold War politics, the result being a conflict-ridden decolonization process followed by the Indonesian invasion of December 1975. To appreciate the significance of the pre-war to post-war transition is to address how World War II and the Cold War led the now-dominant global power, the United States, to position itself strategically in relation to Southeast Asia against a rising Soviet Union and, in the background, communist China. In doing so, the United States had to deal with European colonial powers, including Portugal, and their territories in Southeast Asia.

Although neutral during World War II, the Portuguese had gained favor with the United States for permitting the allies military use of the Azores.[8] The authoritarianism of Portugal's Salazarist state with its large empire and insular economy would appear to be diametrically opposed to United States' post-war liberal empire. But in exchange for various concessions, including ongoing military use of the Azores, the United States assured Portugal in 1946 that "any threat to the territorial security of Portugal would constitute a threat to the security of the Atlantic and the world as a whole, and would therefore represent a problem of paramount interest to the United States."[9] This set the stage for Portugal's admission into the North Atlantic Treaty Organization (NATO) whereby the question of self-determination for the colonies was tacitly shelved. Inside Timor, there was no nationalist movement to challenge the Portuguese as there had been in the Dutch East Indies (Indonesia) and elsewhere in Southeast Asia.[10]

The post-war role of the United States in Europe was an important factor in shaping how the Portuguese would come to frame their mission in Timor. The European Recovery Plan or "Marshall Plan," which Portugal signed on to in 1947, accelerated Portugal's integration into the Atlantic community and made it a recipient of foreign aid.[11] The Marshall Plan also contained the seed of Third World developmentalism in its manner of projecting American business structures, industrial practices, educational principles and scientific knowledge from the United States onto Europe, while promoting the removal of trade barriers and the increase of industrial and agricultural productivity. Accordingly, the American model of science-based progress came to stand as a pattern for what could be achieved in the so-called Third World as ideological divisions drove the polarization of East and West to an extreme.

The massive industry surrounding "development" oriented the relations between the US-led conglomerate of Western nations and the Third World, while the technocentric premises inherent in the emergent global development ideology attained dominance as the way to organize international relations between the "First" and the "Third Worlds."[12] The development agenda was applied principally to political, economic and, potentially, military allies of the United States; but more than that, it became the very means through which alliances were secured. The category of the Third World encompassed countries of Latin America, Africa and Asia-Pacific; their commonality was economic "underdevelopment" and poverty, of which both the prevalence of disease and traditional "underproductive" agriculture were construed as central components.

Some aspects of the new development agenda were swiftly absorbed by Portugal. The Portuguese superimposed the new conceptual map—underdevelopment as problem, development as goal, and technology transfer as means[13]—upon the old notion of the civilizing mission. They did not, however, adopt the development agenda as did the other countries that figure in this volume, where budding nationalist elites deployed it to distinguish their path forward from the long history of colonial oppression. In the case of Timor, development came to serve Portuguese colonialism just as its repertoire of concepts facilitated Portugal's deceptive image of the colony as a modern development state, not despite the persistence of colonialism but by virtue of it.

A succession of five-year "Development Plans" from 1953 onwards became instrumental to Portugal's modus operandi. As a form of organizing knowledge, the Development Plans appealed to the centralizing tendencies of the *Estado Novo* and were broadly applied to all of Portugal's African and Asian colonies. From now on, all development planning would be directed, administered and financed from Lisbon; the role of science, scientific expertise and scientific institutions would be pivotal; and the colonies would be subject to standard criteria for evaluating underdevelopment and specifying technological intervention. Accordingly, Portugal worked to improve its metropolitan scientific institutions and strengthen the links between these and their counterparts in the colonies; data, collected in Timor, Angola or Mozambique, would henceforth be analyzed in Lisbon. The development-oriented activities of the post-war period thus contrasted notably with the sluggish and intermittent activities of the interwar years, which tended to rely on the charisma of outstanding governors.

Given Portugal's enthusiastic uptake of the new development terminology, one could easily overlook the fact that Portugal had little time for development's ideological content of liberal capitalism, decolonization, democracy and human welfare. (The ideals of democracy and human welfare could, of course, be quickly forgotten if client states began to lean too far left; indeed, one could say that democracy and human welfare had to be carefully calibrated to serve capitalism.) In particular, the welfare of colonial subjects, including the Timorese, was destined to become a contentious issue internationally. The Portuguese had won infamy regarding forced labor, prison labor and the general health of the populace.[14] Historically, it had concealed or denied systemic abuses, but the cocoon-like nature of its colonies fractured in the post-war era of rising global scrutiny. Even the United States, once consoled by the anticommunism of the Salazar regime, frowned at the fascist Portuguese Empire.

More troubled by, and troubling to, Portugal was the United Nations. In 1952, Portugal balked at the prospect of a United Nations Educational, Scientific and Cultural Organization survey mission entering its overseas territories. One high official of the Ministry of Foreign Affairs objected:

> Particularly in respect to bodies associated with the United Nations, we have every reason to suspect that such inquiries into the so-called "dependent countries" will serve as a pretext for malicious criticisms whose aim is to smite the colonial nations. The issue lies not in the facts as such, but in the interpretations that will ultimately be derived from them.[15]

The said United Nations survey never took place. Portugal, then, could stall outside "interference" into its colonies in the form of official inquiries, but it could not prevent the mounting anecdotal evidence regarding the highly repressive and censorial style of the Portuguese colonial system.[16] Naturally, Portugal could not manage much more than to make democratic gestures towards its "provincial" governments, so outsiders would explain its oppressive style as a product of the unique mix of metropolitan dictatorship and colonialism.[17] Portugal's effort to join the United Nations was hindered by a number of Western countries while Portugal continued to justify itself by adapting the old "civilizing mission" language to the political pressures, moral imperatives and sociotechnical imagery of new developmentalism. Extolled were the icons of modernity—cities, hospitals, roads, plantations—and the benefits they delivered to the indigenes.[18]

Portugal was eventually admitted to the United Nations in 1956 when it ratified the Forced Labor Convention of the International Labor Organization (ILO). The same year, however, a high Portuguese official of Foreign Affairs, Dr Carlos Abecassis, traveled to Timor to assess the living and working conditions of the indigenous people. Appalled at how the Timorese suffered under heavy taxes, compulsory sale of produce at low prices, conscripted labor and routine whipping, he instructed the governor to terminate corporal punishment and other abuses.[19] Yet the labor regime with corporal punishment continued and Portugal concocted technicalities to contest the constraints imposed by the ILO convention.[20] The United Nations became the principal forum through which critics, particularly African and South Asian member states, expressed their alarm at Portuguese misconduct. Dissenting voices in the United Nations reached a crescendo by the mid-1960s and economic sanctions were imposed at the worst possible time: Portugal's colonial wars in Africa had broken out.[21]

This post-war and Cold War context set the stage for Portugal's strategy of a selective appropriation of what development meant over the final quarter century of Portuguese colonialism in Timor. It challenges us to see through Portuguese hubris, particularly in what concerns their fostering of the impression of theirs as a benevolent and altruistic presence aimed at improving the lot of the Timorese people. And yet it also requires us to examine the way Portuguese selectively embraced many technical components of development. At the strictly local level, improving the Timorese lot had everything to do with neutralizing or even eliminating what was commonly seen as the cult of animism. But what was animism, how pervasive was it, and what did it have to do with health?

Animism and Traditional Medicine

By the time British anthropologist David Hicks landed in Portuguese Timor in 1966, illness and witchcraft in the indigenous or "uncivilized" parts of the world had long drawn the attention of anthropologists (Figures 1.1 and 1.2). Hicks conducted his fieldwork amongst one of the island's many ethnolinguistic groups, the Tetum. Although the Tetum residing around the south-coast township of Viqueque turned out to be too acculturated for Hicks's liking, he remained there for the convenience of a health post—which not coincidentally was located in a prioritized, lowland development zone—in case he, his wife or their baby fell ill. Hicks's primary research concern was animism, and to the extent that he succeeded in disentangling its many expressions from Portuguese influences (for example, Catholicism), his first research monograph, *Tetum Ghosts and Kin* (1976), shows just how much animism, health and medicine were bound up with each other.[22]

Hicks explored the way disease among the Tetum was typically traced to spirits. Disease resulted when an alien spirit entered the body (usually at night and through the mouth, nostrils or ears) and, in so doing, pushed out the victim's soul, thus displacing it. If the soul could not reoccupy the body, the malignant force prevailed and led to the victim's death; if, in contrast, the soul managed to reinsert itself and expel the occupying spirit, the victim recovered. Hicks discovered that sickness-inducing spirits were often hermaphroditic witches who traversed the realms of the living and the dead. No village was without "a witch or two." They infected bodies not necessarily out of malice but because of wrong doing: a misdemeanor or act of non-conformism was enough "to prompt a witch to pay the guilty person a nocturnal visit."[23]

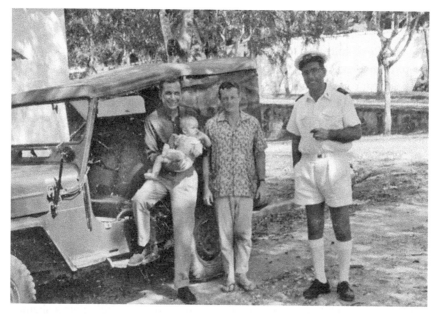

Figure 1.1. David Hicks (center) is paid a surprise visit by Ruy Cinatti (left, nursing Hicks's baby). Cinatti had initially helped Hicks secure his research visa from Portugal. On the right in uniform is the local administrator, José Teles. Viqueque, August 1966. © Maxine Hicks.

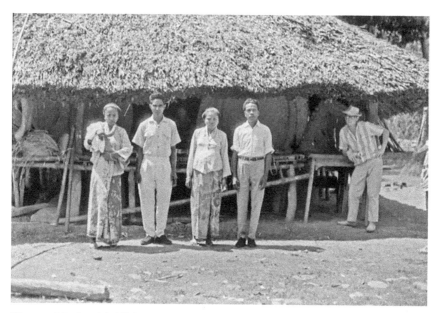

Figure 1.2. David Hicks (right) with villagers posing for a photo in 1967. © Maxine Hicks.

Hicks's animistic disease etiology went further. Illness could equally arise from revenge exacted by the souls of the dead. This tended to happen within the first year of a kinsman's death, when his or her dead soul was likely to linger, creating trouble for living kinsmen, harassing and haunting them and even making them sick or damaging their crops. The Tetum and indeed Timorese method for dealing with capricious dead kin was to propitiate them with ritual offerings: rice, betel and chicken among others. As Hicks put it, "to ignore the needs of ghosts invites sterile unions, sickness and death."[24] The ultimate goal of what Hicks called "rituals of separation" was to drive the offending ghost out of "the secular world" (for example, the village). A rite that took place exactly one year after a deceased's death (and physical interment) constituted a major ritual of separation whose goal was to oblige the dead soul to join the deadly ancestors at a respectable distance from human habitation.

Hicks's ethnography extends to the way individual sickness would invite the focused attention of a shaman. For the price of three little pigs a shaman would determine whether the illness had been caused by a witch or a ghost. The diagnosis proceeded as follows: after masticating and spitting out betel, the shape and shade of the spittle would tell the shaman whether the culprit was ghost or witch. If ghost (generally dead kin), he would recommend a sacrifice; if witch, he would grapple with the power of the witch on the spot to expel the alien spirit from his patient's body. When the shaman's powers proved greater than those of the witch, the patient would be cured. If not, the patient died.[25]

Hicks mentions the shamanic use of the bark of the St Domingo tree as a key ingredient for a medicine applied to wounds.[26] Otherwise, he pays short shrift to traditional medicines used to treat the numerous illnesses of Timor. Portuguese colonials and researchers, however, conducted a few studies into traditional plant medicines: "Timorese Medicinal Plants" appeared as early as 1902 and "Contribution to Medicinal Plant Knowledge in Timor" [my translations] was published in 1968.[27] In the latter study, pharmacologist Fausto Moreira identified 40 medicines across three ethnolinguistic groups (Tetum, Mambai and Kemak).[28] The medicines were derived from parts of plants to treat a range of dermatological, rheumatological, gastroenterological and other conditions. In some cases, the methods deployed to extract or process medicines were described. The author noted that his list was but a fraction of the traditional medicines available. He emphasized the role of specialized shamanic knowledge in collecting, preparing and applying medicines, and he pointed out that remedies were not simply possessed by biophysical properties but also exuded magical properties (Figure 1.3). As Moreira noted:

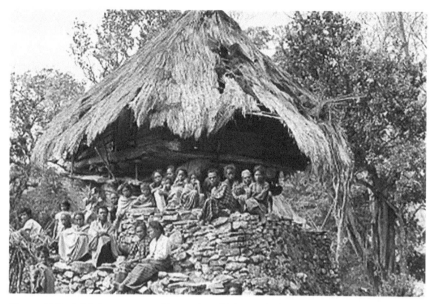

Figure 1.3. A Makassae sacred house in which magic is performed, November 1973. © Shepard Forman and Leona Forman.

> The knowledge of the shamans (*matan dooc*) is vast but hidden. It is not easy to penetrate the secrets about the Gods. In many cases, medicinal plants are considered *lulic* (sacred) and they can only be collected for the purpose of curing ailments, and very few know their applications.[29]

Abel Guterres (who after the Indonesian invasion of 1975 became active in the Timorese "resistance in exile") also noted the connection between animism and medicine. He recalled from his childhood years in Baguia (a remote highland village of Baucau district on the slopes of the awe-inspiring and enchanted Mt Matebian) the old men who "knew more of these [medicines] and also of the animist religious secrets passed down through the person whose ancestor knew it." Medicines, however, were not only the province of specialists:

> We used mainly traditional medicines, leaves and plants. Once I was bitten by a venomous green snake. My whole leg was swollen. My mother heated pawpaw leaves on the fire and put the juice on the bite and cured me. This finger I cut badly but it healed quickly because I put the sticky juice of a special root on it. All village people know the common cures. For diarrhea you drink the thick water the rice was cooked in; if you eat anything poisonous you quickly eat coconut which soaks up the poison so you can vomit it up.[30]

As far as spirit causality and biophysical causality existed as separate categories, they were not equivalent. "Efficient cause is not sufficient cause," wrote
American anthropologist of Timor, Shepard Forman, after observing at his field
site that while a stray spark caused a devastating village fire, behind the spark
lay a malevolent supernatural force (Figure 1.4).[31] Spirits, in other words,
trumped physics. As a rule, the more serious the adversity (medical or otherwise), all the more responsible were the spirits. (A mild sniffle or a stubbed
toe are less likely to be attributed to spirits.) Modern colonial medicine, in effect, sought to turn the tables such that efficient cause would really become
sufficient cause. Eventually, physics would override spirits, or so the Portuguese hoped.

Colonial Medicine and the Colonial Construction of Animism

In the 20th century, two shifts played a key role in establishing the peculiarly
Timorese Cold War medical landscape that ensued after the Japanese occupation (1942–45). First was the turn-of-century pacification of the native
kingdoms that enabled the Portuguese to consolidate their control over the

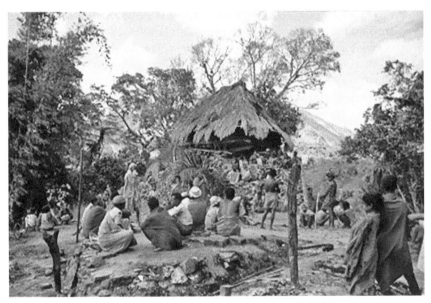

Figure 1.4. After a fire at a sacred site, July 1974.
© Shepard Forman and Leona Forman.

colony and exert more influence over animism. Second, increased colonial control ensured that modern medicine could, by degrees, be delivered to the native population, which in turn highlighted the value-laden intersection between scientific medicine and animistic superstition. Indeed, the 20th-century expansion of medical facilities was pitted against the inadequacies and evils inherent in animistic medicine.

The ethnographic writings of Captain José Martinho, who spent 25 years on the island, exemplify these changes. At the time of his arrival in Timor in 1909, he noted that 450,000 indigenous inhabitants were attended to by only three doctors and a few nurses. After the final pacification war of 1911–12, medical assistance "became more effective." Medical personnel began to travel to districts and "the treatment and cure of ulcers and swellings, from which thousands of Timorese suffered . . . produced a revolution in the mentality of the native." The "empirical science of the shamans began to wane," the captain pronounced. By 1925, he went on, over 50 medical staff, including pharmacists, indigenous nurses, midwives, trainees and helpers, served the sick. Accordingly, "little by little the natives abandoned their shamans . . . and their trade ceased to be lucrative." The Captain predicted that "eventually, the existence of these healers will be but a memory of a long-lost tradition." His story was a common one that would carry over to the post-war period without much alteration: the rationality of science, by its very truth and efficacy, would prove its worth over superstition.[32]

Considerable colonial infrastructure had been destroyed during the Japanese occupation (especially as a result of allied bombing) so a reconstruction effort, including of medical facilities, ensued after Portuguese repossession. By this time, the old colonial storyline of the civilizing mission was becoming mixed up in the new post-war discourse of development. Development of the post-war—indeed the Cold War—period differs in one crucial respect from the "civilizing" interventions of the pre-war decades. Post-war development was acutely conscious of the urgency to legitimize Portuguese colonialism to an international audience and post-war multilateral institutions (for example, the United Nations) amidst the broader waves of decolonization.

The most enthusiastic exponent of post-war development in Timor was the Portuguese captain Hélio A. Esteves Felgas. In his volume *Timor Português*, published in 1956, his glowing account of health infrastructure mirrored that of the other sectors (for example, agriculture and education). By the mid-1950s, he lauded, Timor had four public hospitals and one private one (to serve a large plantation). There were 47 health clinics across the 13 districts and 109 medical staff, including one dentist for approximately 14 million teeth (if my calculation is correct). Felgas insisted that the "high budget accorded to the Health Services in Timor stands as ample proof of the good will that exists to improve the physical condition of a population whose weakness has been visibly accentuated with the difficulties and deprivations suffered during the foreign occupation."[33]

Felgas obfuscated the fact that the budget accorded to health was meager, which in turn was a tiny fraction of a meager total budget.[34] But in the face of growing international scrutiny on Portuguese colonialism in general, he ceded some ground and acknowledged, in a roundabout way, that the Timorese were not such a healthy bunch. His strategy here was the usual one, namely to lay the blame on Timorese primitivism and native mentality: although "our assistance to the natives is free" and "the only wish of the doctors is to treat them," the natives regularly "refuse treatment."[35] More hospitals, doctors and nurses could not alone remedy the health of the population, he stressed, as if hinting at their actual shortfall. The underlying issue, presumably, was that the natives were still not sufficiently civilized to overcome their "instinctive repugnance" of hospitals.

Felgas pointed to a vicious circle inherent in native psychology. The health services, the Captain began, do not find out early enough when a given native is sick, and by the time he gets to hospital not even the best physicians can save him.[36] (Note that the entire native collective was represented by the masculine pronouns "he," "him" and "his," which included women.) The high percentage of those who died in hospital justified the native's aversion for the place: he would avoid admitting himself to hospital because he suspected he would die there, which he usually did for turning up when it was already too late.[37] Added to this problem, the native was averse to undressing and receiving a good scrubbing. Nor did he appreciate the bed he was put into, and often crept out of it and lay on the nice cool floor until such a time as the nurse returned and ordered him back up. The native, finally, failed to understand the nature and duration of treatment, observation and recovery, and he could not fathom why he was kept there like a prisoner when he had always enjoyed his freedom. The discipline, the cleanliness and the stench of disinfectant, and probably the doctor's freaky features, implements and dress, reinforced his decision never to step foot inside a hospital ever again. If the education of the ignorant native was generally touted as the solution to problems that were thought to spring from Timorese primitivism, Felgas proposed that no amount of instruction could break the vicious loop.

Felgas deemed it better to place the sick native alongside his family in new huts that approximated the best of his existing huts, constructed in "indigenous townships" close to the hospital but suitably distant from "the smells, the discipline and the magnificence of the hospital edifice that so frightens him." Although this would appear to hinder the process of civilizing, Felgas was adamant that it would actually accelerate it, for "something will be gained (better construction, greater cleanliness etc.)." He reassured his readers that this hut-beside-the-hospital system had been adopted in Portuguese Africa and it boasted numerous other advantages, not least enabling hospitals to be smaller with beds reserved for those most in need and for those who actually appreciated hospitalization. (The Portuguese frequently branded the Timorese as ungrateful, which they demonstrated by noting that the Timorese did not possess a word for "thank you" until the Portuguese gave them one—*obrigado*.) Felgas advanced another strategy whereby the native's aversion to hospitals could be used to strengthen his participation in vaccination campaigns, since "if the native verifies that a simple injection prevents his admission to hospital, he will be the first to present himself for one."[38]

Felgas conceded that more nurses were needed in rural areas to identify the sick in a timely manner. Portuguese nurses were unaffordable, so it is no surprise that Felgas would insist these should be native nurses as "only they could understand their own race." But, Felgas warned, they should not be the type of nurses who live in huts similar to the native's huts with little hygiene. Rather, the huts needed to be dignified ones, with decent latrines and not littered with rubbish, thus setting an example for the ordinary native.

Raising the ongoing specter of shamanism in a manner not unlike José Martinho had done, Felgas concluded that when the benefits of following the nurses' treatments are recognized, alongside technical knowledge and a pharmaceutical kit, with constant visits to villagers in their huts since the natives rarely visit a health post, the nurses will gain the authority of the old shamans.[39]

Felgas's prognosis did not come to naught, as most Portuguese prognoses did. Although accurate counting was not a Portuguese strength, by 1965 there was said to be 88 practicing Timorese male nurses and 12 non-Timorese practicing doctors.[40] But where were they, and did they ever gain the authority of the "old shamans"?

Colonial Medicine, Malaria and the Agricultural Frontier

In 1969 and 1970, fifteen years after the publication of Felgas's *Timor Português*, German geographer Joachim Metzner criss-crossed the districts of Baucau and Viqueque atop a Timorese pony. The resultant monograph, *Man and Environment in Eastern Timor* (1977), makes it clear not only that shamanic medicine was never replaced in Portuguese Timor, but also that many of Felgas's claims and projections were spurious. Metzner regretted that medical assistance had remained inadequate and barely touched the rural population. He found that only two doctors served the 140,000 people who inhabited the districts of Baucau and Viqueque. As in the other districts, the population had remained widely dispersed and often inaccessible to outside authorities. Nothing, in other words, had come of earlier ideas to condense the rural population into nuclear villages or *aldeamentos indígenas*, thereby replicating aspects of European town planning and facilitating the alternative modes of hospitalization and care that Felgas had envisaged. It is not simply that the Portuguese lacked the resources to undertake large-scale relocation into modern indigenous villages. The Timorese would have resisted any attempt at moving too far away given their strong ties to sacred sites and the burial grounds of their forefathers; for the very same reasons, animism remained strong.[41]

These at once medical and animist questions played out illustratively in relation to Timor's most serious disease, malaria. Its prevalence along the coastal lowlands explained the low population density there compared to the uplands; animism had obviously not prevented them from noticing the correlation between altitude and the incidence of the disease. None of this is to suggest that the Timorese had no traditional applications for what they called *isin malirin*, or "cold body," in the form of rituals, shamanic consultations and medicines; a potion derived from the bark of *Strychnos zigustrina* or *ai baku moras* (in Tetum) was one. However we construe the efficacy of traditional medicine, population density in the coastal regions could be 30 times lower than in the foothills and mountains.[42]

Because lowland alluvial soils along the south coast were particularly fertile, the lack of an indigenous labor force there posed a real problem to the Portuguese, whose sights were set on wet rice development. After pacification (1912) up until the Japanese invasion (1942), attempts to colonize the south and expand rice production had been sporadic and ineffective. From 1960, the Portuguese provided incentives in the form of land, housing, agricultural machinery and chemical inputs to entice highland farmers to settle down south. Typically, enough farmers succumbed to malaria to convince them all that local spirits would prefer not to deal with them and that the land was sacred (Tetum: *lulik*). Farmers did not, Metzner reminds us, report to a health authority, if indeed one was in the vicinity; nor did they await the tardy arrival of a nurse to the village, if indeed one would ever appear. Rather, they packed up then and there and returned to the safety of the mountains.[43] Disease and superstition came together to constitute a single issue for the authorities longing for development.

In order to understand the significant development changes in Timor of the 1960s and 1970s, we must briefly backtrack to consider the way agricultural research and extension in key crops well beyond Timor's shores were rapidly evolving, and the political context in which that was occurring. Prompted by the United States' concerns about China and contagious communism in the early years of the Cold War, rice development had become a central part of the US-led development industry's vision for a well-fed, placid and secure Southeast Asia.[44] When China was beginning to assert its credentials as a net-exporter of rice in the early 1950s, an article in *Foreign Affairs* was indicative of American anxiety that in

> a restless Asia, revolutionary in mood, caught between two opposing ideological and political forces, the question of the supply of this commodity upon which life itself is based has far-reaching political implications. The major problem in the struggle to keep south and southeast Asia free of communist domination is the standard of living of their peoples and the development of their economic resources. There is urgent need for efforts to help the peoples [there] understand that the pretense of plenty and prosperity in China is a myth . . . and they be made to realize that increased production and a higher standard of living are possible in their own countries without the adoption of totalitarian methods. The struggle of the "East" versus the "West" in Asia is, in part, a race for production, and rice is the symbol and substance of it.[45]

The United States government, American philanthropies and the Philippine government established the International Rice Research Institute (IRRI) in 1962. This belonged to a broader effort to create a network of International Agricultural Research Centers (IARCs) based on a number of key crops (wheat, maize, potato, rice), modeled on the Mexican Agricultural Program (MAP).[46] Leading to what became heralded as the Green Revolution, the breeding of high-yielding varieties and their attendant technological packages (that is, chemical inputs and irrigation technology) were usually accompanied by land-reform, infrastructure development (for example, dams), credit and specialization of knowledge.[47] These sociotechnical practices were exported throughout Asia and took the shape of social engineering, going beyond production itself to include agro-industrial and consumption regimes.

The uptake of rice varieties emanating from IRRI was bound to differ in Portuguese Timor from elsewhere in Southeast Asia. Timor was atypical since rice was not already the principal staple. Rather, it was maize. The vast majority of people inhabited precisely those areas that were ecologically inappropriate for the cultivation of wet rice. If the Portuguese post-war agricultural research body, the Overseas Agronomic Research Mission,[48] was to aggressively promote rice cultivation in Timor, it could not do so through an extension strategy of substituting local varieties for "improved" ones simply because the rice that did exist was traditional dry rice grown in uplands on a limited scale, cultivated predominantly for ceremonial (and animist) purposes. In other words, people lived in the wrong places and planted the wrong crops in order to implement a broad scale rice development program without rearranging other agro-social circumstances, including demographic ones. More than for most other parts of Southeast Asia, rice development in Portuguese Timor would have to rest on a more ambitious and trickier undertaking to extend the agricultural frontier and move people accordingly.

The Agronomic Research Mission was encouraged by the specific vari-etal prospects from the IRRI as much as by the general rice bias of the emergent development imaginary for Asia. The Mission began to investigate the land through the lens of rice cultivation. Scientists confirmed that the best agri-cultural lands were the uncultivated lowland strips of the north and south coast. They held that the total area of rice cultivation should be expanded by 25,000 hectares with a corresponding reduction in the supposedly environmen-tally deleterious cultivation of maize involving shifting agriculture on poor soils; the highlands should be set aside mainly for coffee.[49] Research into hydrological resources using aerial photography resulted in a number of irrigation developments north and south along the main rivers.[50] Initially, 7,000 hectares of additional rice cultivation land resulted. High-yielding vari-eties of rice from the Philippines—IR5, IR8, IR22 and IR24—were tested against local varietal controls, including "Java." The new varieties were found to increase yield as much as tenfold under controlled conditions of transplant-ing, weeding and application of fertilizers, herbicides and pesticides.[51]

Just as the research that led to the Green Revolution was gaining pace internationally, so too was research into malaria; indeed, as becomes clear in Annick Guénel's essay in this volume on malarial control in Vietnam, West-ern research into tropical diseases shared the underlying fear of communism with the Green Revolution.[52] By the early 1950s, malaria had become one of WHO's primary global health preoccupations. Portugal first participated in a WHO conference on malaria in 1954;[53] the WHO, in fact, would manage to dispatch a team of experts to three Portuguese African colonies in 1962.[54] I suspect that the WHO would have encouraged the Portuguese to participate in the malaria eradication program that the WHO initiated in 1956 in Indonesia, including in islands that surrounded Portuguese Timor (Sumba, Flores, Solor) and, significantly, in West Timor.[55] While post-colonial Indonesia had became cautiously open to foreign technical assistance, as Vivek Neelakantan demon-strates later in this volume,[56] Portugal manifested something akin to what Xiaoping Fang, also in this volume, refers to as China's resistance to the "international epidemic surveillance network" in the post-war years up until 1972.[57] It is therefore not coincidental that in 1956, the course of action Portugal pursued instead was to have its own Institute of Tropical Medicine inaugurate the Medical Study Mission for Timor, which continued until 1962.[58] The Mission was to investigate malaria across the entire territory down to the last of the 404 villages; it would conduct entomological and epidemiological studies covering distribution and vectors of the disease against the *natural* variables of climate, topography and altitude.[59] WHO involvement was negligible, for the only WHO officials permitted a visit were two public health administrators (one from Manila, the other from Jakarta) in 1960.[60]

In the half-a-dozen or so scientific papers that the Mission produced on malaria between 1956 and 1962, the clear implication was that the research would lead to a plan of action. The titles of three articles began with "Studies on malaria with a view to establish a plan to combat the disease";[61] it was as if a broader audience was being placated. Had a combat strategy emerged, one would further assume from the terms and coverage of the research that it would have spawn interventions targeted to areas of highest prevalence across the whole territory, all other things being equal.[62] No such plan of action to combat malaria ever materialized as it did practically everywhere else in Southeast Asia, and in this respect malaria was no different from all the other ills that afflicted the colony. After 1962, one could be forgiven for thinking that such was the impact of the research alone that malaria had just vanished from Portuguese Timor altogether, and did so right at a critical moment too, when outside calls on Portugal to decolonize had reached fever pitch. All the while, in fact, malaria was surging. Only after unearthing unpublished reports from the Timor Health Services as well as an obscure unpublished dissertation was Metzner able to confirm that between 1950 and 1970 annual malaria contagions had increased from 3.25 percent to 10.87 percent (or 66,368 souls) of the population.[63] Metzner suspected what the Portuguese could not possibly admit to, namely, that this rising infection rate was *unnatural*—"man-made"—and, as in other parts of the "Third World," had been created precisely by the expansion of wet rice agriculture.[64] It should come as no great surprise, then, that in the highly malarial districts of Baucau and Viqueque specifically, Metzner and his pony detected very little in the way of medical facilities, nothing resembling a mosquito net, much less a general antimalarial campaign—at least until such a time as they trotted into Uato Lari.

Uato Lari of the southern coastal region, it turned out, was the one administrative post with a malaria program in full swing.[65] It was here in Uato Lari where modern medicine and modern agriculture intersected most forcefully, and it was here that the Portuguese managed to overcome the double hurdle of malaria and superstition in what Metzner describes as one of the few successful agricultural development undertakings of the post-war period.

Marshy and mosquito-infested Uato Lari had always been very thinly populated relative to the uplands given hyperendemic (51–75 percent) malaria levels. Prior to 1963, there had been some regular field rice cultivation (squeezed between the swamps, equally infested by snappy crocodiles), albeit with minimal paddy. In 1964, the Agricultural Services convened with local administrators, chiefs and village elders to arrange for the opening of 2,500 hectares of paddy. One thousand five hundred smallholder peasants, drawn partly from the foothills above, were enrolled, each of whom received a concession of one or two hectares of land. In the first few years, however, malaria remained high and labor shortages persisted. These problems were resolved with the opening of a health post offering antimalarial treatment. With medical facilities in place, a rice-savvy seasonal labor force with their own field-puddling buffalo could also be enticed to hike from the uplands to the lowlands.

Soon there were 600 seasonal migrants, mostly from Quelicai. Production increased sharply over successive years and further expansion ensued, particularly after the introduction of IR8 in 1968. The Portuguese vaunted a net rice export of 650 tons, up from a mere seven tons in 1961. On the basis of the 1969 figures, Metzner estimated that of a total population of nearly 13,000, each person would have derived a revenue of 112 *escudos* were the benefits shared equally. (Reflecting well-established patterns, however, some chiefs owned paddy areas greater than 100 hectares.) Health facilities and malarial treatment had been central to this transformation.[66] The case concurs with what an abundance of studies internationally have shown, namely that wet rice cultivation was always associated with higher exposure to malarial transmission, and that this rice-malaria relationship can be reversed by targeted antimalarial policies and interventions.[67]

Conclusion

Portugal was bound to continue good old-fashioned Portuguese imperialism in the post-war, and this can be seen most clearly in the ongoing campaign against indigenous animism. It was the Cold War—not simply the post-war— that altered the distribution of intervention in Timor. From about the 1860s and particularly after pacification (1912) up until the Japanese occupation (1942), the Portuguese had been more focused on developing the highlands than the lowlands. The prevalence of coastal malaria and the paucity of treatment, the lesser focus on rice development and the nonexistence of improved rice varieties explain this bias; highland plantation agriculture (especially coffee) was prioritized while traditional swidden agriculture was discouraged.[68] Lowland wet rice development was, of course, a post-war, but principally a Cold War, phenomenon.

It remains to ask where exactly the Cold War asserted itself most in agro-medical terms? Based on what we know from Metzner in Baucau and Viqueque, it appears that modern medicine shadowed agricultural development, and the case of Uato Lari bears this out. We also know that the major plantation complex in Ermera district, the SAPT (*Sociedade Agrícola Patria e Trabalho*), was afforded its own private hospital; historically, the large government plantations had been similarly endowed with health facilities; and Ermera, the heartland of coffee cultivation, had its own public hospital. Conversely, claims that attested to a wide and equitable distribution of medical services for the indigenous population need to be treated as politically motivated nonsense. It would appear that the 1963 decree that each of the health services' "sub-delegacies" provide a hospital of 20 to 30 beds, a maternity clinic and a health post for every constitutive "administrative post" (roughly equivalent to sub-districts) had not produced any apparent result.[69]

In sum, two logics guided the spread of modern medicine. The first logic was to cater to the health of Europeans, and so health facilities were concentrated in places of European habitation. This, of course, explains why two major hospitals were situated in the northern lowlands, Dili and Baucau, and one in Ermera. The second logic was to cater to the health of indigenous subjects when it became economically advantageous to do so. Accordingly, health facilities accompanied agricultural modernization programs, particularly when underlying demographic objectives were in question. It follows that the Portuguese had little incentive to improve the health of subjects whose primary mode of agriculture was of a subsistence nature; resources were too stretched for that anyway. Indigenous ill-health, therefore, became most visible, and most in need of treatment, where concerns about indigenous labor and agricultural production prevailed. The shortcomings of animism, particularly its opposition to scientific reason, also became visible to the same degree; but where labor and modern agriculture were less at issue, the remedy fell to proselytism; in the mountainous swidden realm it was cheaper to have the clergy save souls than for the state to cure ailing bodies.

The strategic convergence of medicine and agriculture was in fact a common response in colonial and post-colonial Southeast Asia and beyond.[70] Yet we should not overlook the broader Southeast Asian dynamics in which this post-war convergence took place. Portuguese Timor absorbed technologies whose development had been vigorously pursued during the Cold War in order to contain communism; according to the rationale, nourished peasantries were happy peasantries, leaving no energy for proletarian mobilization. Because Portuguese Timor had remained a colony, this did not apply in the standard way. Yet, it did apply in three odd ways. Firstly, it applied because Portugal employed the narratives, imagery and technologies of development—both medical and agricultural—to defer inevitable decolonization and, meanwhile, make it seem that the Portuguese themselves were most qualified to develop Timor, and indeed were doing so with unlikely success. Secondly, it applied because the days of the Portuguese in Timor were numbered; pressure was mounting on the international front, and finally from within Portugal when the Carnation Revolution of 1974 ended dictatorship. Communism (or the perception thereof) would sooner or later pose a more direct "threat" to East Timor, and indeed it did in the last few years of the Portuguese colonial presence with the sudden emergence of a pro-independence party (FRETILIN), which advocated for collectivization and, among other things, science-based medical equity.[71] Thirdly, two other pro-plantation parties, comprised of elites (one aligned with Portugal, the other with Indonesia), arose to counter the pro-independence party's growing popularity. Tensions erupted in a period of civil war in 1975, and both the constitution of parties and the civil conflict show just how much the nationalist tide was governed by Cold War politics before Indonesia invaded in December of that year.

Once East Timor was fully integrated into Indonesia, the Cold War shaped the politics of development in ways that are consistent with elsewhere in Southeast Asia and are thematically represented in the coming chapters of this volume: health and agriculture switched to the Indonesian nationalist model, as addressed by Neelakantan in Chapter 6;[72] foreign aid got involved in complex ways, like in the case of Laos, covered by Kathryn Sweet in Chapter 3;[73] and animistic medicine played a heroic role for the Timorese resistance movement, not unlike what in the next chapter Por Heong Hong tells of "folk healing" during the Malayan Emergency (1948–60),[74] with echoes of the role of "original medicine" in Vietnam, as examined by Nara Oda in Chapter 4.[75] Portuguese Timor, however, presents the Cold War anomaly in Southeast Asia: it presents as an "absence" at least until the 1970s, and it often escapes mention in the Portuguese literature of the day as well as in the extensive historiography that treats the post-war period (1945–75).[76] Yet the Cold War was anything but absent from the mid-1940s throughout the 1950s and 1960s. Paradoxically, Portugal's duplicitous management of Cold War influences—which amounted to vastly exaggerating achievements and the scope of future interventions—enabled it to hang on to Timor for as long as it did, just as it precipitated its sudden end as a Portuguese colony.

NOTES

1. Hans Hägerdal, *Lords of the Land, Lords of the Sea: Conflict and Adaptation in Early Colonial Timor, 1600–1800* (Leiden: KITLV Press, 2012).

2. Douglas Kammen, *Three Centuries of Conflict in East Timor* (New Brunswick, NJ and London: Rutgers University Press, 2015).

3. Christopher Shepherd, *Haunted Houses and Ghostly Encounters: Animism and Ethnography in East Timor, 1860–1975* (Singapore: NUS Press, 2019), pp. 11, 22, 279.

4. James Scott, *The Art of Not Being Governed: An Anarchist History of Upland Southeast Asia* (New Haven, CT: Yale University Press, 2009), pp. ix–xi.

5. Michitake Aso, *Rubber and the Making of Vietnam: An Ecological History, 1897–1975* (Chapel Hill, NC: University of North Carolina Press, 2018), pp. 30–6, 48, 78, 200–3; Tania Murray Li, "Compromising Power: Development, Culture, and Rule in Indonesia," *Cultural Anthropology* 14, 3 (1999): 295–399; Christopher Shepherd and Lisa Palmer, "The Modern Origins of Traditional Agriculture: Colonial Policy, Swidden Development, and Environmental Degradation in Eastern Timor," *Bijdragen tot de Taal-, Land- en Volkenkunde* [Journal of the Humanities and Social Sciences of Southeast Asia and Oceania] 171, 2–3 (2015): 281–311, 281–5; Hélder Lains e Silva, *Timor e a Cultura do Café* (Lisbon: Ministério do Ultramar, 1956), p. 93.

6. Joachim Metzner, *Man and Environment in Eastern Timor: A Geoecological Analysis of the Bacau-Viqueque Area as a Possible Basis for Regional Planning*, Monograph 8 (Canberra: Development Studies Centre, Australian National University, 1977), pp. 154–9.

7. Shepherd, *Haunted Houses*, pp. 5–8, 18, 29.

8. Luís Nuno Rodrigues, "Crossroads of the Atlantic: Portugal, the Azores and the Atlantic Community (1943–57)," in *Atlantic Community and Europe 1: European Community, Atlantic Community?* ed. V. Aubourg, G. Bossuat and G. Scott-Smith (Paris: Éditions Soleb, 2008), pp. 456–67.

9. Rodrigues, "Crossroads," p. 464.

10. Douglas Kammen and Jonathan Chen, *Cina Timor: Baba, Hakka, and Cantonese in the Making of Timor-Leste*, Monograph 67 (New Haven, CT: Yale University Southeast Asia Studies, 2020), pp. 9, 135, 151–2. By way of contrast, see Neelakantan, "Mobilizing Applied Medical Knowledge in Indonesia: Soekarnoist Science and Asian–African Solidarity in the 1950s," Chapter 6 in this volume.

11. Rodrigues, "Crossroads," p. 463.

12. Arturo Escobar, *Encountering Development: The Making and Unmaking of the Third World* (Princeton, NJ: Princeton University Press, 1995), pp. 1–5.

13. Jonathan Crush, ed., *Power of Development* (London: Routledge, 1995), pp. 8–15.

14. Christopher Shepherd, *Development and Environmental Politics Unmasked: Authority, Participation and Equity in East Timor* (London: Routledge, 2014), pp. 86–7.

15.   Ministerio dos Negocios Estrangeiros, "Informação sobre o oficio no. 15, de 16 de Abril do Ministerio dos Negocios Estrangeiros, sobre o Inquérito a Realizar pela UNESCO nos Territórios Ultramarinos" (25 April 1951. AHU MU GM mç 1939–1951, Lisbon: Arquivo Histórico Ultramarino), p. 2.

16.   Antonio de Figueiredo, *Portugal and Its Empire: The Truth* (London: Victor Gollancz, 1961).

17.   Anders Ehnmark and Per Wästberg, *Angola and Mozambique: The Case against Portugal*, trans. Paul Britten-Austin (London and Dunmow: Pall Mall Press, 1963).

18.   Hélio A. Esteves Felgas, *Timor Português* (Lisbon: Agência Geral do Ultramar, 1956). See also Fernando Alves Aldeia, "Timor na Esteira do Progresso. Discurso Proferido na Sessão de Abertura da Assembleia Legislativa e da Junta Provincial, em Dili, no dia 14 de Maio de 1973," [Speech Delivered at the Legislative Assembly in Dili, 14 May] (Lisbon: Agência Lusitânia, 1973), p. 2. Icons of progress—hospitals, plantations, rice fields, grain storage facilities, schools, roads, churches, monasteries, convents and monuments—are put on show in Boletim Geral do Ultramar, "Apontamentos para a Monografia de Timor," *Boletim Geral do Ultramar* 41, 480 (1965): 71–113.

19.   Ernest Chamberlain, "The 1959 Rebellion in East Timor: Unresolved Tensions and an Unwritten History," in Proceedings of *Understanding Timor-Leste*, ed. M. Leach, N.C. Mendes, A.B. da Silva, A. da C. Ximenes and B. Boughton (Melbourne: Swinburne Press/Timor-Leste Studies Association, 2010), pp. 174–9; Filipe Temudo Barata, *Timor Contemporâneo: da Primeira Ameaça da Indonésia ao Nascer de Uma Nação* (Lisbon: Equilíbrio Editora, 1998), pp. 2–3; Christopher Shepherd and Andrew McWilliam, "Divide and Cultivate: Plantations, Militarism and Environment in Portuguese Timor, 1860–1975," in *Comparing Apples, Oranges, and Cotton: Environmental Histories of the Global Plantation*, ed. Frank Uekotter (Chicago: University of Chicago Press, 2014), pp. 139–66.

20.   William Gervase Clarence-Smith, *The Third Portuguese Empire, 1825–1975: A Study in Economic Imperialism* (Manchester, UK: Manchester University Press, 1985), chapters 6–7.

21.   Ehnmark and Wästberg, *Angola.*

22.   David Hicks, *Tetum Ghosts and Kin: Fieldwork in an Indonesian Community* (Palo Alto, CA: Mayfield Publishing Company, 1976). There are several more recent, usually jargon-saturated, treatments of animism and medicine in the anthropological literature on Timor, whose interpretations of animism would differ and today might be considered more complete. I have stayed with Hicks since the ethnography was conducted during the period in question, the language is accessible to non-anthropologists, and I follow a relativist meta-ethnographic methodology.

23.   Hicks, *Tetum Ghosts*, pp. 24–30, 111.

24.   Hicks, *Tetum Ghosts*, p. 27.

25. Hicks, *Tetum Ghosts*, p. 112.

26. Hicks, *Tetum Ghosts*, p. 34.

27. João Cardoso, Jr, "Plantas medicinais da Ilha de Timor," *Subsidios para a Materia Médica e Terapeutica das Possessões Ultramarinas Portuguezas*, vol. 1 (Lisbon, 1902), pp. 233–6; Fausto Moreira, "Contribuição para o Conhecimento das Plantas Medicinais do Timor Português," *Revista Portuguesa de Farmácia* 28 (1968): 13–18.

28. Moreira, "Contribuição," pp. 15–16.

29. Moreira, "Contribuição," p. 17.

30. Abel Guterres, "Life Was Good and Easy," in *Telling East Timor: Personal Testimonies, 1942–1992*, ed. Michele Turner (Kensington, NSW: The University of NSW Press, 1992), p. 65.

31. This story is recounted in the superb ethnographic narrative: Shepard Forman, "Spirits of the Makassae: The Vengeful Dead Hasten an Anthropologist's Departure," *Natural History* 85, 9 (1976): 12–18.

32. José Simões Martinho, *Problemas Administrativos de Colonização da Província de Timor* (Oporto: Livraria Progredidor, 1945), pp. 231–5.

33. Felgas, *Timor Português*, pp. 367–8.

34. See L.M. Moreira da Silva Reis, "Timor-Leste, 1953–1975: O Desenvolvimento Agrícola na Última Fase da Colonização Portuguesa," MA thesis (Lisbon: Universidade Técnica de Lisboa, 2000). A decade later, for the period 1965–67, only 7,500 *contos* was accorded to health. See Boletim Geral do Ultramar, "Apontamentos," pp. 90–1.

35. Felgas, *Timor Português*, p. 368.

36. Felgas, *Timor Português*, p. 369.

37. I have no data on the ratio of male to female hospital admissions.

38. Felgas, *Timor Português*, p. 370.

39. Felgas, *Timor Português*, p. 371.

40. Boletim Geral do Ultramar, "Apontamentos," p. 86.

41. Joachim Metzner, "Malaria, Bevölkerungsdruck und Landschaftszerstörung im Östlichen Timor," *Methoden und Modelle der Biomedizinischen Forschung. Beihefte de Geogr. Zeitschrift* (Wiesbaden: Franz Steiner Verlag, 1976), p. 128; Metzner, *Man and Environment*, p. 19.

42. Metzner, "Malaria," pp. 123–4.

43. Metzner, *Man and Environment*, p. 246; Reis, "Timor-Leste," pp. 108–10; Christopher Shepherd and Andrew McWilliam, "Cultivating Plantations and Subjects in East Timor: A Genealogy," *Bijdragen tot de Taal-, Land- en Volkenkunde* [Journal of the Humanities and Social Sciences of Southeast Asia and Oceania] 169 (2013): 152–5.

44. Robert S. Anderson, Edwin Levy and Barrie M. Morrison, *Rice Science and Development Politics: Research Strategies and IRRI's Technologies Confront Asian Diversity, 1950–1980* (New York: Oxford University Press, 1991); Elta

Smith, "Imaginaries of Development: The Rockefeller Foundation and Rice Research," *Science as Culture* 18, 4 (2009): 461–82.

45.   J.K. King, "Rice Politics," *Foreign Affairs* 31, 3 (1953): 453–60.

46.   Bruce H. Jennings, *Foundations of International Agricultural Research: Science and Politics in Mexican Agriculture* (Boulder, CO and London: Westview Press, 1988); Christopher Shepherd, "Imperial Science: The Rockefeller Foundation and Agricultural Science in Peru, 1940–1960," *Science as Culture* [Special Issue]: *Postcolonial Technoscience* 13, 14 (2005): 113–37.

47.   Smith, "Imaginaries," pp. 461–7.

48.   The MEAU or *Missão de Estudos Agronómicos do Ultramar* [Overseas Agronomic Research Mission] was formed in 1960 from what had previously been the *Brigadas de Estudos Agronómicos de Timor* [Brigades for Agronomic Research in Timor].

49.   Hélder Lains e Silva, "Programa de Desenvolvimento Agrícola 1965–1975," *Comunicação* 47 (Lisbon: MEAU, 1964), pp. 1–4.

50.   These were: Seiçal, Laclo, Uato-Carbau, Atabai, Maliana, Natar-Bora, Ue-Berec, Quirás, Merno (Maliboca) and Lete-Foho. See reports: M. Pais de Ramos, "Timor: Seus Recursos Hidroagrícolas," MU/T/Cx, 82, 5, n.d. (Lisbon: Arquivo Histórico Ultramarino). Ministério do Ultramar, Direcção dos Serviços Hidráulicos, "Recursos Hidroagrícolas da Província de Timor. Elementos para um Programa de Acção," MU/T/Cx, 82, 6 (Lisbon: Arquivo Histórico Ultramarino, 1965).

51.   Agência Geral do Ultramar, *Timor: Pequena Monografia* (Lisbon: Agência Geral do Ultramar, 1970 [1965]), p. 117; M. Mayer Gonçalves, A.P. Silva Cardoso, N. Sui Siong and M. Si Min, "Melhoramento da Cultura do Arroz em Timor. Introdução e Selecção de Variedades e Primeiros Ensaios de Adubação," *Comunicações* 84 (Lisbon: MEAU, 1974).

52.   Annick Guénel, "Building a 'Socialist Health System': Soviet Assistance in Malaria Control in the Democratic Republic of Vietnam during the Cold War," Chapter 5 in this volume.

53.   A. Pedroso Ferreira, "Estudos sobre a Endemia Malárica em Timor, com Vista a Estabelecer-se um Plano de Luta contra a Mesma: 1—Considerações Biogeográficas," *Anais do Instituto de Medicina Tropical* 18, 1–2 (1961): 109.

54.   Boletim Geral do Ultramar, "Relatório dos Peritos da Organizacão Mundial de Saude que em 1962 se deslocaram às Provincias Ultramarinas de Guiné, Angola e Moçambique, a Convite do Governo Português," *Boletim Geral do Ultramar* 39, 456–7 (1963): 115–22.

55.   Metzner, "Malaria," pp. 136–7.

56.   Vivek Neelakantan, "Mobilizing Applied Medical Knowledge in Indonesia," Chapter 6 in this volume.

57.   Xiaoping Fang, "The Cholera Pandemic, the Chinese Diaspora and the Cold War Politics in Southeast Asia and China during the 1960s," Chapter 7 in this volume.

58. A. Pedroso Ferreira, "Relatório Anual da Missão Permanente de Estudo e Combate de Endemias de Timor: 1959," *Separata dos Anais do Instituto de Medicina Tropical* 17, 3 (1960): 908–10.

59. See, for example, J. Fraga Azevedo, A. Franco Gândara and A. Pedroso Ferreira, "Missão de Estudo a Timor II—Contribuição para o Conhecimento da Endemia Malárica na Província de Timor," *Anais do Instituto de Medicina Tropical* 15, 1 (1958): 35–52.

60. Ferreira, "Relatório," p. 925.

61. I am referring to three articles that appear in one volume of *Anais do Instituto de Medicina Tropical*, the first of which is cited above as Ferreira, "Estudos," p. 109. The second and third articles focus on epidemiological and entomological aspects of malaria.

62. The evidence for this assumption is the conspicuous silence that surrounds the topic.

63. Metzner, "Malaria," pp. 123–5.

64. Metzner, "Malaria," p. 128. On the rice-malaria relationship in Sub-Saharan Africa, see Kallista Chan, Lucy S. Tusting, Christian Bottomley, Kazuki Saito, Rousseau Djouaka and Jo Lines, "Malaria transmission and prevalence in rice-growing versus non-rice-growing villages in Africa: a systematic review and meta-analysis," *The Lancet Planetary Health* 6, 3 (2022): 257–69; on the relationship between colonial policy and the rise of a host of diseases, including malaria, see Ken de Bevoise, *Agents of Apocalypse: Epidemic Disease in the Colonial Philippines* (Princeton, NJ: Princeton University Press, 1995).

65. An "administrative post" corresponds roughly to today's "subdistrict." Baucau had six administrative posts, and Viqueque had five, of which Uato Lari was one.

66. Metzner, *Man and Environment*, pp. 228–35.

67. Chan et. al, "Malaria Transmission." Note that the incidence of malaria can also be reversed by rice farmers' own responses, enabled by rice sales which in turn enable them to purchase, for example, mosquito nets or insecticides. Failing to understand this relationship led to what used to be called "the paddies paradox," whereby wet rice farming increased mosquito vectors but which, in turn, did not increase disease transmission.

68. Silva, *Timor*, pp. 86, 146–9.

69. The five sub-delegacies were Lautém, Viqueque, Manatuto, Cova Lima and Maubisse. Boletim Geral do Ultramar, "Apontamentos," pp. 86–8.

70. See Aso, *Rubber*; also, Chapter 5 in this volume, Guénel, "Building a 'Socialist Health System'."

71. See FRETILIN [Frente Revolucionária de Timor Leste-Independente], *Manual e Programa Políticos* (Dili, 1974).

72. Vivek Neelakantan, "Mobilizing Applied Medical Knowledge in Indonesia," Chapter 6 in this volume.

73. Kathryn Sweet, "Health Sector Contestation in Cold War Laos, 1950–75," Chapter 3 in this volume.

74. Por Heong Hong, "Tool of Domination and Act of Benevolence: Medicine and Healthcare during the Malayan Emergency, 1948–60," Chapter 2 in this volume.

75. Nara Oda, "More Eastern than Traditional: The Making of *Đông y* in the Republic of Vietnam during the Cold War," Chapter 4 in this volume.

76. Two exceptions are: Kammen and Chen, *Cina Timor*; Shepherd, *Development.*

Tool of Domination and Act of Benevolence: Medicine and Healthcare during the Malayan Emergency, 1948–60

Por Heong Hong

Introduction

Was medicine a tool of domination or an act of benevolence during the Malayan Emergency (1948–60)? Both are equally correct. However, each description has its historiographical as well as epistemic implications, and they tend to be mutually exclusive when it comes to writing about the place of healthcare during that episode of conflict. In one strand of historical narratives about the Malayan Emergency, medicine is narrated either as stories of "battling for people's hearts and minds" or official triumphalist accounts of disrupting medical supplies to the communists.[1] Both the inclusion/provision and exclusion/deprivation of healthcare are narrated as war strategies against the communists. Underlying this triumphalist account, often uncritical of the colonial authority, is the benevolent assumption of healthcare services which benefit the general public. In contrast, the other description, informed by a Foucauldian approach and post-colonial critics, often portrays biomedicine as a tool of domination by the authorities.[2] The second perspective tends to treat actors involved in healthcare provision and medical services and those who receive treatment as undifferentiated and homogenous. More often than not, patients and healthcare users are portrayed as passive and without a voice.

As an attempt to connect both perspectives and being aware of their shortcomings, this chapter reconstructs the history of medicine during the Malayan

Emergency by pulling together three disparate bodies of literature—Malaya's history of counter-insurgency, the history of public health and the history of military medicine. Drawing from government reports, newspapers, personal memoirs, oral histories conducted by other researcher and one interview by the author, this chapter situates Malaya's healthcare and medicine against the backdrop of several rivaling forces in the post-war and Cold War context by taking into account perspectives of European and local actors. On the one hand, the more militant anti-imperialist movements led by the communists were pressing for independence; on the other hand, the nationalists were pushing for Malayanization in the public sector and medical services. New Villages (NVs henceforth)—militarized and transitional communities—were set up to regulate people's everyday activities and to cut off food and medical supplies to the Malayan communists. Facing multiple post-war challenges, the British government had to adjust the military tone of its anti-communist strategies to one that projected medical benevolence. In reality, the government budget largely went to anti-communist military warfare, economic services and urban infrastructure, leaving health services scant resources. However, the government encouraged the voluntary and missionary sectors, largely drawn from the missionaries who fled communist-controlled China in 1949, to fill the healthcare void in the NVs and other resettlement areas, shaping the medical landscape in Malaya. Outside of the NVs and the Orang Asli jungle forts, the British colonial government largely neglected the healthcare needs in the predominantly Malay rural areas. Hence, I argue that healthcare, available only to those who conformed to colonial authority, was an "instrument of war" disguised as "medical benevolence" during the Malayan Emergency. Nonetheless, local actors were not passive; they remained critical of the authority. Meanwhile, an international collaborative research network on military medicine was formed between the US, Australia and British Malaya to conserve the fighting strength of the anti-communist forces and to study tropical diseases. In contrast, the communist guerillas relied on self-acquired healing knowledge to keep healthy and treat illnesses.

While the colonial government was preoccupied with its anti-communist warfare, local nationalist elites were divided into two camps, those engaged in a less militant anti-colonial movement and those who were more militant, such as the communist insurgency. The moderate nationalists pressed the colonial government to Malayanize civil and medical services, and to establish a second medical college to train more local doctors. Saturated with modernization and self-determination discourses, the Malayanization movement aimed to drive the expatriates out of the country. Nonetheless, there were too few medically trained local experts to fill the void left behind by the departing expatriates.

In spite of their good intention to improve healthcare in Malaya, the movement paradoxically contributed to the shortage of medical manpower in public health.

This chapter is divided into eight sections. The first narrates the post-war context and the place of healthcare in the colonial authority's counter-insurgency strategy. The situation of inadequate healthcare in concentration-camp-like NVs unfolds in the second section, followed by stories of medical missionaries who fled communist-controlled China to provide healthcare in the NVs. The fourth section describes how healthcare provision was visualized and instrumentalized as a psychological weapon against the communists, and this is followed by sections on healthcare in the Orang Asli settlement and the predominantly Malay rural areas. Importantly, both communist guerillas and counter-insurgency soldiers needed healthcare too, and their stories are recounted in the seventh section, which is succeeded by a section on the nationalists' struggle to remove expatriates from the government medical services.

Briggs Plan: The Birth of New Villages

In the aftermath of World War II, Malaya was placed under the seven-month rule of the British Military Administration (BMA) until the establishment of the Malayan Union on 1 April 1946. A series of post-war healthcare service assessments and rehabilitations were undertaken by the Civil Administration, which replaced the BMA in 1946. The colonial army and the Red Cross societies supplied essential equipment and drugs to the hospitals, which were dilapidated and poorly equipped during the Japanese occupation.[3]

Between 1946 and 1948, while the British civil government was engaged in repairing Malaya's economy and other sectors, the Malayan Communist Party (MCP) was active in installing governments in several local areas, consolidating its national organization and laying plans to seize power from the British.[4] On 16 June 1948, the killing of three European plantation managers by the MCP in Sungai Siput, Perak, prompted the colonial government to declare an emergency in July 1948. This led to the eruption of an anti-communist war, which lasted for 12 years until 1960.[5] During the early years of the emergency, the counter-insurgency campaign was at its weakest position, despite a rapid build-up of security forces and large amounts of expenditure to support the anti-communist operation. The total cost of defence, police and counter-insurgency operations rose from $82 million in 1948 to $296 million in 1953, with 1952 and 1953 being the most expensive years. The sum amounts to $225,000 a day in 1948 and $811,000 a day in 1953.[6] The colonial authority blamed ethnic Chinese settlers in the rural areas and the Orang Asli in the jungle for their support of the communists.[7]

It was not until mid-1950 that British General Harold Briggs, Director of the anti-communist campaign, came up with a resettlement plan to deprive the communists of several essential supplies which they obtained from the Chinese settlers, items such as food, medicine, clothing, money and also intelligence. The resettlement plan, also called the Briggs Plan, moved over 1.2 million people from the unguarded remote areas to 600 settlements fenced with double layers of barbed wire and guarded by the British security forces.[8] The plan aimed to disrupt the communist influence of the Chinese settlers, many of whom were thought to be communist sympathizers. Police searched people every time they entered or left the resettlement areas to deter them from passing food and medicine to the communists. Curfew was also imposed to allow the movement of villagers only during prescribed hours. Hence, the birth of the NVs, which witnessed the extension of state power into the everyday lives of the Chinese settlers.[9] This, however, by no means suggests that all ethnic Chinese were at the receiving end of state surveillance. A significant number of ethnic Chinese were recruited and trained to become a type of Home Guard, which, in Leon Comber's words, was "virtually a Chinese army made up mostly of KMT (Kuomintang) supporters, with some Chinese secret society supporters," or the eyes and ears of the colonial authority in the NVs.[10]

Lack of Healthcare in the NVs

A year after the implementation of the Briggs Plan, the "Member System" was introduced in the Federal Executive and Legislative Council in April 1951. The Member of Health was a quasi-ministerial portfolio under the newly instituted Member System, a predecessor of post-independence Malaya's cabinet. Personalities with nationalist leadership were given political responsibility through the Member System as they were viewed by the colonial government as a "convenient antidote" to communism.[11] Compared to their militant communist counterparts, the nationalist leaders were much preferred by the British for their moderate anti-colonialist approach which was more in line with the colonial commercial and industrial interest. The Member System was thus an institutional platform created by the British for nationalist leaders to participate in carefully controlled popular politics in the face of rising nationalism in post-war Malaya.

Lee Tiang Keng,[12] the first Member of Health (1951–55), sent a memorandum to all state governments in July 1951, urging them to provide static dispensaries in NVs with a population over 3,000 and mobile dispensaries to those with less than 3,000 settlers. These dispensaries were to be staffed by hospital assistants.[13] Lee's memorandum only fell on deaf ears, as the colonial government was preoccupied with anti-communist warfare and reluctant to commit further to healthcare provision. Despite being disregarded, Lee and other Malaysian Chinese Association (MCA) leaders and members continued to play a role through their engagement in charitable activities and their funding for voluntary and missionary healthcare in NVs throughout the emergency period. Various speeches delivered by Henry Gurney, the British High Commissioner from 1948 to 1951, repeatedly mentioned that the formation of the MCA and its community services in the resettlement areas were welcomed by the government. He viewed the MCA as providing the ethnic Chinese with an alternative to communism.[14]

The government's budget allocation clearly suggests its lack of commitment in expanding healthcare. Of the total $680.6 million allocated for the Federation in the 1951–55 period, $155.6 million went to agricultural development and $394.5 million to urban infrastructure, leaving merely $15.3 million or 2.25 percent to healthcare.[15] For the resettlement fund, of the $7 million disbursed for the year of 1950, $3.8 million went to building grants and subsistence allowances paid to people uprooted from their home and livelihood. The remaining $3.2 million was spent on public works, for example, roads, drains, latrines and the construction of wells, but there were hardly any funds for social or health services. In the following year, only $2.4 million out of a total $41 million resettlement fund was allocated to educational, medical and health amenities. In 1952, the resettlement budget dropped to $19 million, of which only $0.89 million went to medical and health facilities. Despite the meagre allocation for social and health services, the total cost of the emergency increased to $208 million in 1953, as a result of the expansion of the armed forces.[16]

In April 1952, the problem of healthcare in the NVs was raised again, this time by the Malaya Branch of the British Medical Association (MBBMA). The MBBMA expressed its concern over the "gross inadequacy of medical services in the resettlement areas," described the resettlement areas as "a new risk to public health, threatening epidemics which may endanger, not only the areas themselves, but also the adjacent populations," and urged the government to provide static dispensaries to all camps with a population greater than 1,000 people. H.M.O. Lester, then Director of Medical Services in the Federation, however, disagreed with the suggestion on the grounds that there were insufficient fully trained hospital assistants to man the dispensaries.[17] Lester's response to the MBBMA's recommendation was not completely baseless, as there were severe healthcare manpower shortages in the congested NVs. Two states with the largest number of NVs faced a serious shortage in healthcare facilities. In 1958, 56 NVs in Perak and 29 NVs in Pahang were not covered by any health services.[18]

Medical Benevolence: The Arrival of Missionary Healthcare

Given the lack of interest by the colonial government to expand healthcare services in the NVs, a void was created. However, the void was soon filled by a large army of foreign missionaries, estimated to be over 7,000 people, who were forced to leave China after the communists took over the country in October 1949.[19] In her memoir, Kathleen Carpenter, a missionary from the Church Missionary Society who opened up clinics and served in Jinjang NV and Salak Selatan NV, Kuala Lumpur, during the emergency period, recollected:

> In 1951 when these new villages were being established, the leaders of the various Churches in Malaya saw in them a great challenge. For the first time it was possible to reach these people, who had formerly been inaccessible, scattered as they were in small groups throughout the jungle. It was felt that in this, their hour of need, the villagers might be specially open to the message of God's care and love for each individual, and that the challenge of the claim of God on their lives might prove to them a greater challenge than that of Communism. The Bishop of Singapore therefore wrote first to the Church Missionary Society, later to the Church of England Zenana Missionary Society, and again to the Anglican branch of the Overseas Missionary Fellowship (formerly the China Inland Mission) inviting them to send missionaries who could no longer work in China, but who knew and loved the Chinese, to work in the new villages of Malaya.[20]

"The High Commissioner and those in authority gave much support and encouragement," said Carpenter. The foreign missionaries from China were invited, first by Henry Gurney and later by Gerald Templer,[21] to serve in the NVs. Given their years of service in China and with their command of Chinese dialects and medical skills, Henry Gurney saw their value in serving the healthcare needs in the predominantly Chinese NVs. He likened each missionary to "a brigade of troops" against the communists.[22] After the assassination of Henry Gurney in 1952, it became even clearer to the Colonial Office that communism could not be defeated by military means alone. The Secretary of State for the Colonies, Oliver Lyttelton, informed the House of Commons that "we cannot dissociate the economic, social and political problems of this area [Malaya] from the military problem."[23] There was thus a shift in the anti-communist strategy from a military oriented one, to one that was fringed with social services to win the "hearts and minds" of the people, via the "after care" services in the NVs. In a 90-minute policy review, Gerald Templer told the Federal Legislative Council:

The battle will be a long one, and in the main it must and will be won in the hearts and minds of the people. We must be on our guard against recrudescence of full-scale and widespread terrorism. Our security forces and our Emergency precautionary measures are an insurance against this.[24]

The missionary contribution in the NVs' healthcare services was significant, but unevenly distributed. In February 1954, the Malayan Christian Council already had 125 resident workers in 65 NVs and 150–200 voluntary workers in 43 NVs, while the Catholic Church had 56 workers in 176 NVs. In total, over 400 missionaries from more than a dozen missionary boards came to serve in 333 NVs during the emergency period. Even though not all missionaries were engaged in providing health services, half of all clinics in Perak, which has a total of 155 NVs, were run by church or missionary groups.[25]

These missionaries were drawn to Malaya largely because they already had command of Chinese dialects, which they picked up while serving in China. Proficiency in these dialects facilitated their work in the predominantly Chinese NVs. Even though they welcomed the colonial government's invitation to serve in the NVs, they were not monolithic. Some shared the British government's view, seeing their missionary work as combating the communist insurgency; some worried that working under the government might be perceived in the wider community as their being agents of Western imperialism, and feared that being perceived as such might endanger the lives of some missionaries. The difference was also informed by linguistic and cultural identities and historic divergence between different denominations. The support of the English-educated urban leaders for missionary work in the NVs was lukewarm as such work was perceived to be communally oriented; competition also existed between existing Malaya-based churches and the newly arrived foreign missionaries who were expelled from China.[26] Despite the differences among the missionaries over what kind of relationships they should maintain with the colonial authority, clinics and medical services provided opportunities for "unobstructed evangelism." In some missionary-run clinics in Pahang, the walls were decorated with posters, and medicine packets carried Christian messages in Chinese.[27] It was a shared goal among the missionaries that they had a duty to Christianize, if not to civilize, the non-Western societies. Consider the memoir of G.D. James, an India-born and Singapore-based missionary of the Malaya Evangelistic Fellowship, who recollects his service in Malaya during the Malayan Emergency:

The world population is increasing at a tremendous rate of 50 million each year. And half the people of the globe have no chance of hearing the gospel

even once if missionary work is to be carried on at the rate it is done at present . . . in 1960 there were 2,850,000,000 people in the world, and it is
expected that at the end of this century the population will have swelled to
6,950,000,000; and about half of this will be Asians.[28]

Nevertheless, one particular event is worth highlighting to illustrate the
"dilemma" facing the colonial government in providing healthcare in the NVs.
In 1953, the China Inland Mission proposed to the government that it set up a
60-bed hospital to serve several of the NVs. H.M.O. Lester, then Director of
Medical Services in the Federation, turned down the proposal on the grounds
that it was likely to increase government spending and it might also invite religious objections in a multi-religion society.[29] Given that the priority was
placed on anti-communist warfare and maintaining industrial and economic
activities, the real concern behind the refusal might be the reluctance of the
government to spend more on healthcare.

One of the funding sources that helped the missionaries to build clinics
came from the MCA. Over a period of two and a half years, from early 1950
to July 1953, the MCA raised a total of 4 million Malayan dollars through
selling lottery tickets.[30] Being offered a legitimate platform by the colonial government to fund, mobilize and organize missionary healthcare, the MCA was
crucial for engaging ethnic Chinese in providing social services. In so doing,
it also hopefully directed the Chinese away from participating in other political
activities unwelcomed by the British.

Turning to voluntary organizations' contributions was another strategy
by the colonial government to overcome insufficient healthcare in the NVs. To
avoid duplication, a Coordinating Committee, chaired by the Chief Secretary,
was set up. The committee consisted of local representatives of the British Red
Cross Society, St John's Ambulance Brigade, Women's Voluntary Services,
Boy Scouts Association, the MCA, the Central Welfare Council, and churches
and missionary bodies.[31]

Healthcare Provision in the New Villages and Psychological Warfare

Despite inadequate healthcare facilities in the NVs, anti-communist propaganda painted a positive image of the resettlement plan and highlighted the
provision of healthcare services in the NVs; as Templer recognized, the "after
care" of the resettlement villages was crucial to win the "hearts and mind" of the
villagers.[32] At the early stage of the Briggs Plan, there was no reference to
the resettlement areas as "new villages." Some newspaper coverage and

commentaries simply used "resettlement villages" as a neutral and descriptive term, or sometimes a somewhat ideologically loaded term "free town" (a town "free from communists" and "free from worries") to refer to the resettlement areas.[33] There was, however, a turn in strategy beginning from 19 March 1952, when Templer first coined the term "new villages" to refer to the resettlement areas in his speech to the Legislative Council.[34] After that, "New Village" was used interchangeably with "resettlement villages." Some NVs were selected, via newspaper coverage, to showcase the benefits and advantages of living in a "new born" town equipped with electricity, water supply, agricultural land, place of worship, roads and drains, and health services.[35] Healthcare provision was often highlighted as one of the welfare services in the NVs. The image of "new born town" was created not only to justify the resettlement plan; it was also a tool of psychological warfare intended to weaken the will and morale of the communists by contrasting "comfortable lives" in the NVs to the hardship and miseries of being guerillas in the jungle.

Apart from painting a positive image of the NVs, anti-communist leaflets printed in Chinese characters with pictures of "surrendered communists" receiving good-quality healthcare were also distributed to deter people from joining the communists and to force the communists to give up their political struggle (see Figures 2.1 and 2.2). "Operation Shoe" was one such psychological war effort waged against the communists. Around July 1957, leaflets were dropped in Labis, Johor, appealing to the 50,000 people in the area to deny the communists food and medicine.[36] The message of the propaganda was plain and simple: stay away from communists, and give up armed struggle, and you can enjoy healthcare services. In short, both the provision and the deprivation of healthcare were equally crucial in managing and governing people's political affiliation and allegiance.

Although it was the colonial government's strategy to control people's political leaning through healthcare provision, not a single case of attack by the communists had been made on the 25 Red Cross teams operating in Malaya then, indicating that the voluntary health service was positively received by the communists.[37] The villagers too were not hostile to government healthcare. At the very beginning, they viewed the government mobile clinics with suspicion, but then their trust in these services grew when they realized the nursing staffs were genuine.[38] Importantly, as argued by James Scott, the subordinate class may appear to be conforming and consenting in front of authority, but they tend to keep their hidden transcript and offstage speeches to sustain an everyday resistance to the power of domination.[39] A large number of oral histories conducted by Tan Teng Phee in several NVs reaffirms Scott's notion of "weapons of the weak." Despite the inconveniences and hardship caused by

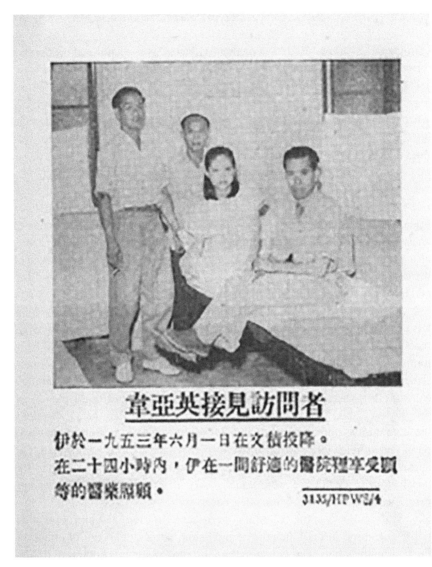

Figure 2.1(a). Anti-communist leaflet in 1953: Wei Ya-Ying Received Visitors. She surrendered on 1 June 1953. Within 24 hours, she could enjoy healthcare of superior quality.

你們需要一位醫生嗎？

如果你們受了傷，你們會獲得好的醫藥治療嗎？

你們的答案當然是不幸的「沒有」，你們只能夠希望或祈禱你們會好一點或者是早一點死去。

政府當局對於任何一位保安隊伍的人員在受傷後都予以最完善及必要的醫藥治療。

政府當局也希望將這同樣的醫藥治療去照顧任何一位受傷及需要援手的馬共人員。

如果你們患了病或受了傷，去和民衆接洽，叫他們帶你們到最近的醫站或兵站去。

跑到公路上來，揮手停止一輛汽車然後乘車到警站去。

我們允諾給予你們那你們自己組織所不能給你們的一切東西。

立刻爭取醫藥治療。

不要棄之不理，不然就太遲了！

3135/HPWS/4

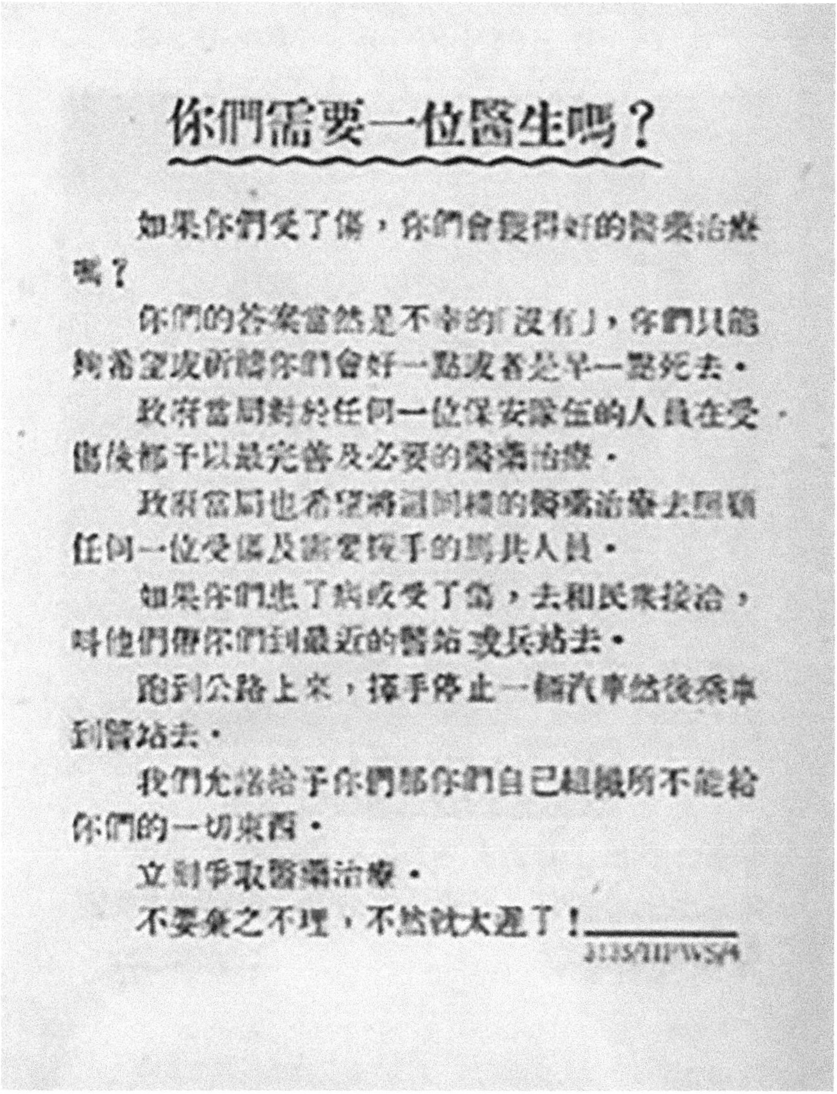

Figure 2.1(b). Anti-communist leaflet in 1953: Do You Need a Doctor?
If you get injured, do you get good medical treatment? Your answer is certainly an unfortunate "no." You can only pray that you would get better or die early. The government offers every single injured member of the security forces necessary and comprehensive medical treatment. If you fall sick or get injured, you can get in touch with the public, ask them to direct you to the nearest clinic or police station. You can also stop any car and ask for a lift to the police station. We promise to give you everything your organization is unable to provide. Get your medical treatment now. If you do not bother to get it, it might be too late. Source: http://www.psywar.org/product_MY3135HPWS04.php [accessed 20 April 2013].

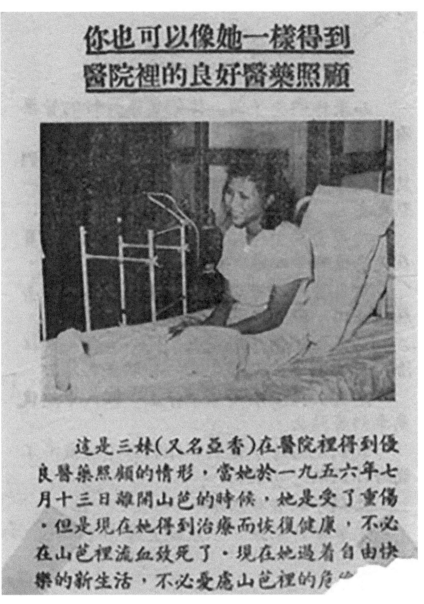

你也可以像她一樣得到
醫院裡的良好醫藥照顧

這是三妹(又名亞香)在醫院裡得到优
良醫藥照顧的情形‧當她於一九五六年七
月十三日離開山芭的時候，她是受了重傷
‧但是現在她得到治療而恢復健康，不必
在山芭裡流血斃死了‧現在她過着自由快
樂的新生活，不必憂慮山芭裡的危

Figure 2.2. Anti-communist leaflet in 1956: You Can Also Get Good Healthcare Like Her. This is San Moi (also named Ya Xiang). She gets good healthcare service at the hospital. She was seriously injured while she left the jungle to surrender on 13 July 1956. Now she has recovered, after getting medical treatment. She will not die of bleeding in the jungle. She is happy and free in her new life, no longer needs to worry about the danger of living in the jungle. Source: http://www.psywar.org/product_MY3135HPWS4.php [accessed 20 April 2013].

the resettlement and everyday surveillance, most villagers remained critical of the colonial authority.[40]

Jungle Forts and Healthcare for the Orang Asli

Apart from the ethnic Chinese resettled into the NVs, the Orang Asli was another community caught in the war between the British government and the communists. Before World War II, there was no policy by the colonial government on the "welfare" of the aborigines. The British left the aborigines to lead their own lives in the jungle, or placed them under the authority of Malay rulers. In the aftermath of World War II, a federal protector of aborigines associated with the Department of Social Welfare was appointed. However, the colonial government's interest in the aborigines soon changed into a security and military concern during the Emergency. The colonial authority realized the political importance of the aborigines, who possessed skills in jungle living. A department that aimed "to cater for the needs of the aborigines" was created in 1950 and headed by Peter D.R. Williams-Hunt, a British major and a trained aerial photographic interpreter who married a Semai woman in the early 1950s while doing ethnographic research among the Orang Asli after the war. The department was later renamed Department of Aborigines (DOA, or Jabatan Hal Ehwal Orang Asli in Malay) and tasked with the responsibility to curb communist influence by winning the hearts of the Orang Asli through the provision of various social and healthcare services.[41]

Compared to the resettlement of the ethnic Chinese, the scale of aboriginal resettlement was not as massive, but the lives of the resettled native people were no less disrupted and uprooted. In areas where the communists operated freely, the aborigines were forcefully evacuated and brought to camps in Pahang, Perak, Kelantan, Negeri Sembilan and Johor respectively. Social dislocation, malnutrition, dissatisfaction over the new environment and immobility caused illnesses and higher death rates among those resettled.[42] Though there is no comprehensive data on the aboriginal morbidity and mortality rates, some fragmented data gathered by ethnographers and medical doctors in certain camps give us a picture of the health conditions of the resettled natives. In the Semai-occupied Bukit Betong resettlement camp in Pahang, 217 deaths were recorded among the 2,200 resettled population in the period from November 1949 to January 1951. Twenty-four out of the 217 who died were less than 50 years of age, indicating that aging was not the cause of death. Causes of death included dysentery and malaria. Overcrowdedness in resettlement areas made shifting agriculture no longer possible and the environment become more prone to dysentery epidemics.[43] In another large camp in 1951 the death rate was astonishingly 204 per thousand.[44]

Disheartened by the decaying scenes of the resettled Orang Asli communities, Williams-Hunt suggested the establishment of "jungle forts," wide natural areas equipped with various facilities, to replace resettlement camps. Apart from providing "visible evidence of Government" and protection of the Orang Asli from communist influence, the DOA also extended medical facilities, education and welfare services to the forts. Pamela Gouldsbury, a European jungle nurse, recalled in her memoir that for Williams-Hunt,

> it was possible to break the Communist guerrillas' domination of the groups, thus freeing large areas of the jungle from the terror they caused and denying the guerrillas freedom of movement and safety for their food cultivation and camps . . . with the aborigines on our side we would be able to supply the security forces jungle patrols with an endless stream of information as to guerrilla movements in addition to guides to take them through the jungle.[45]

Despite Williams-Hunt's premature death in an accident in June 1953, the DOA was reorganized to provide education, welfare and medical services, and 12 forts were established by the end of the same year. The department grew from under 20 to over 200 personnel. Special medical centers exclusively for the Orang Asli were started beginning from the early 1950s. A 12-bed hospital was set up in Kuala Lipis, Pahang, and later expanded to a larger one and relocated to a forested area in Gombak, near Kuala Lumpur, in 1957.[46] In 1954, an Intelligence Section was created in the DOA for the "collation, evaluation, synthesis and dissemination of intelligence obtained from aborigine sources and technical supervision of departmental intelligence activities and training." Some aborigines were recruited into a military unit, called "Senoi Pra'aq," to patrol the jungle forts and nearby areas, given their lack of trust of the Malays, by whom the police force was dominated. The Senoi Pra'aq greatly resembled the Chinese Home Guard in the NVs: both were ethnicized armed forces guarding their own communities. It was estimated that the number of Orang Asli under communist domination dwindled from several thousand in 1953 to only 250 in 1958.[47]

British historian Anthony Short attributed the success of the British government in winning the "hearts and minds" of the native people to the provision of medical services:

> Perhaps the greatest of the positive attractions which [the British] government offered to aborigines were the medical clinics. In one year alone, the ten forts between them treated over fourteen thousand new

aborigine patients; and as many aborigine medicine men trained as Medical Assistants they were able to more than double the range or remedies for poor hygiene, minimal nutrition and the high incidence of disease, particularly yaws.[48] More and more families made their way to the jungle forts and were treated by government as refugees while their new cultivation areas, opened up close to the forts, matured. On discovering that they were provided immediately with rations, that government were prepared to continue this up to a period of nine months, and that they would not be locked up let alone killed, as a result of seeking government protection, aborigine confidence in the guerrillas waned.[49]

Like what their Chinese counterparts encountered in the NVs, the resettled aborigines were also subject to political surveillance and state discipline, as a price they had to pay for gaining access to the DOA's healthcare and other social services. Laced with rhetorics of "welfare," medical services were a tool of the colonial authority to govern and control political leanings of the aborigines and their relations with other communities. However, it is important to note that both the communities of Orang Asli and ethnic Chinese were not homogenous; they were just as divided. The pro-regime segments worked as the eyes and ears of the state, such as the Senoi Pra'aq and the Chinese Home Guard.

Inter-Racial Mortality Discrepancy and Rural Health

Obviously, the predominantly Malay rural areas did not benefit from the expansion of healthcare in the NVs, provided by the missionaries or otherwise. The "luxury" of the predominantly Chinese NVs inevitably invited protests from political leaders of other races. Some Malay state representatives insisted that "[healthcare] facilities in the NVs and towns should not be greater than those already provided for Malay villages which had not had the 'luxury' of being resettled."[50] Indeed, the inter-racial discrepancy in both infant mortality rate and maternal mortality rate (see Tables 2.1 and 2.2) reveals the relatively poorer state of rural health. In 1951, a Malay correspondent from the *Straits Times* also conveyed dissatisfaction among the Malays over how their community had been neglected. Pleas were made to improve living standards, better roads and better health services.[51] In 1953, Dato Onn bin Ja'afar, the then Malay Member for Home Affairs and Chairman of the Rural and Industrial Development Authority (RIDA), protested the perceived lack of urgency accorded to Malay kampongs: "To give a square deal to the Malays, the money is essential and it must be found, Emergency or no Emergency."[52] The most commonly found disease in the predominantly Malay East Coast states during the counter-insurgency period was gastroenteritis.[53] The outbreak of gastroenteritis

Table 2.1. Infant mortality rate (per 1,000 live births) in the Malayan Union (1946–47) and Federation of Malaya (1948–59), by racial group, 1946–59

Year	Malay	Chinese	Indian	All
1946	118	64	92	92
1947	129	70	99	102
1948	111	67	89	89
1949	93	64	85	81
1950	121	74	114	102
1951	108	82	103	97
1952	101	70	109	90
1953	98	61	92	83
1954	100	59	83	83
1955	97	53	78	78
1956	95	47	72	74
1957	96	47	76	75
1958	101	49	74	79
1959	84	41	63	66

Sources: MURMD (1946–47); FMRMD (1948–59). Note: The marked increase of infant mortality amongst the Malays in 1947 may be associated with the epidemic outbreak of smallpox in the predominantly Malay rural area in 1946 and 1947.

Table 2.2. Maternal mortality in the Malayan Union (1946–47) and Federation of Malaya (1948–59), rate by racial group, 1946–59

Year	Malay	Chinese	Indian	All
1946	9.3	3.5	8.2	6.7
1947	9.9	3.2	7.7	7.0
1948	8.4	3.2	5.5	5.8
1949	7.2	3.0	5.0	5.3
1950	7.0	3.3	5.2	5.3
1951	NA	NA	NA	5.7
1952	NA	NA	NA	5.2
1953	NA	NA	NA	4.7
1954	NA	NA	NA	4.8
1955	NA	NA	NA	4,2
1956	NA	NA	NA	4.0
1957	NA	NA	NA	3.2
1958	NA	NA	NA	2.8
1959	NA	NA	NA	2.1

Sources: Malayan Union Report of the Medical Department (1946–47) and Federation of Malaya Report of the Medical Department (1948–59).

was an annual occurrence in Kelantan between 1954 and 1958. Yaws was another disease identified as "a disease of the rural population particularly Malays" in the post-war years.[54] Given the "lag" in rural health development, foreign funding and assistance poured in through international platforms, such as the World Health Organization (WHO) and United Nations Children's Fund (UNICEF), in the early post-independence years.[55]

Interestingly, the discrepancy between the aim and the actual achievement of the rural health plan opened up a space for political mobilization. Apart from insufficient facilities, deficiency in education, hygiene knowledge and health literacy were frequently cited as a factor contributing to poor health in these areas. In 1958, Mohamed Idris, Kelantan Minister for Works, called on Malay teachers to give more hygiene lessons to their students, so that the pupils and their families "could live longer." "I made a startling discovery when I interviewed applicants for appointments as Malay teachers, 20 percent, had no parents. This showed that Malays in the kampongs did not know much about hygiene," appealed Mohamed Idris.[56] Dato Abu Bakar bin Baginda, Selangor Menteri Besar, attributed rural people's inability to work long in the field to their lack of hygiene and health knowledge. He urged the teachers to extend this knowledge to the rural people.[57] Not only teachers, but also youths became a target of mobilization.[58] A gendered space too was carved out for Malay girls and women in the rural health movement. They were called on to participate in domestic science and to make sure the menfolk, their children and themselves had balanced diets.[59] The Women's Institute, a multi-objective campaign formed by urban educated women, started a nationwide campaign to teach rural folk fundamental hygiene at the government's suggestion.[60] Rural health was thus a discursive space that allowed the Malay leaders to "speak for," to mobilize and to regulate the predominantly Malay rural folk.

As far as maternal mortality rates were concerned, there was improvement in people's health situation over the 12-year counter-insurgency period (see Table 2.2). Increased attendance in Infant and Child Welfare Centers and more home visits by nurses and midwives over the same period were another two indicators of improved health services (see Table 2.3). Nevertheless, it is an undeniable fact that healthcare had been a tool of the colonial government to discipline and govern its population's political leanings. Local nationalist leaders, such as Onn Ja'afar and Abu Bakar Baginda, were quick in learning to appropriate the rhetoric of welfare and the importance of healthcare to critique the colonial authority, and to make use of hygiene and health education to mobilize and build their communities. As a tool of the Cold War, and to win hearts and minds, the rhetoric of "medical benevolence" and "healthcare" had paradoxically become a tool of the local elites, especially those trained in

Table 2.3. Attendance in Infant and Child Welfare Centers and volume of home visits by nurses and midwives, 1946–59

Year	Attendance	Home Visits
1946	320,000	112,000
1947	420,000	200,000
1948	583,755	245,003
1949	633,638	271,553
1950	873,249	310,092
1951	838,074	348,337
1952	983,385	419,939
1953	1,087,204	500,866
1954	1,192,413	470,510
1955	1,346,683	460,036
1956	1,433,538	529,156
1957	1,461,844	528,712
1958	1,494,701	617,581
1959	1,715,519	765,636

Sources: MURMD (1946–47) and FMRMD (1948–59).

Western medicine and across all ethnic backgrounds, to push for more welfare. The colonial authority risked losing their support if they did not respond to these calls (discussed further in the section on "Malayanization").

Medicine, Military Forces and the Guerrillas

While the delivery of medical care to ordinary people was driven by the need to win the hearts and minds of people, the application of medicine in war zones was structured by the imperative to conserve fighting strength and to avoid the outbreak of epidemics among the troops. Consisting of Gurkha, East African, Australian, New Zealand and Fijian contingents, the anti-communist forces were well taken care of by the colonial authority. In addition to injuries and wounds, falling prey to disease was a common encounter among those who fought in the tropical forest. "I was a captain then and in one year, I lost 50 soldiers—30 died and 20 were wounded. I got malaria 13 times from going in and out of the jungle," recollected Akanit Muansawad, a Thai general who fought with the Malayan communists at the Thai-Malaysian border during the Malayan Emergency.[61]

Fighting in the jungle meant exposure to the risk of injury and contracting tropical diseases. It was, however, also perceived as an opportunity for medical research and intervention by medical experts. John William Field, a malariologist who headed the Institute for Medical Research (IMR), Kuala Lumpur, from 1949 to 1955, viewed "war as the locomotive of medicine." Commenting on the impact of the Malayan Emergency on medicine, J.W. Field said:

> The opportunities for medical investigation must often await the course of events. Jungle operations against Communist terrorists, the excellent hospital facilities of the Army in Malaya, and the deployment of many keen young doctors throughout the country, have brought unique opportunities. The medical services of the Army have taken ample advantage of this situation in their research on jungle diseases, sometimes with the co-operation of the Institute [for Medical Research], particularly at the Kinrara Military Hospital. Much of the early experimental work on the antibiotic treatment of typhus, the proof of resistance to proguanil in the gametocytes and pre-erythrocytic forms of P. falciparum, the first isolation of Japanese B virus from a human infection, and more recently the work on jungle fevers has been made possible by this harmonious and most useful collaboration.[62]

An international and local collaborative network of medical infrastructure was formed between four British Military Hospitals,[63] the IMR, laboratories in the University of Malaya, general hospitals in Malaya and army medical units from abroad, such as the US Army Medical Research Unit and the army doctors of the Royal Australian Air Force. While medicine benefits from war, the military too seem to gain from medicine in return. New discoveries during World War II, for example chloromycetin, an antibiotic which was found to be an effective treatment for scrub typhus, in return benefited the anti-communist troops in the late 1940s. For example, two Gurkhas affected by scrub typhus in 1949 were successfully treated with the newly discovered antibiotic, which their communist counterparts in the jungle had no access to.[64] The overall survival rate for casualties who made it to hospital alive had greatly improved from 92.9 percent in 1948–49 to 95.7 percent in 1952.[65]

Hiring non-Europeans as combatant forces was a common practice in the British colonies, as European troops were often too expensive to employ.[66] Yet, the presence of "foreign bodies" was at once perceived as potential "pathogenic agents." For instance, the entry of a Fijian troop in 1950 alarmed the IMR authorities when bancroftian filariasis was found among some soldiers in the troop. Filariasis was then known to be caused by at least two parasitic worms, wuchereria bancrofti and brugia malayi.[67] Only brugia malayi was common in Malaya, while wuchereria bancrofti was usually found in immigrants from India and China. In spite of the fact that bancroftian filariasis was thought to be rarely locally transmitted in Malaya, its presence still caused alarm among the IMR and the medical authorities. The whole Fijian battalion was then subject to periodical examination to avoid outbreak and contamination of the anti-communist forces, even though the troop had already been medically screened and treated for diseases and infection prior to their departure for Malaya. In 1952, some 725 blood films from the 1st Battalion Fijian Regiment were examined for microfilariæ.[68] It was reported that dissecting mosquitoes to find filarial larvae was not as challenging as doing the same to find malarial infections:

> Dissecting mosquitoes to find filarial larvae does not demand the skill required to find malarial infections. Instead of carefully extracting the stomach and salivary glands, the mosquito has merely to be pulled to pieces bit by bit with needles.[69]

In addition to cautious medical arrangements against "potentially pathogenic foreign bodies," the alerted medical authorities also cast their watchful eyes over the potentially pathogenic environment of the tropical forest. Extensive studies were conducted to prevent local infectious diseases and potential vectors from infecting or weakening the anti-communist forces. In July 1953, with the support of Colonial Development and Welfare Funds, the IMR established a small laboratory in Kuantan to conduct research on brugia malayi, as Pahang was found to be the most infected territory. The kampongs chosen for the experiment were located along the lower reaches of the Pahang River where the population was heavily infected. A blood survey was conducted on a total of 4,500 persons; over 3,000 mosquitoes of the Mansonia species, which was thought to be the vector, were dissected.[70]

The presence of chronic visceral schistosomiasis among East African soldiers also caused concerns for the medical authorities when a troop was brought to Malaya. The only form of schistosomiasis known to be endemic in Malaya then was cercarial dermatitis caused by schistosoma spindale or what the local people refer to as "sawah itch," but a different species of parasitic worm, schistosoma haematobium, was found in the bodies of the troop. The fact that these worms were "excreting ova" did not escape the microscopic gaze of IMR researchers, who were worried about the likelihood that the disease might become established in the country. The IMR sent batches of local snails, the potential intermediate host, to Arthur Anantharaj Sandosham at the University of Malaya, who jointly conducted experiments with the Army Pathological Laboratory in Singapore to ascertain whether the larva of s. haematobium would develop in these local snails.[71]

The presence of venereal disease (VD) also raised the concern of the military authorities. This was the case with both the British Army and the Royal Australian Air Force. In the first six months in Malaya, over 400 VD cases per

1,000 troops per year were recorded among the Australian force in 1956. The disease was at once perceived as a consequence of immoral behavior, a wastage of manpower, a medical issue as well as an issue of national reputation. "Neither the public at large, nor political leaders could accept a high rate of VD among the soldiers. The reason for this probably lies in the inability of the Australian public to reconcile its heroic image of its young serving men with what it sees as immoral behavior leading to the disgraceful disease of VD," said O'Keefe.[72] Apart from imposing disciplinary methods against soldiers who concealed their venereal infection, anti-vice squads were designated in all bars, hotels and restaurants to dissuade soldiers from risking contracting the disease, and free condoms were freely available as a prophylactic measure.[73] Another form of medical intervention in keeping the fighting strength of anti-communist forces was dietary intervention. Sometimes the military authorities took the initiative to consult the IMR regarding ration scales of nutrition[74] or to request a full analysis of the ration scales for the Imperial Gurkha Troops[75] and the nutritional components of food ration packs distributed for police on jungle assignments.[76]

In contrast to the medical services the anti-communist forces enjoyed, the communists largely relied on self-acquired healing knowledge, which they gained through their lived experience in the jungle. A shortage of antibiotics was common; most of the time the guerrillas had to make use of medicinal herbs to treat illnesses and wounds caused by gun shots and explosive blasts and to induce abortion in the jungle. However, there was a small team of medically trained guerrillas to take care of their injured members. Consider the story of a former communist medical officer Nana, a Malaya-born and UK-trained nurse who joined the MCP and eventually trained as a medical officer during the Vietnam War under the supervision of Phạm Ngọc Thạch:

> When I first joined the guerrillas, I was the only doctor and there were no other medical officers. I got really panic, when I first heard the sound of landmine explosion and carried out my first ever surgical operation in a makeshift "operation hut." But gradually, I got used to it. Sacrifices and injuries were almost inevitable, whenever my comrades went out to detect and inspect landmines. Injuries caused by landmines were very common, and there were many cases of amputation. Therefore, we have a team who were trained to make prostheses.[77]

Taken together, the military-medicine relations during the Malayan Emergency was one of mutual influence and mutual benefit: medicine benefits from war, war benefits from medicine. On the guerrillas' front, despite the paucity of drugs and facilities, they were creative enough to make use of local healing knowledge and makeshift "operation hut" made of local materials.[78]

Healthcare, Anti-Colonialism and Malayanization

In the preceding sections, I have illustrated how insurgency and counter-insurgency jointly shaped the healthcare landscape in the predominantly Chinese NVs and displaced the communities of Orang Asli. In contrast to the NVs, healthcare was underdeveloped in the rural areas. Running parallel to the insurgency was a strand of less militant anti-colonialism, comprised of local elites of various ethnic origins and occupational backgrounds. Among them were local physicians, civil servants and local elites. Compared to their MCP counterparts, these elites were given legitimate platforms to proclaim their vision of building a new nation, of which healthcare and medicine formed a significant aspect.

During the Japanese occupation, lasting from 15 February 1941 to 9 September 1945, the healthcare services in Malaya were placed under the Civil Medical Institution. The medical works were carried out almost entirely by locally recruited staffs, who worked for the previously British-controlled Malayan Medical Services, as the Europeans fled Malaya following the fall of Singapore.[79] In the absence of colonial personnel, local medical graduates, who had been denied equal treatment and fair opportunity of promotion during pre-war British rule, were given the opportunity to be "solely responsible for the medical and health care services of the population under very difficult circumstances."[80] The exposure to new ideological forces during Japanese occupation between 1941 and 1945 gave birth to "the generation of 1945."[81] The experience gained through greater access to more senior public service posts had injected new confidence among Asians in countering the European racial discrimination and imperialism.

When the British colonial government returned to Malaya after World War II, it faced mounting pressure to employ more Asians in administrative posts. On 5 June 1951, the King Edward VII College of Medicine Alumni Association (KECOMAA) submitted a memorandum to E.R. Pridie, Medical Adviser to the Colonial Office, protesting against the Malayan government's move in maintaining two parallel lists of seniority between European expatriate doctors and locally trained doctors.[82] Some locally recruited doctors had even resigned due to the "[g]overnment's failure to offer them a 'square deal', compared with the expatriate officers." They criticized the government for creating an "artificial shortage" of doctors in the Federation and Singapore.[83]

Facing both the militancy of the MCP and the less militant push from the local nationalist elites to Malayanize the civil services, the British government chose to suppress the former and work with the latter. A Malayanization Committee was set up in 1954 in Kuala Lumpur to look into the replacement of expatriates with locally recruited officers in the state administration, including in the health services.[84] Among the issues debated in the committee was the rate by which the Malayanization scheme should proceed. The committee had reasoned that the replacement "should take place only as normal attrition occurred." Any accelerated replacement, the British argued, might saturate the bureaucracy with less competent applicants. Expatriates should be retained until fully qualified Malayans were available to fill the posts. Nevertheless, any expatriate retirement scheme based on normal attrition was apparently not well received by the nationalists.

With a heightened sense of anti-colonialism as well as nationalism, or what Baratham Ramaswamy Sreenivasan, Chairman (1955–56) of the Malayanization Committee, called a "desire to determine their own progress,"[85] the local medical elites worked together with other native elites from various occupational backgrounds to Malayanize the state administration. Thamboo John Danaraj, the founding Dean of the Faculty of Medicine of the University of Malaya, also expressed such nationalistic aspirations when recollecting and reflecting the need for establishing local medical education three decades later:

> [The Malayan] people were eager for knowledge and demonstrated their enthusiasm for establishment of schools and higher centres of learning by petitions supported sometimes by funds. But there was little appreciation of the urgency of local needs nor support of local aspirations by British officialdom. Instead, there was apathy, inevitable delays and numerous obstacles. Local persistence occasionally bore fruit and there were some expatriate visionaries like Sir Alexander Carr-Saunders whose boldness set the pace for future University development. Brought up under the colonial system and closely involved in attempts to establish higher education, I came to the inevitable conclusion that self-determination is essential for progress. Then, if nationals make mistakes, they have to live with them![86]

Despite the warning of possible incompetency, if replacement was over-paced, policies and plans were made to speed up local recruitment. In 1956, a year after the first general election, the Minister of Health and Social Welfare, Leong Yew Koh, insisted that his department "want[s] to get on with Malayanization because the local people can best understand and appreciate the habits, customs and psychology of those they must meet in connection with the department's work," while proposing to the Federation's planning committee that they provide 60 scholarships over a five-year period to send suitable candidates from the University of Malaya to Britain for training.[87]

Led by the fact that there was a shortage of local experts in many areas, including in healthcare, the Federation government realized that it was unlikely

Table 2.4. Medical posts and unfilled posts, 1948–59

Year	Medical Posts	Filled	Unfilled	Held by temporary officer
1948	300	213	87	37
1949	305	199	106	35
1950	330	196	134	39
1951	338	228	110	56
1952	339	185	154	88
1953	342	218	124	88
1954	376	219	157	103
1955	402	236	166	84
1956	393	266	127	57
1957	447	291	156	45
1958*	436	350	86	51
1959**	467	369	98	23

Source: FMRMD (1948–59).

to fill all the medical posts in the government service with local doctors and turned to recruiting foreign doctors from elsewhere in Asia. Around June 1956, efforts were taken to recruit 30 doctors from India to work on a three-year contract.[88] Foreign aid also played a role in training local experts at this stage. In 1955, 15 nurses and 3 X-ray assistants underwent training in Australia under the Colombo Plan, while 12 doctors, 12 nurses, 6 male nurses and hospital assistants, 1 X-ray assistant and 1 sanitary inspector undertook post-graduate training in the United Kingdom.[89] Table 2.4 shows medical posts in the government service between 1948 and 1959. The number of vacancies peaked in 1955, with 166 out of 402 unfilled, and was sharply reduced to 86 in 1958 when a large number of doctors were recruited from India.[90] Among the 350 filled posts, 202 were permanent, 97 on contract and 51 temporary. In 1959, among the 369 posts, 239 were permanent, 107 on contract and 23 temporary. By the end of 1959, only 48 posts or 13 percent were filled by expatriate officers and the rest were filled by Asians, including 238 Malaysians. In a review of rural health services a decade after independence, L.W. Jayesuria, the Deputy Director of Medical Services, admitted that "Malayanization" of the medical and health services contributed to the shortage of medical manpower.[91]

The push for Malayanization by the nationalist elites was not the only factor that contributed to the "problem" of insufficient modern medical manpower. Equally significant was the increasing acceptance of Western medicine among the Asian community. The 1955 International Bank for Reconstruction and Development's (IBRD) report Economic Development of Malaya (EDM) indicated that: "Professional staff is insufficient and, as has long been appreciated might happen, all racial groups in the population now increasingly accept and expect 'western medicine', and have begun to demand clinic and hospital services exceeding the capacity of the available resources."[92] While the EDM's description could have been an attempt to claim the "triumph" of Western medicine over other traditions of healing practices and to justify its application in non-Western society, the increased attendance in Infant and Child Welfare Centers (Table 2.3) appears to support the successful promotion of Western medicine in Malaya. The proposal to build a second university in Malaya to train more local physicians in the post-war years and the Malay leaders' appeal to increase modern health service in rural areas during the counter-insurgency period were also signs of increasing demand among the locals, especially among the elites. All these jointly contributed to insufficient modern medical manpower.

In addition to differences between European doctors and Asian doctors, the contestation over the racial structure of the state medical services also reveals tensions between the government medical officers and doctors in private practice. This was disclosed in the 1954 Report of the Committee on the Malayanization of the Government Service that local medical officers "prefer[red] medical and surgical work to [public] health work" as they would be "better equipped for private practice on retirement and that medical and surgical specialists have opportunities for earning fees which do not come to Health Officers." In the 1956 FMRMD, Angus Alexander Cameron,[93] the Acting Director of Medical Services, also blamed the private practitioners for the shortage of medical manpower in the public service:

> Recruitment of expatriate doctors and nursing sisters from overseas is at a standstill. During the year, 25 medical officers were recruited and 30 house doctors were recruited as medical officers on completion of their 12 months statutory service. Although the recruitment of local doctors has been given high priority, and has been given preference over the recruitment of others, doctors continue to enjoy lucrative private practice and are not unduly anxious to join Government services. Some who are already established in general practice have responded to an appeal to do part-time duty in the hospitals. To overcome this shortage it was decided to recruit doctors and, possibly, nurses (qualified) from India and other adjoining countries, but at the end of the year the scheme had not yet been finalized.[94]

The perceived insufficiency of modern medical manpower and the tensions between the government medical officers and the doctors in private practice prefigured a series of contestations between the private and public health sectors, which were to prevail in the post-independence years.

Concurrently, there were attempts by practitioners of Western biomedicine to delegitimize Asian and indigenous healing practices. Yet, no conscious and collective effort was taken by the latter to contest the hegemonization of biomedicine until the 1980s, which is beyond the time frame of this article.[95]

Conclusion

After World War II, Asians in Malaya were injected with a new confidence that they were capable of self-rule and self-determination. They came to fight colonialism on different fronts and their aspiration to establish a nation of their own was expressed in different ways. All these anti-colonial efforts came to shape the healthcare services in Malaya before independence. On the more militant front, the communist struggle and the anti-communist war pushed healthcare towards one that was dominated by missionary healthcare in the re-settlement areas. Healthcare was instrumentalized as a psychological tool to regulate the political leanings of the people in these resettlement zones. Dictated by the security concern to suppress communist activities, the colonial government's budget largely went on military spending, leaving scant resources for the healthcare needs in the predominantly Malay rural areas. Nevertheless, rural health and hygiene programs were put into place to engage, mobilize and regulate the rural population and the Malay communities. Overall, there were some improvements in the population's health during the counter-insurgency period as compared to the time of Japanese occupation, but it was not without social cost, as people's everyday lives were deeply regulated, if not disciplined to identify with the colonial state, through the provision and deprivation of healthcare services. Healthcare during the counter-insurgency period was thus intrusive as well as exclusive. It was a tool of domination by the colonial state and an act of benevolence and kindness by those who genuinely served and cared for people on the ground. Nonetheless, local actors were not passive, and many remained critical of the colonial authority. Importantly, both communist guerillas and anti-communist troops were concerned with keeping their fighting forces healthy, the former largely relying on self-acquired healing knowledge, while the latter were taken care of by state-sponsored medical care. The Malayan Emergency, through international medical research collaboration, had paradoxically improved healing and lifesaving knowledge while taking the lives of many. Both the international military medicine research network and the influx of missionary healthcare suggest the impact that the international Cold War had on the local medical landscape.

On a less militant front, the nationalist leaders were engaged in the Malayanization movement to decolonize the racial composition of the state administration and healthcare by replacing expatriates with local experts. Despite their good intention, the movement was caught in a self-created dilemma due to insufficient local healthcare experts, exacerbating the existing problem of medical manpower shortage, and the nationalist elites stretched between the urgency to expand rural healthcare and the need to increase medical manpower. Without decolonizing healing knowledge, Malayanization was a work of biomedicine hegemonization and domination by nationalist elites, which went unchallenged for several decades until the 1980s.

NOTES

1.   Kumar Ramakrishna, *Emergency Propaganda: The Winning of Malayan Hearts and Minds, 1948–1958* (London: Curzon Press, 2002); Lee Kam Hing, "A Neglected Story: Christian Missionaries, Chinese New Villagers, and Communists in the Battle for the 'hearts and minds' in Malaya, 1948–1960," *Modern Asian Studies* 47, 6 (2013): 1977–2006; Phua Kai Hong, *The Development of Health Services in Malaya and Singapore* (University of London: Unpublished Thesis, 1987); Anthony Short, *In Pursuit of Mountain Rats: The Communist Insurrection in Malaya* (Singapore: Cultured Lotus, 1975).

2.   David Arnold, *Colonizing the Body: State Medicine and Epidemic Disease in 19th Century India* (Los Angeles: University of California Press, 1993); Lenore Manderson, *Sickness and the State: Health and Illness in Colonial Malaya, 1870–1940* (Cambridge: Cambridge University Press, 1996); Michel Foucault, *Power/ Knowledge: Selected Interviews and Other Writings 1972–1977* (Brighton, Sussex: The Harvester Press, 1980).

3.   *Malayan Union Report of the Medical Department (MURMD)* (Kuala Lumpur: The Government of the Malayan Union, 1946).

4.   Cheah Boon Kheng, *Red Star Over Malaya: Resistance and Social Conflict during and after the Japanese Occupation, 1941–1946*, 4th edn (Singapore: NUS Press, 2012); Christopher Bayly and Tim Harper, *Forgotten Wars: The End of Britain's Asian Empire* (London: Penguin, 2007); Timothy N. Harper, *The End of Empire and the Making of Malaya* (Cambridge: Cambridge University Press, 1999); John Kerry King, "Malaya's Resettlement Problem," *Far Eastern Survey* 23, 3 (1954): 33–40.

5.   Despite deteriorating conflict, the term "emergency," instead of "war," was used to allay business and insurance concerns. See Lee Kam Hing, *A Matter of Risk: Insurance in Malaysia, 1826–1990* (Singapore: NUS Press, 2012).

6.   All currency in Malayan dollars, unless otherwise specified. Richard Stubbs, *Counter-Insurgency and the Economic Factor: The Impact of the Korean War Prices Boom on the Malayan Emergency* (Singapore: Institute of Southeast Asian Studies, 1974), p. 13.

7. A Malay term for "aboriginal people."

8. The number of people who were relocated and resettled has always been contested, with different researchers' estimates ranging from half a million to over a million. The figure shown here is taken from Ray Nyce, *Chinese New Villages in Malaya Community Study* (Kuala Lumpur: Malaysian Sociological Research Institute, 1973). See also Timothy N. Harper, "The Politics of Disease and Disorder in Post-War Malaya," *Journal of Southeast Asian Studies* 21, 1 (1990): 88–113; Loh Kok Wah, *Beyond the Tin Mines: Coolies, Squatters and New Villagers in the Kinta Valley, Malaysia, c.1880–1980* (London: Oxford University Press, 1988); Short, *In Pursuit of Mountain Rats*; Tan Teng Phee, *Behind Barbed Wire: Chinese New Villages During the Malayan Emergency, 1948–1960* (Petaling Jaya: Strategic Information and Research Development Center, 2020).

9. Kathleen Carpenter, *The Password Is Love* (London: The Highway Press, 1958), pp. 16–17; G.D. James, *Missionary Tours in Malaya* (Singapore: Malaya Evangelistic Fellowship, 1962), p. 50; Short, *In Pursuit of Mountain Rats*, pp. 405–9; Tan Teng Phee, *Behind Barbed Wire*.

10. Leon Comber, "The Malayan Emergency: General Templer and the Kinta Valley Home Guard, 1952–1954," *Journal of the Malaysian Branch of the Royal Asiatic Society* 85, 1 (302) (June 2012): 45–62.

11. Martin Rudner, "The Draft Development Plan of the Federation of Malaya 1950–55," *Journal of Southeast Asian Studies* 3, 1 (1972): 63–96.

12. A Burma-born medical doctor and founding member of the Malayan Chinese Association (MCA), which later became a member party of British handpicked ruling coalition Alliance.

13. Phua, *The Development of Health Services*, p. 273.

14. Henry Gurney, *Communist Banditry in Malaya: Extracts from Speeches by the High Commissioner Sir Henry Gurney* (Federation of Malaya: Department of Public Relations, 1949).

15. Rudner, "The Draft Development Plan."

16. Loh, *Beyond the Tin Mines*, pp. 136–9.

17. "Doctors Debate 'Lack' of Medical Services: Resettlement Areas Threat to Health," *The Straits Times*, 12 April 1952, p. 4.

18. Nyce, *Chinese New Villages*, p. 171.

19. "Missionaries with Nowhere to Go," *Singapore Free Press*, 22 July 1955, p. 4.

20. Carpenter, *The Password Is Love*, p. 18.

21. British High Commissioner in Malaya, from 15 January 1952 to 31 May 1954.

22. Harper, *The End of Empire*, p. 185.

23. As cited in Rudner, "The Draft Development Plan," p. 68.

24. "Templer's Progress Plan: The Door to M[alayan]C[ivil]S[ervice] will now be open to non-Malays," *The Straits Times*, 20 November 1952, p. 1.

25. Harper, *The End of Empire*, p. 185; Lee, "A Neglected Story," p. 1977; Nyce, *Chinese New Villages*, p. 171.

26. Harper, *The End of Empire*, p. 186; Lee, "A Neglected Story," p. 1986; John Roxborogh, *A Short Introduction to Malaysian Church History: A Guide to the Story of Christianity in Malaysia and How to Go About Discovering the History of Your Church* (Kuala Lumpur: Seminari Theoloji Malaysia and the Catholic Research Center, 1989).

27. Harper, *The End of Empire*, p. 185.

28. James, *Missionary Tours*, p. 155.

29. Lee, "A Neglected Story," pp. 2001, 2003.

30. "Give—Don't Gamble," *The Straits Times*, 4 July 1953, p. 9; "Lottery Ban Was Breach of Faith, Says MCA," *The Straits Times*, 8 August 1953, p. 7.

31. E.H.G. Dobby, "Resettlement Transforms Malaya: A Case History of Relocating the Population of an Asian Plural Society," *Economic Development and Cultural Change* 1, 3 (Oct. 1952): 163–89; Phua, *The Development of Health Services*, p. 277.

32. Kumar, *Emergency Propaganda*, p. 127.

33. "A Town Is Born," *The Straits Times*, 31 August 1950, p. 9.

34. Kumar, *Emergency Propaganda*, p. 126; Loh, *Beyond the Tin Mines*, pp. 136–9.

35. "Resettlement Area Becomes a Town," *The Straits Times*, 7 April 1952, p. 9.

36. "Operation Shoe," *The Straits Times*, 11 July 1957, p. 6.

37. Phua, *The Development of Health Services*, p. 280.

38. Tan, *Behind Barbed Wire*, pp. 209–10.

39. James Scott, *Weapons of the Weak: Everyday Forms of Peasant Resistance* (New Haven, CT: Yale University Press, 1985).

40. Tan, *Behind Barbed Wire*.

41. Alun Jones, "The Orang Asli: An Outline of Their Progress in Modern Malaya," *Journal of Southeast Asian History* 9, 2 (1968): 286–305; Gordon Means, "The Orang Asli: Aboriginal Policies in Malaysia," *Pacific Affairs* 58, 4 (1985): 637–52.

42. Ivan Polunin, "The Medical Natural History of Malayan Aborigines," *Medical Journal of Malaya* 8, 1 (1953): 62–171.

43. Polunin, "Malayan Aborigines," p. 160.

44. Jones, "The Orang Asli," p. 297.

45. Pamela Gouldsbury, *Jungle Nurse* (London: Jarrolds Publisher, 1960), p. 82.

46. Colin Nicolas and Adela Baer, "Healthcare for the Orang Asli: Consequences of Paternalism and Non-Recognition," in *Health Care in Malaysia: The Dynamics of Provision, Financing and Access*, ed. Chee Heng Leng and Simon Barraclough (New York: Palgrave, 2009), pp. 119–36.

47. Jones, "The Orang Asli," pp. 299–300.

48. Yaws is a contagious disease caused by bacterial infection, which affects the skin, bones and joints.

49. Short, *In Pursuit of Mountain Rats*, pp. 451–2.

50. Dobby, "Resettlement Transforms Malaya," p. 177.

51. "How Do the Malays React to It?" *The Straits Times*, 27 June 1951, p. 6.

52. As cited in Phua, *The Development of Health Services*, p. 266.

53. Gastroenteritis refers to inflammation of the gastrointestinal tract, usually caused by viral infection.

54. FMRMD 1950–58.

55. L.W. Jayesuria, *A Review of the Rural Health Services in West Malaysia* (Kuala Lumpur: Ministry of Health, 1967).

56. "Teach Hygiene and Save Lives," *The Straits Times*, 28 August 1958, p. 2.

57. "Illiteracy Blamed for Poverty in Rural Areas," *The Straits Times*, 22 December 1962, p. 6.

58. "Back-to-Land Plan to Save 'Food Bowl', '4-H' Clubs for Youths Urged," *The Straits Times*, 6 July 1951, p. 7.

59. Lenore Manderson, *Women, Politics, and Change: The Kaum Ibu UMNO, Malaysia, 1945–1972* (Oxford: Oxford University Press, 1980).

60. "Health campaign for kampongs," *The Straits Times*, 11 February 1958, p. 4.

61. "Thai Ex-Generals Pay Final Respects to Chin Peng," *The Malay Mail*, 20 September 2013. Available at: https://www.malaymail.com/news/malaysia/2013/09/20/thai-ex-generals-pay-final-respects-to-chin-peng/528589 [accessed 23 August 2023].

62. *Annual Report of Institute for Medical Research (ARIMR)* (Kuala Lumpur: Institute for Medical Research, 1954).

63. Each in Perak's Kamunting, Pahang's Cameron Highland, Kuala Lumpur's Kinrara and Singapore.

64. *Annual Report of Institute for Medical Research (ARIMR)* (Kuala Lumpur: Institute for Medical Research, 1949), p. 5.

65. Brendan G. O'Keefe, *Medicine at War: Medical Aspects of Australia's Involvement in Southeast Asia, 1950–1972* (New South Wales: Allen & Unwin, 1994), p. 7.

66. Bayly and Harper, *Forgotten Wars*, p. 325.

67. A different parasitic worm *brugia timori*, common in Lesser Sunda Islands of Indonesia, was identified as the third causative agent in 1977.

68. *ARIMR 1950*, pp. 210–2; *ARIMR 1952*, pp. 4–7.

69. *ARIMR 1950*, p. 221.

70. *ARIMR 1953*, p. 4.

71. *ARIMR 1952*, pp. 4–38.

72. O'Keefe, *Medicine at War*, pp. xxvii–xxviii.

73. O'Keefe, *Medicine at War*, pp. xxvii–xxviii.

74. *ARIMR 1952*, p. 51.

75. *ARIMR 1954*, p. 52.

76. *ARIMR 1957*, p. 47.

77. Nana, face-to-face conversation with the author, 6 October 2016. She returned to Malaysia a few years after the 1989 Hat Yai Peace Agreement. She only managed to obtain PR status, despite being born in Malaya. Without a medical license, she could only work as an ordinary helper in a community clinic in Kuala Lumpur and later practice Chinese medicine.

78. The communist narrative in this section is imbalanced due to difficulty of accessing interview with the communists, who remain demonized today, and the archival materials in China.
79. *MURMD 1946*.
80. Thamboo John Danaraj, *Medical Education in Malaysia: Development and Problems* (Subang Jaya: Pelanduk, 1988).
81. Harper, *The End of Empire*.
82. "Posts Kept for European Doctors, Protest Memo for UK Adviser," *The Straits Times*, 5 June 1951, p. 7.
83. "Govt. Has Caused Lack of Doctors," *The Straits Times*, 23 August 1952, p. 5.
84. For more discussion about Malayanization of state bureaucracy, see Robert O. Tilman, *Bureaucratic Transition in Malaya* (Durham, NC: Duke University Press, 1964), pp. 63–81.
85. Sreenivasan, B.R. "The Role of Physicians in Developing Countries," in *Proceedings of the Conference on Medical Education*, 3–6 August 1965 (Faculty of Medicine, University of Malaya, 1965), pp. 22–5. Dr B.R. Sreenivasan was also the first president of the Singapore Medical Association (SMA), formed on 15 September 1959 through the merging of the Malaya Branch of the British Medical Association and the KECOMAA.
86. Danaraj, *Medical Education*, p. 22.
87. "Social Welfare Dept. Will Be [Malayanized] First," *The Straits Times*, 15 February 1956, p. 8.
88. "Doctors for the Federation," *The Straits Times*, 11 June 1956, p. 20.
89. *FMRMD 1955*, p. 8.
90. *FMRMD 1955*.
91. Jayesuria, *A Review of the Rural Health Services*, p. 3.
92. International Bank for Reconstruction and Development, *The Economic Development of Malaya* (Singapore: International Bank for Reconstruction and Development, 1955), p. 400.
93. A.A. Cameron was born in Dumbarton, Scotland, in 1909 and graduated as a medical doctor in Glasgow University in 1933. He joined the Malayan Medical Service in 1937 and was appointed the first Director of Medical Services of independent Malaya. His remit included the training of his Malay successor. He retired in 1959 and began a new career in his home country.
94. *FMRMD 1956*, p. 5.
95. This is in contrast to the overt competition between indigenous medicine and biomedicine in China, which started in the early 20th century. Regarding the competition and politics of different healing traditions in Malaysia, see Carol Laderman, "The Politics of Healing in Malaysia," in *Women and Politics in Twentieth Century Africa & Asia*, ed. V.H. Sutlive, N. Altshuler and M.D. Zamora (Williamsburg, VA: College of William and Mary, 1981), pp. 143–58, and H. Heggenhougan, "Bomohs, Doctors and Sinsehs: Medical Pluralism in Malaysia," *Social Science and Medicine* 14B (1980): 235–44.

CHAPTER 3

Health Sector Contestation in Cold War Laos, 1950–75

Kathryn Sweet

Introduction

The Lao prime minister, Prince Souvanna Phouma, a French-educated political neutralist, suffered a heart attack in July 1974. It came just months after the negotiation of a ceasefire to the long-running Lao conflict and the formation of a third coalition government, and therefore caused considerable concern among regional and international governments. The complex nature of Laos' political situation within Cold War Southeast Asia was highlighted by the diverse mix of medical personnel who gathered at Souvanna Phouma's bedside. The prime minister's American son-in-law observed:

> In addition to the two Lao doctors there were a leading heart specialist from Bangkok, whom the Thai government had rushed to the scene, and a young brilliant American cardiologist from Clark Field in the Philippines, who represented the contribution from the United States government. The French doctor in residence in Laos had been joined by two heart men flown in from Paris. The Soviet Union sent three specialists to tend to the Prime Minister, and three Chinese physicians—an elderly gentleman and two intense women—came from Beijing as an offering from the People's Republic of China. Surely this was a unique moment in the annals of international medicine.[1]

Souvanna Phouma recovered, but was relieved of the prime ministership when the Lao revolutionaries seized power a year later. This chapter does not focus on the health of Souvanna Phouma. Rather, it explores how the political dynamics of the Cold War played out in the Lao health sector, and how foreign aid and the political influence which accompanied it developed and expanded, but also complicated and fractured, the fledgling health sector of post-colonial Laos. The cosmopolitan gathering of medical professionals around Souvanna Phouma's bedside serves simply to illustrate the predicament of the Lao health sector, and the broader social, economic and political environment, after two decades of Cold War jostling and positioning in Southeast Asia.

The Lao health sector experienced rapid, wide-ranging development and expansion during the Cold War years from 1950 to 1975. In the 25 years following the French transfer of the colonial health service, the *Assistance médicale au Laos*, to the Royal Lao Government in April 1950,[2] the number of health facilities more than doubled, numbers of Lao health staff increased more than tenfold, and Lao nationals began to qualify as medical doctors, pharmacists and registered nurses for the first time. Higher-level medical and health training institutions were established in-country and nationwide health coverage expanded considerably.

The health sector's rapid development and expansion was accompanied by significant divergence and fracturing, a direct result of Laos' position within the Cold War politics of Southeast Asia and the provision of separate, and frequently non-complementary, streams of foreign aid from regional and international powers. The Lao conflict lasted 30 years from 1945 until 1975, but most notably involved the First Indochina War of 1946–54 and the Second Indochina War of 1964–73. In just over a decade following the French handover, three major civilian health services, two military services and a modest private sector emerged from the smallest and most simply structured of Indochina's colonial health services. These multiple health services, funded by foreign aid, developed in divergent ways, with fractured skills, training and service delivery rather than consolidation of scarce financial, human and technical resources of newly independent Laos.

Laos experienced a more complicated journey from colony to post-colonial nation than many. Its turbulent political evolution throughout the period from 1945 to 1975 was heavily influenced by the political interests and alliances of regional and international powers. Following a short-lived period of independence in 1945–46, the nationalist *Lao Issara* (Free Lao) movement split ranks in 1950: one side returned from exile in Thailand to join the Royal Lao Government, accepting arrangements for a graduated pathway to national independence agreed with France, while the other side—known alternately as the *Neo Lao Issara*, the *Pathet Lao* and from 1956 as the *Neo Lao Hak Xat* (NLHX)—rejected the arrangements and relocated from Thailand to Vietnam, where it aligned with the revolutionary Viet Minh movement. The split within the *Lao Issara*, recognized internationally at the 1954 Geneva conference on Indochina, led to the territorial and administrative division of Laos into two zones from 1954 until 1975.[3] While Laos achieved full independence from France in 1953, this was not recognized by the revolutionaries who continued their political struggle until the 1973 ceasefire and their assumption of power in 1975. While the split within the *Lao Issara* was more likely to have been prompted by personality differences than Cold War rivalries, the resulting political and financial support to the two political factions and their respective zones, and for a brief period a third neutralist faction, was firmly shaped by Cold War policies. The global capitalist camp perceived non-aligned Laos to be at risk of succumbing to communism, while the fraternal socialist camp was concerned that Laos was being unduly influenced and exploited by global capitalism.

Both zones of Laos relied heavily on foreign aid to deliver healthcare and other public services. Then, as now, foreign aid was provided within a larger framework of political relations and influence. As a non-aligned nation, the Kingdom of Laos (and its Royal Lao Government zone) received financial, technical and military assistance from donor nations across the political spectrum, but predominately from the United States and France. For its part, the revolutionary NLHX relied on financial and in-kind assistance from a range of socialist nations, most notably North Vietnam, China and the Soviet Union. Health sector development, maintenance and expansion was enabled in large part by this flow of international technical assistance contributions, which funded development projects, overseas scholarships, construction of new and upgraded health facilities, as well as supplied foreign medical advisors and health workers to supplement the Lao health workforce. Characteristic of foreign aid globally, assistance to Laos was rarely provided in a coordinated manner, and national needs and local capacities were infrequently prioritized. The split in health services created by Laos' political and territorial divisions was further exacerbated by the different nature of health sector assistance received by the two territorial zones from their disparate donors, which impacted on staff training, construction standards, use of medical supplies and, presumably, health outcomes.

This chapter provides a much-needed context for the diverse health infrastructure, staffing, and professional and technical standardization inherited by the Lao People's Democratic Republic (Lao PDR) regime, and the Ministry of Health's subsequent challenges when confronted with the task of uniting the fragmented health services into a uniform national healthcare system. It shows how the Cold War manoeuvres that played out in Laos in the 1950s and 1960s resulted in widespread fragmentation of the nation's fledgling health sector at a time of rapid expansion and development, and posed awkward challenges for its development for decades to come.

The research is informed by official documents from the Lao National Archives Department in Vientiane, Lao PDR, the World Health Organization (WHO) Western Pacific Regional Office in Manila, the Philippines, the National Archives and Records Administration in Washington DC, United States, as well as United States Agency for International Aid (USAID) documents. Sources include several Lao-language biographies and autobiographies of Lao health workers, which have appeared in recent years and have provided scholars with more insight into the less frequently documented revolutionary health services.[4] The chapter occasionally refers to the intersections and overlaps between civilian and military services, but for the most part focuses on civilian health services. Access to information and sources relating to the military health services remains restricted in both Lao PDR and the United States.[5]

Health Services in the Royal Lao Government Zone

The Royal Lao Government's Ministry of Health (*kasouang sathalanasouk*) was Laos' leading health service during the 25 years from 1950 until 1975.[6] It closely resembled the colonial health service, the *Assistance médicale au Laos*. It inherited the vast majority of colonial health facilities and staffing, and remained a francophone entity throughout this entire period. The ministry represented Laos to the WHO, and received the bulk of foreign aid provided for health sector development. Foreign aid, delivered within the political framework of Cold War influence and alliances, fueled the rapid development and expansion of the ministry, albeit from a very low baseline. However, expansion of the Ministry of Health service was held in check by the establishment of the Royal Lao Government military and police forces, whose separate health services siphoned staff and resources away from the civilian service. As the conflict in Laos progressed, further limitations on expansion were experienced as government health facilities in rural areas were overrun by the advancing revolutionary forces.

In the immediate post-colonial period, the Ministry of Health required strengthening and consolidation to both maintain healthcare in urban areas and to expand into unserved rural areas. It faced staffing vacancies left by the departure of Vietnamese medical assistants and the reassignment of French doctors from colonial managers to international advisors, as well as budget shortfalls. Foreign aid plugged many of Laos' financial, material and human resource gaps, when most of its scarce resources were being directed to the war effort rather than to nation-building. As a result, Laos relied on foreign aid to support the construction and maintenance of health facilities, medical equipment and supplies, and professional education and training in-country and abroad. Aid was commonly delivered in the form of development projects, international technical advisors and overseas scholarships.

French influence continued to predominate in the health sector in the post-colonial period, with assistance provided through France's civilian and military aid missions. While the United States was the largest overall foreign aid provider to Laos at this time, the majority of American assistance was directed to the military and police forces and to public works, and not to the health sector.[7] French assistance was complemented by francophone technical advisors from United Nations agencies. The WHO provided the bulk of assistance from the United Nations agencies through several long-running development projects with the Ministry of Health.[8] Notably, until the 1973 ceasefire, WHO assistance in Laos was directed to the Royal Lao Government and not to the NLHX or populations in the Liberated Zone.[9] The Ministry of Health also received aid from the Colombo Plan—funded by the United Kingdom, Japan and Australia, among others—and from the early 1960s, modest volumes of aid from socialist nations led by the Soviet Union. A handful of international non-government organizations (NGOs), such as CARE, Catholic Relief Services, International Voluntary Service, and Tom Dooley's Operation Laos/MEDICO, also provided ad hoc assistance to the ministry.

The number of medical facilities under Ministry of Health management more than doubled during the period 1950–75. Health facilities opened in areas distant from the major towns, although sources reveal little about staffing, supplies or the quality of healthcare services provided. Official statistics demonstrate, however, the ministry's desire to expand biomedicine into rural Laos. At handover from France in 1950, Laos was reported to have one hospital in each of the six major towns, six smaller *infirmeries-ambulances* in lesser provincial towns such as Salavanh and Attapeu, and 64 rural dispensaries.[10]

Following consolidation, the health network began to expand in the 1960s. The number of main hospitals under Ministry of Health management remained constant, but the number of *infirmeries-ambulances* more than doubled by 1966, and the number of rural dispensaries increased from 64 in 1950 to 148 in 1973.[11] Growth was not incremental, though, because dispensaries opened and closed as territory was gained or lost in the ongoing fighting between government and NLHX forces. Nor did growth necessarily correlate with quality of service; visiting a dispensary in northern Namtha province in the late 1950s, American aid worker Dooley reported that it had "nothing in the way of medicines, not even aspirins, quinine or adhesive tape."[12]

Vientiane's Mahosot Hospital emerged as the nation's largest and most advanced health facility. As Royal Lao Government development centered on Vientiane, Mahosot surpassed the bed capacity of Luang Prabang and Pakse provincial hospitals, with capacity rising from 52 beds in 1950 to 394 in 1973.[13] Vientiane also hosted the ministry's new specialist health centers for tuberculosis, ophthalmology and dermatology.

France and the United States funded the bulk of the ministry's infrastructure: construction of new and upgraded hospitals and dispensaries along with specialist wings and medical and health training facilities at central and provincial levels. France funded an extension to Luang Prabang hospital in the 1950s and new buildings for the Royal Medical School in Vientiane in the late 1960s.[14] For its part, the United States funded construction of a new nursing school at Mahosot Hospital, the Maternal and Child Health Center in Vientiane, Maternal and Child Health wings in five provincial hospitals, and the renovation of similar wings in an additional ten sites.[15] A noted historian of Laos, Martin Stuart-Fox, concluded that hospital construction was one of the successes of USAID's assistance to the Royal Lao Government.[16] Medical equipment and supplies, including pharmaceuticals, were provided by France, the United States, Australia and Canada, among others.

As health facilities increased, so did the number and professional diversity of health workers at all levels of Laos' health sector. At handover in 1950, Laos' non-European health staff was reported to comprise one doctor,[17] eight Indochinese doctors,[18] four public health assistants (*assistants indochinois de médecine sociale*), four registered midwives, 220 nurses, and an unspecified number of low-level rural birth attendants (*accoucheuses rurales*).[19] There were no Lao medical specialists, dentists, radiographers or laboratory assistants. Moreover, in-country training was available for midwives, nurses and rural birth attendants, but no other health professions.

Overseas scholarships were integral to expanding and up-skilling the health workforce. Most scholarships in the 1950s were provided by France, WHO and the Royal Lao Government. France was the preferred destination for high-level medical education, and French the predominant language of instruction. The recipients of Lao and French scholarships studied medicine, midwifery, pharmacy and dental surgery in France,[20] whereas WHO scholarship recipients studied to be assistant doctors and assistant dental surgeons at the Royal School of Medicine in Phnom Penh. By 1966, Lao medical students were scattered across seven countries, determined by the availability of scholarships. The majority were in France, but others studied in the Soviet Union, Thailand, Czechoslovakia, Australia, Canada and Japan. In the same year, there were nine pharmacy students and two dental surgery students in France, six dental students in Phnom Penh, five midwifery students in Saigon, and ten nursing students in Thailand.[21] This state of affairs marked the beginnings of the diverse patchwork of professional training and foreign language proficiency that dogged the health workforce for decades.

In addition to overseas scholarships, the range of in-country professional training expanded considerably. The opening of the Royal School of Medicine in Vientiane significantly augmented the existing Practical Nursing School and the Midwifery School at Mahosot Hospital.[22] The medical school offered courses with assistance from France and the WHO. From 1957/58, a four-year course for assistant doctors (*médecins assistants*) was offered.[23] Curricula for assistant dental surgeons and assistant pharmacists were added in 1965 and 1966 respectively.[24] Courses in nursing and midwifery at the Mahosot-based nursing and midwifery schools were upgraded in the 1960s with WHO assistance. The establishment of provincial-level auxiliary nursing and midwifery schools in the mid-1960s in the towns of Luang Prabang, Savannakhet and Pakse, also with WHO assistance, increased the numbers of staff at auxiliary level. Finally, in-country training for doctors, registered nurses and registered midwives was introduced at the medical school in 1969, although training for pharmacists and dental surgeons remained unavailable in-country until after 1975.[25] Laos' first cohort of 25 medical students embarked on a seven-year medical (*doctorat en médecine*) course at the renamed Faculty of Medicine at Sisavangvong University in Vientiane in October 1969, and did not graduate until after the establishment of the Lao PDR.[26] The gradual introduction of professional courses, commencing at assistant-level, made sense in the low-resource context of Laos, where limited funding was matched by few Lao nationals with sufficient teaching qualifications to conduct the courses, and a limited supply of eligible students.[27]

Lao staff with high-level qualifications were in demand to manage the various departments of the Ministry of Health, provide technical direction, and work with the mounting number of international donors. However, there was an imbalance between supply and demand, due to the small number of medical graduates produced overseas, and further exacerbated by their employment choices. Concerned about a professional brain drain, USAID reported that, in 1968, two-thirds of qualified Lao doctors remained overseas rather than returning to Laos.[28] Of those who returned, many opted to join the military health service rather than the civilian Ministry of Health, possibly attracted by higher salaries and more rapid advancement opportunities. An American report from 1971 states: "With only 36 Laotian doctors in the country [a veiled allusion to those remaining abroad], 17 are in the military and the remaining 19 work as administrators in the RLG [Royal Lao Government] government . . ."[29]

For the most part, Lao staff clustered in the middle and lower ranks of the professional health hierarchy, due to low completion rates within the formal education system. They were employed as assistant doctors and nurses, assistant pharmacists, assistant dentists and laboratory technicians. The Ministry of Health was therefore compelled to rely on an international mix of health professionals: Lao assistant doctors complemented by foreign doctors, pharmacists and dental surgeons to meet the increased staffing demands of its expanding health network. Provincial hospitals and outreach services typically made do with assistant doctors, as fully qualified doctors were rarely assigned outside Vientiane. As such, one could assume that assistant doctors in Laos were assigned a level of responsibility similar to doctors in other countries.

Foreign doctors outnumbered Lao doctors in the Royal Lao Government zone for most of this period, as did foreign registered nurses. France provided many of the doctors and medical advisors, including the majority of international instructors at the medical school.[30] In the early 1960s, France provided 12 instructors: five from its civilian budget and seven from its military budget.[31] The French Military Mission contributed skilled personnel who served as technical specialists at Mahosot Hospital and major provincial hospitals until at least 1973.[32] They were complemented by the provision of francophone WHO technical advisors in a variety of roles. Britain and Japan provided small numbers of medical staff to assist provincial health facilities, presumably with some linguistic barriers. During the 1960s, British doctors served in Xayabouly, Salavanh, Luang Prabang and Thakhek provincial hospitals.[33] Japan operated a mobile clinic in the Vientiane Plain area in the 1960s, and later supplied doctors to Savannakhet provincial hospital and Tha Ngone dispensary on the outskirts of Vientiane,[34] while Swiss technical advisors assisted Luang Prabang hospital in the 1970s.[35] Medical teams from non-aligned India assisted hospitals in Vientiane and Paksanh during the mid-1960s.[36] High numbers of Filipino doctors served in a parallel heath network of American-funded Operation Brotherhood hospitals (discussed later in this chapter).

The high proportion of foreign doctors and advisors working within the ministry, and the project funds accompanying them, created a delicate situation that at times resembled the power relations of the colonial period. By the 1970s, the extent of foreign involvement and particularly the high level of international staffing seems to have become quite sensitive for the Ministry of Health, as staffing demographics became a regular feature of annual statistical reporting. From 1970, the ministry made overt efforts to show that the number of Lao staff outnumbered foreigners. It boosted the proportion of Lao doctors by statistically combining the numbers of civilian and military doctors, and merging the professional classifications of doctor and assistant doctor.[37] This sensitivity is likely to have been linked more to the control rather than the receipt of international assistance, on which it continued to be highly reliant.

Laos' nursing cadre also increased significantly during the period 1950–75, in part because it had the lowest educational prerequisite: completion of primary school. The number of Royal Lao Government civilian nurses increased almost four-fold, from 220 in 1950 to 801 general nurses and 29 registered nurses in 1973.[38] Two developments in the nursing profession are noteworthy during this period. Firstly, the upgrading of nursing to a profession and the introduction of auxiliary and registered nurses offered an element of career progression. Secondly, the proportion of female nurses rose within the first decade of independence from 23 percent in 1950 to 70 percent in 1959, a steep increase likely hastened by the number of male nurses electing to join the military health service.[39] The overall number of trained staff in the Ministry of Health increased more than six-fold between 1950 and 1973, from 260 to 1,644 staff (or 2,514 staff if one includes those employed in the military's medical service), and expanded to include a much wider selection of health-related professions.[40]

Many of Laos' key health developments during this period, such as yaws eradication, malaria prevention, mother and child health, and nursing education, were enabled by internationally funded development projects. The WHO supported the Yaws Eradication Project in three southern provinces from 1953.[41] Project activities were undoubtedly successful: WHO reported it had reached approximately 94 percent of the population in the project area. At the same time, WHO overstated its achievements by claiming to have taken "medical care to many remote areas for the first time," when in fact the project was preceded by 60 years of activity by the colonial health service.[42] A visiting WHO monitoring team noted in 1965 the limitations in the Ministry of Health's capacity for continuation of activities promoted by the project. Re-surveys had not been feasible since project end, due to the withdrawal of WHO's project staff, and the Royal Lao Government's "limitation in personnel and the demands of other health problems."[43]

A six-year regional project in malaria eradication, co-funded by WHO and the United States, began in 1956 to address what continued to be cited as the leading health issue in Laos.[44] In 1957, malaria accounted for 73.6 percent of all hospitalized cases, as well as 35.4 percent of hospital deaths.[45] The malaria project relied heavily on technical advisors from the United States and Thailand. It facilitated the establishment of the National Service for Malaria Eradication within the Ministry of Heath, and a number of provincial field stations. Like the yaws project, it required a large contingent of local field technicians, some of whom quite possibly transferred from the yaws project to the malaria project.[46] DDT spraying commenced in southern Laos in 1957 and in the north in 1959. By then, the program claimed to have coverage of almost half the total population. However, the ministry was unable to sustain the activity and spraying ceased in 1961, coinciding with the end of American funding and increasing rural insecurity.[47] A second WHO-supported malaria project, which also included DDT spraying, began in 1969 in locations around the Nam Ngum Dam construction site north of Vientiane, and in internal refugee camps on the Vientiane Plain inhabited by people displaced by the American bombing.[48] It expanded into a National Malaria Program after 1973 with the support of the coalition government.[49]

The commencement of the WHO's Maternal and Child Health Project in 1959 marked a different type of development engagement, which required long-term education and behavior change rather than the more straightforward vaccination or spraying campaigns. The project, which extended until 1976, aimed to develop effective maternal and child health services as an integral part of Laos' general health program.[50] It was complemented with a Nursing Education Project from 1962. The project supported the establishment of a National Maternal and Child Health Service in 1960, followed by a National Maternal and Child Health Center which collaborated with the maternity and pediatric wards at Mahosot Hospital.[51] Maternal and Child Health centers were progressively opened at the larger provincial hospitals.[52] The provincial Maternal and Child Health centers and maternity wings were constructed by USAID, and supported by four provincial auxiliary nursing and midwifery schools mentioned above. Vaccination rounds were integrated into a broad set of basic rural healthcare services, alongside maternal and child health services.

WHO also piloted a Rural Development in Public Health Project from 1961 to 1967, in cooperation with a larger rural development project implemented by the United Nations, UNICEF, UNESCO, International Labour Organization, Food and Agriculture Organization and the Colombo Plan. Efforts were made to improve the quality of primary healthcare provided by rural dispensaries. WHO nurses and public health advisors performed health education, especially home sanitation, nutrition promotion, and mother and child healthcare. However, the ongoing conflict in Laos "limited project activities and delayed the signature of an overall agreement."[53] Therefore, rather than expand into more remote areas, the project contracted in the early 1970s into a series of peri-urban community health centers in the area immediately surrounding Vientiane.[54]

The efforts of WHO advisors, as well as the advisors of many donor nations, were diminished by weak government structures and staff capacity. A WHO health planning advisor in 1961 cited a "lack of organisational machinery, inadequate coordination between government agencies, the relative unfamiliarity of national staff with the planning process, lack of budgetary and material resources and, in certain instances, internal instability" as limitations on health development efforts.[55]

The cessation or continuation of foreign aid projects influenced not only the functioning of the Lao health sector but also its structure. For example, the National Malaria Department, established in the mid-1950s when the WHO and USAID funds for anti-malaria activities were available, stood vacant when external funding later dried up. In contrast, the National Maternal and Child Health Department established in the early stages of the WHO-funded Maternal and Child Health Project in the 1960s was maintained until the change of regime, in part because WHO funding remained constant.

The Ministry of Health also regulated a private health sector, which emerged in the first decade of independence and grew rapidly. It comprised medical clinics, dental surgeries and pharmacies, heavily concentrated in Vientiane. Doctors, assistant doctors and dentists applied to open clinics and/ or to treat patients privately, while nurses and merchants applied to open pharmacies.[56] In 1962 Khamsone Sassady reported a total of 14 private medical practitioners nationwide, of whom ten were Lao, three French, and one Vietnamese.[57] By 1973, numbers had risen to 106 private practitioners nationwide.[58] Chinese residents were strongly represented in dental and pharmaceutical businesses.[59]

Lao and foreign commentators alike considered that the private sector placed pressure on the ministry's health service; the relationship between the two was effectively a zero-sum game. Khamsone observed in the early 1960s that the director of studies at the Royal School of Medicine juggled his responsibilities between the school, the main hospital and his private practice.[60] Several years later, USAID officials commented in seeming frustration that most Lao doctors "devoted 80% or more of their time to private practice."[61]

The rural population of Laos were the losers. By 1973 a staggering 87.5 percent of all Lao doctors (civilian and military) in government service and 61 percent of all assistant doctors were based in Vientiane.[62] Inevitably the provinces had become less attractive for Lao professionals during the years of internal conflict and bombing, although most of the main towns remained firmly within the Royal Lao Government zone. The ministry's Vientiane-centrism compromised its ability to provide healthcare to the rural population, which elicited criticism from USAID concerning its "relative indifference to the health problems in remote areas,"[63] and generated fuel for NLHX propaganda campaigns to the rural population.

Operation Brotherhood and the USAID-Funded Village Health Program

The United States government, frustrated at a perceived lack of capacity and responsiveness within the francophone Ministry of Health, decided to establish and support a parallel health service in provincial areas of the Royal Lao Government zone. The aim of the Village Health Program, as the service was administratively known, was to provide healthcare to Laos' rural population and, importantly, to military and paramilitary combatants in the developing conflict.[64] Funded through USAID's Public Health Division from 1963 to 1975, the Village Health Program comprised facilities operated by USAID itself, and facilities operated by the Filipino NGO Operation Brotherhood,[65] which had been deploying medical teams into Laos under the banner of "Asians helping Asians" since 1957.[66] As the conflict in Laos continued into the late 1960s and early 1970s, Village Health Program activities shifted from a focus on the health of combatants and their family members, to one that encompassed the increasingly large refugee populations that were a product of relentless bombing and land battles.

The Village Health Program was not a mere NGO program that complemented government services. It almost matched the Ministry of Health in size, in terms of the numbers of health facilities, Lao staff and patients. Operation Brotherhood and the Village Health Program have frequently been dismissed as tools of the Central Intelligence Agency in Laos. Certainly, the 1971–72 inquiry of the US Government Accounting Office disclosed that the Operation Brotherhood contract was partly funded by the Central Intelligence Agency:

> The costs of the Operation Brotherhood Project since its inception in 1963 have been borne by USAID/Laos. Starting in fiscal year 1972 the CIA [Central Intelligence Agency] is sharing these costs based on a predetermined formula.[67]

Military historian Timothy Castle cites high-ranking USAID officials describing USAID's operations and its funding arrangements in Laos as "unprecedented" and "unique."[68] And while the political processes surrounding the cost-sharing arrangements were of concern to American lawmakers, there was no suggestion that such arrangements compromised in any way the quality of medical care provided on the ground.

Operation Brotherhood operated multiple health facilities in rural Laos. Initially, its teams were based in the small hospitals (*infirmeries*) and dispensaries of the Ministry of Health, in locations that had experienced some level of healthcare during the colonial period. These sites tended to be in smaller provincial towns or army garrisons, with which Operation Brotherhood staff coordinated closely. In the early 1960s, the NGO began to build and operate its own facilities, including a teaching and referral hospital at That Luang in Vientiane. In all, Operation Brotherhood established a long-term presence in seven locations and made shorter-term contributions in another 12 locations.[69]

USAID operated fewer hospitals but considerably more dispensaries than Operation Brotherhood. The USAID health facilities were based in remote rural locations chosen for their strategic importance in the escalating conflict. Many facilities were accessible only by air or by foot, which added considerably to the cost of providing services and replenishing supplies. The number of USAID dispensaries varied from month to month, as many were located in contested areas that were liable to be overrun by revolutionary forces. USAID reports indicate that it operated approximately 150 dispensaries in 1964, considerably more than the 106 operated by the Ministry of Health in 1966, and 250 in 1972 compared to the ministry's 148 in 1973.[70] However, as the number of Ministry of Health dispensaries slowly rose, those of USAID gradually reduced from 1972. Some were captured by the NLHX, others were handed over to the Ministry of Health, and others closed because the ministry was unable to staff and/or supply them.[71]

It is unclear from the available sources how many hospitals USAID ran at any time. In 1964 the agency reported running nine "bamboo hospitals," although it is not possible to assess whether these were facilities of considerable size and capacity, or simply glorified dispensaries.[72] USAID hospitals were often established adjacent to landing strips, termed Lima Sites, scattered throughout rural Laos, which allowed for the air transport of people, equipment and supplies for military and civilian purposes. The Sam Thong hospital, established in 1963, treated large numbers of Hmong and other ethnic minority groups near the fighting, and served as a medical training center for local recruits. When captured by NLHX forces in March 1970, the hospital had 250 beds, and X-ray, laboratory and surgical capacity, placing it on a par with Vientiane's Mahosot Hospital in patient capacity if not in staffing terms. Staff and patients had been transferred to a newly built USAID hospital further south at Ban Xone prior to the capture of Sam Thong.[73]

The Operation Brotherhood and USAID facilities worked hand in hand as an integrated network. USAID dispensaries referred patients to Operation Brotherhood's rural hospitals, which transferred serious cases to its Vientiane hospital, or to the capital's military hospital. Moreover, Operation Brotherhood medical and nursing staff filled gaps in USAID facilities, and provided medical training for its Lao staff.[74]

Operation Brotherhood began work in Laos with all-Filipino teams, and gradually added Lao staff to its payroll.[75] The Filipino staff consisted of doctors, surgeons, dentists, nurses and health administrators, as well as community development teams of social workers, nutritionists and agricultural extension workers. Filipino staff numbered 44 at the close of 1957, its first year of operations in Laos, and had almost tripled to 129 in 1974.[76] USAID's staffing structure appears to have been similar, with a small core of international staff supported by a much larger number of Lao trained by the two organizations. References to American doctors and nurses assisting the Lao teams at rural USAID facilities appear from the early 1960s.[77] By 1973, the Village Health Program had approximately 650 Lao staff employed by USAID and another 550 employed by Operation Brotherhood.[78] These statistics indicate that the Village Health Program network's Lao staff comprised nearly 50 percent of the Royal Lao Government zone's total civilian health workforce. The Village Health Program trained and categorized its Lao staff according to an American-style system. Operation Brotherhood conducted training programs for its own nurses and nursing aides in Vientiane from 1959. At least 148 practical nurses were trained from 1961 to 1969. When the training program began, Operation Brotherhood produced the most highly qualified nurses in Laos.[79] However, from 1969 the Ministry of Health, with WHO support, offered superior education with the introduction of its three-year courses for registered nurses. From then on, Operation Brotherhood ceased nurse training as its own hospital network was slated for integration into the Royal Lao Government health service, and the ministry trained nurses itself. The NGO continued, however, to offer on-the-job training for nursing aides and other health personnel. USAID employed many ethnic minority medics trained at the Sam Thong hospital, who did not meet the minimum educational level required under either the Royal Lao Government or Operation Brotherhood services.[80] It is unclear to what extent Operation Brotherhood assisted in training these staff, but a 1975 report states that the NGO had "participated very effectively" in the training of almost 2,000 health workers to date, exceeding the number of practical nurses and nursing aides trained for its own facilities.[81] Training activities under the Village Health Program appear to have declined as plans to handover operations to the Royal Lao Government gradually progressed. When United States officials visited Laos in 1971 to gather information for a Government Accountability Office report, they found very few obvious training activities taking place.[82]

The main focus of the Village Health Program was curative medicine, although some aspects of public health were also addressed. Vaccinations were provided, as were mother and child health services, and family planning services were offered from the early 1970s. The Senate committee report of

1970 found that "A significant portion of USAID-funded medical supplies provided under the Village Health Program is made available to military combatants, paramilitary forces and their dependents, and other groups," but USAID emphasized the opposite.[83] Many non-combatants could have been classified as dependents of combatants, or within the vague classification of "other groups." Such comments suggest the possibly intentional obscuring of the situation. It is also interesting to consider why the Village Health Program network regularly claimed a larger share of patients than the Ministry of Health. For example, the Government Accountability Office reports that in 1970 Operation Brotherhood treated 20,831 in-patients at its seven hospitals and a further 26,887 in 1971.[84] For the same years, the ministry reported 17,897 and 27,452 hospitalizations respectively. However, its figures purport to contain those of the Operation Brotherhood hospitals, which were now integrated on paper if not in reality into the Ministry of Health network of facilities.[85] Such discrepancies suggest problems with statistics, but also hint at the lack of correspondence between the two health networks.

The US Senate inquiries of the early 1970s hastened the unraveling of the Village Health Program network by drawing the American public's attention to USAID's refugee relief and health programs. USAID officials confirmed in 1976 that their approach had focused less on developing a health service, and more on immediate political objectives: "From the inception . . . the [US] Mission was concerned about the severe lack of trained health personnel particularly at the professional and middle levels, but the urgent need for immediate medical services caused by the expanding insurgency, had to receive priority attention."[86] The report continues:

> The Health Development Project [of which the Village Health Program was part] despite its name was not a development project in the sense of building a lasting institutional base for a long-term health delivery system. It was created and expanded as an expediency in response to humanitarian military and political needs. In terms of providing acute medical care for insurgent and refugee areas, it was highly successful.[87]

The Government Accountability Office questioned the network's focus and funding. Its 1971 report observed: "The statement of goals of the Village Health Program are so vaguely worded making it practically impossible to show progress or the lack of progress."[88]

From 1967, USAID instructed Operation Brotherhood to begin a phased transfer of administrative and financial responsibility for its facilities to the Ministry of Health. The transfer proved problematic due to the Royal Lao Government's insufficient funds and staffing levels. In 1971 the Government

Accountability Office team observed: "The administrative function of the hospitals was transferred to the Royal Lao Government, on paper, in 1967, however the Filipino personnel actually operate the hospitals."[89] The deadline for transfer was extended until 1975 because of the Lao government's resource limitations. The Government Accountability Office report also expressed the opinion that neither USAID nor the Royal Lao Government could afford the "luxury" of an expedient medical program like the Village Health Program. It recommended a shift in focus to more long-term training of personnel and institutional development.[90] The recommendations were not implemented.

USAID advised Operation Brotherhood in 1969 of the Royal Lao Government's requirement to phase out and transfer its Lao staff to the Ministry of Health, but few were willing to transfer: Lao staff still numbered 550 in 1974.[91] The program's phase-out plan was hampered not only by the reluctance of Lao staff to transfer to the Lao government's lower wages,[92] but also by the lack of correspondence of staff skills and training. Their professional classifications of "practical nurse," "nursing aide" and "medic" did not accord with French-style classifications used by the ministry. Furthermore, their technical training had emphasized use of English terminology over French, and they were more familiar with American than French pharmaceuticals.[93]

The Health Sector in the Liberated Zone

Laos' other territorial zone, the revolutionary NLHX's Liberated Zone, hosted two health services, a military service and a civilian service, from the mid-1950s. A Lao People's Army commemorative history suggests that a military health service (*senahak*) was formally established within the revolutionary forces in the northeast region of Laos in November 1954.[94] This service provided healthcare to the revolutionary armed forces and political cadres, as well as to civilians in what became known as the Liberated Zone. A civilian health service under the direction of the Central Health Committee (*Khanakama-kane Sathalanasouk Sounkang*) split from the original military service in 1965.[95] The split followed the disintegration of Laos' second coalition government (1962–64) and the revolutionary leadership's move from its base in Xieng Khouang to the cave complex of Viengxay in Xam Neua province,[96] where the NLHX began to formalize its administrative and technical services with assistance from North Vietnam. In theory, the Central Health Committee was responsible for civilian healthcare, whereas the military service remained responsible for battlefield medics and rear-area military hospitals. However, frequently it is difficult to distinguish in archival sources between the military and civilian health services, suggesting that the distinction was neither clear nor consistent.

The operation of the Liberated Zone's civilian health service is perhaps more interesting than that of the Ministry of Health, because it inherited very little from the colonial administration, and was compelled to build its staffing and facilities from the ground up. The NLHX operated in remote, mountainous regions with much lower population density, greater ethnic diversity and lower education levels than did the Ministry of Health. Moreover, it operated within a zone of sporadic and escalating conflict, in which the resistance leadership and rural communities were obliged to frequently relocate to escape aerial bombing and/or land battles. Despite the unfavorable conditions, the NLHX managed to establish a basic health service. It included a modest network of health facilities and village-based first aid, medical training schools, and some elements of primary healthcare outreach. From the late 1960s the civilian Central Health Committee aimed to provide clinical healthcare, control contagious diseases, promote mother and child health, produce and distribute pharmaceuticals, rehabilitate traditional medicine and train health staff.[97] The focus on pharmaceutical production and the use of traditional medicine was motivated by necessity, to keep costs as low as possible, and to avoid the difficulty of delivering pharmaceuticals to remote and potentially insecure areas. Pharmaceutical production also accorded with the NLHX's policy of scientific development, and brought traditional medicine practitioners into the official health sector, which swelled the numbers of health workers in the Liberated Zone.

No budget details of the NLHX health service or its international donors were available for consultation in the Lao National Archives. However, it likely had very low operating costs, as staffing and pharmaceutical expenses were kept to a minimum in line with the Party's self-sufficiency policy. NLHX cadres and soldiers received no or low salaries, and the administration was responsible to meet their basic food, clothing and accommodation needs.

Similar to the various health services in the Royal Lao Government zone, both NLHX services are presumed to have been heavily reliant on foreign aid as the NLHX had no obvious income stream of its own, and was often at war during the period from 1950 to 1975. However, it is reasonable to assume that the volume of foreign aid received by the NLHX was significantly less than that received by the Royal Lao Government. North Vietnam was the main donor to the NLHX's military and civilian health services, partly because it served as a conduit for Soviet support.[98] Most international support is likely to have been received in kind, in the form of technical advisors, scholarships, medical equipment and supplies, pharmaceuticals, construction materials and fuel.

A handwritten note in the Lao National Archives lists thousands of kilograms of pharmaceuticals received from North Vietnam, China, and several East European countries in 1968–70.[99] From the early 1970s, Cuba also provided assistance, sending a medical brigade to work in the NLHX's headquarters at Viengxay.

Organizationally and politically, the Liberated Zone's civilian health service bore the imprint of its foreign benefactors. The organizational structure comprised health committees at each level of the administration from central to village level. Health committees were also to be formed within workplaces, in accordance with the socialist model where one's workplace or work unit took care of all livelihood matters, including healthcare. A special department responsible for the healthcare of the revolutionary leaders was staffed by North Vietnamese doctors and Lao assistants.[100] In 1970 the Central Health Committee was re-organized with the assistance of North Vietnamese advisors. Meeting minutes reveal that two of the four committee members had technical (that is, medical and healthcare) responsibilities, while the remaining two were assigned political responsibilities, highlighting the dual focus of a communist health service.[101] From the early 1970s, the Central Health Committee reported statistics that seemed intent on proving its parity with the Royal Lao Government's Ministry of Health, reminiscent of Cuba's competitive health policy vis-à-vis that of the United States.[102] And finally, a note on the sources. Official sources concerning the NLHX health services are notable for their focus on policies and plans, but not for their reporting of the actual situation.

The Central Health Committee developed a formula for the distribution and size of health facilities. Ideally, each province was to have a 30–50 bed hospital, each district a 15–20 bed hospital, and each sub-district (*tasseng*) a small health facility of 5–7 beds.[103] By 1975, the NLHX claimed that the number of health facilities under its control rivalled that of the Royal Lao Government, an impressive achievement given its limited resources. It is likely, however, that the definitions and levels of quality were not comparable. For example, in one instance a former NLHX health worker referred to a hospital (*hongmoh*) consisting of only two beds, signaling the vast variation in definitions which existed across the various health services in Laos.[104]

Central Health Committee reports cite rapidly rising numbers of health facilities throughout the Liberated Zone, although reported numbers differ and often make no distinction in terms of size or function. A report from 1970 lists 13 hospitals in 1967, 51 in 1968 and 81 in 1969.[105] In Attapeu province, the military and civilian hospitals were co-located, while in other provinces they were separate.[106] A number of villages in the Liberated Zone received drug kits comprising basic medicines to compensate for the absence of a nearby health facility, a practice that continues in the Lao PDR to this day.

The NLHX's health network was a patchwork of facilities inherited from the colonial health service, those established by the NLHX itself or with North Vietnamese assistance, those captured from USAID, Operation Brotherhood, or the Royal Lao Government, and those built by villagers. The regroupment area assigned to the NLHX by the Geneva Conference of 1954 contained two colonial *infirmeries-ambulances* and six rural dispensaries in Xam Neua and Phongsaly provinces. However, it is not known how many of these facilities continued to function after French handover to the Royal Lao Government in 1950.[107]

The NLHX constructed hospitals, dispensaries, small pharmaceutical factories and medical schools in areas under its control. The North Vietnamese forces also constructed facilities within Lao territory, which they operated themselves. Such facilities provided medical care for Vietnamese troops and civilian advisors, as well as training for Lao health staff and treatment of the local population. The Central Hospital in Xam Neua was staffed with North Vietnamese advisors and trainers as early as 1954.[108] In Xieng Khouang, a hospital operated by the North Vietnamese Red Cross was handed over to the coalition government in 1962.[109] In addition, there was a complex network of small NLHX military hospitals.[110] Three Vietnamese and two Lao "rudimentary" hospitals in Namtha were reported by a Vietnamese defector in 1966–67, and another mentions a hospital and training school in Oudomxay.[111] In southern Laos, sources mention a large hospital staffed by 30 North Vietnamese personnel and a joint Pathet Lao–Vietnamese hospital near the Lao–Cambodian border in 1964,[112] as well as a hospital and training school in Phine district on Route 9, and Hospital 48 in Nong district of Savannakhet, on the Hồ Chí Minh Trail.[113] The revolutionaries established military Hospital 101 in Xieng Khouang province in 1962, and Hospital 102 in Viengxay in 1964.[114]

The status of NLHX health facilities, and the reliance on Vietnamese assistance for both construction and operation, became clearer after the Central Health Committee's formation. Acknowledging Vietnamese assistance in numerous rural locations, a 1971 report complained that "some Vietnamese advisors do not have sufficient confidence in the abilities of their Lao counterparts, making plans and implementing health initiatives without consultation."[115]

A retired Lao surgeon who worked in the NLHX's Liberated Zone recalls three hospitals operating in the Viengxay area during the 1960s and 1970s: one for Party leaders, one for the military and one for civilians.[116] In 1969 an official order advised that construction of the temporary Central Hospital (*Hongmoh sounkang*) was complete; patients would be accepted for midwifery,

ear/nose/throat, internal medicine, pediatrics, laboratory and traditional medicine services. Patients were to bring with them medical referral papers,
blankets, mosquito nets, clothing, a bowl and spoon, and 15 days of food
rations.[117] The 50-bed hospital, also known as Hang Long Hospital, was located
in a cave for protection from American bombing. It was replaced in 1972 by
the Lao-Vietnam Friendship Hospital, a 100-bed facility also known as Xieng
Louang Hospital, which had been carved from the rock walls of a large cave.
Wards had doors at either end, but no windows.[118]

The NLHX gained territory and health facilities as the Lao conflict progressed. However, it is not known to what extent the Central Health Committee
was able to staff and supply newly acquired facilities beyond appropriating
abandoned pharmaceuticals and basic medical equipment and supplies. The
number of health staff working in the Liberated Zone before the mid-1960s is
unknown, but from the late 1960s NLHX statistics challenge the assumption
that the Royal Lao Government employed more staff. In 1970 the Central Health
Committee gave a breakdown of its staffing by profession and by region, but
there was wide divergence in the figures. A total 2,093 staff were reported by
profession, 53 of whom were responsible for politics (*kane-meuang*), but the
statistics reported only 999 when calculated by region.[119] It is not possible to
guess which figures are likely to be more accurate.

Sources suggest that health staff were recruited and trained by the NLHX
from at least 1954, possibly earlier.[120] The NLHX recruited rural teenagers into
the revolutionary movement from their villages.[121] In addition, trained health
staff sometimes chose to join the revolutionaries, including a number of graduating medical students returning from studies in France and the Soviet Union
on scholarships offered to the Royal Lao Government. NLHX and Royal Lao
Government health staff were briefly merged during the first coalition government of 1957–58, but after that remained separate until the third and final
coalition government of 1974–75.

As with the United-States-funded Village Health Program, the categories of health worker in the Liberated Zone were quite different to those of the
Royal Lao Government. Professional classifications were reduced to a simpli-
fied three-level hierarchy of high-level, mid-level and low-level health workers
(*phet xanh-soung, xanh-kang, xanh-tonh*), often with little reference to technical
focus. Sometimes a distinction was made between medical workers, pharmacists, midwives, nurses and traditional medicine practitioners, but not always.

Despite significant social, cultural and economic differences in the areas
under their administration, many situations experienced by the civilian
Central Health Committee mirror those of the Ministry of Health. For example, the NLHX relied upon international doctors due to the limited number of

Lao doctors for most of this period. Many of the clinical doctors and medical teachers were Vietnamese, some recruited from among sympathetic immigrants in Thailand and Laos, and others from North Vietnam.[122] By 1971 there were Vietnamese advisors in almost every medical department of the Central Health Committee.[123] This situation confirms that the Filipino nationals of Operation Brotherhood were not the only Asians helping Asians in the Lao health sector.

Professional distribution of staff in the Liberated Zone looks very similar to that of the Ministry of Health. In 1970 there were 18 high-level doctors (of similar rank to the ministry's *docteurs en médecine*) and one high-level pharmacist employed by the NLHX, 117 mid-level doctors (similar to *médecins assistants*, although their training appears to have been one year shorter) and a much larger group of 1,297 low-level health workers, who had similar (but not identical) training to the ministry's base-level nurses.[124] As in the Royal Lao Government zone, the number of high- and mid-level doctors shot up in the final years preceding the establishment of the Lao PDR.

The NLHX also localized lower-level medical training to supply its health services. The schools taught rural teenagers with low education levels, and relied upon Vietnamese teachers who improvised with teaching materials and learning styles. A Vietnamese medical instructor working in a small team of three in Attapeu recounts a class he taught:

> we carried rice from the village for food, wrote lesson plans and delivered lessons by ourselves. If visual aids were not available, we hunted forest animals and brought them to class. For example, for lessons on anatomy, physiology, we hunted animals and conducted surgery to explain from the skeleton, skin and flesh to organs. After having finished the lesson, these animals would be used as food.[125]

He notes that because some students were barely literate, the classes had a strong focus on practical skills rather than theory: "When there were epidemics of malaria, diarrhea [sic], measles, the whole class visited villages to eliminate them and conduct real-life training at the same time. Taking notes was unnecessary."[126]

Several sources note that medical training began with political training. One NLHX health worker spoke of 18 months training at a medical school in Dak Cheung (in present-day Xekong province) in a class of 30 Lao students and 30 young Vietnamese women taught by two Vietnamese women. Before beginning the training, all students studied social and political theory. He says they had to be willing to help other people, not be disgusted by injured patients, and work together and love the Vietnamese "as their siblings" (*pen louk pho dio mae dio kan*).[127] The mix of family and politics arises again in a revolutionary nurse's memoirs. Her medical training began with a question and answer: "Who are the patients? They are your brothers, sisters, fellow-Lao people. The state is your parents. We all live under the same roof."[128]

Provinces were responsible for the training of their own low-level staff. The Center (*Sounkang*) was responsible for training mid-level health workers, and high-level health workers were sent for training in North Vietnam.[129] By 1970 there were a reported 12 low-level medical schools and three mid-level schools in Viengxay, Oudomxay and Savannakhet. Most available information relates to the Viengxay school, as this was the political headquarters of the NLHX. A mid-level military medical school also operated nearby at Na Vit, staffed by Lao graduates of a North Vietnamese medical school.[130] The civilian, mid-level school in Viengxay provided three-year courses to nine cohorts of students, four cohorts of which graduated prior to the change of regime. In addition, the mid-level school in Savannakhet produced at least 36 graduates.[131] In 1970, 142 NLHX students were studying abroad (presumably in North Vietnam): 26 studying high-level medicine, 11 studying high-level pharmacology and another 105 studying mid-level medicine.[132]

An additional category of health workers swelling the NLHX ranks were low-level public health workers, including village-level nurses, "hygiene fighters" (*nakhop anamay*), and mobile and village-based environmental health workers.[133] Basic public health training provided young people with new knowledge, and new roles in their communities. One young village woman recounts her experience as a village-level nurse in Xieng Khouang in the mid-1960s:

> After six months, we were capable of preventing diseases and treating other typical illnesses. We then went out to practise what we had learned, dividing ourselves up among various villages. They told us to eat and live together with the people. Our duty was to take care of the ill and act in such a way that people would believe and support the Neo Lao [NLHX] . . . we didn't take payments for our medical treatments.[134]

The training and employment of public health workers demonstrated the NLHX's policy commitment to preventative and environmental health. When internal refugees returned home after the 1973 ceasefire, the Central Health Committee instructed that they be encouraged to rebuild their villages in accordance with hygienic principles, by digging wells and locating latrines, rubbish pits and animal pens away from houses. An official report from 1974 paints a rosy picture of villages being re-established in perfect accordance with hygienic principles—in contrast to the reality encountered by environmental health teams in the following decade.[135]

In summary, the NLHX managed to create a network of health facilities across many provinces, establish low- and mid-level medical training schools, and employ a cadre of health staff that worked cooperatively with North Vietnamese technical advisors despite limited funding and adverse wartime conditions.

Uniting Laos' Fragmented Health Sector

The political situation was fluid leading up to the eventual establishment of the Lao PDR in December 1975. After the 1973 ceasefire, a third coalition government was formed in April 1974 which paired one Royal Lao Government representative with one NLHX deputy, or vice-versa, in each of the new government's 12 ministries. Dr Khamphaï Abhay and Dr Khamlieng Pholsena, both French-educated, were assigned the positions of Minister of Health and Deputy Minister of Health, representing the Royal Lao Government and the NLHX respectively.

There is scant documentation about the internal changes to the health sector brought about by the coalition government. Documents from WHO and USAID's Public Health Division reveal that behind the third coalition government's public presentation of unity, pro-NLHX staff within the Ministry of Health lobbied for the adoption of socialist-style policies. The provision of free healthcare for ministry staff was one such example, documented in meeting minutes from 1974.[136] In another example, NLHX health workers who had entered the major towns and were working alongside Royal Lao Government staff were advised in 1975 that the ministry's hospitals were places where "the enemy has large amounts of modern scientific equipment. There are things that we do not yet know how to use. If we can remember how it is used, and take good care of it, it will be convenient for our future work in the health sector."[137]

An internal document from July 1975 reveals that the Central Health Committee was planning to assume responsibility for the entire health sector, in the context of the revolutionary movement's nationwide seizure of power, which was gradually gaining momentum over the course of the year. NLHX teams had been despatched to Luang Prabang, Savannakhet, Pakse and Vientiane provinces to generate support for the revolutionary movement among health workers and in the community at large. The document, classified as a "plan," assessed the political situation among health workers:

> Most [Royal Lao Government technical health staff] are the children of [ordinary], exploited people, although some are from the wealthy class that

has aided the enemy . . . It is the capitalists and the American imperialists who have incited them to use their professional skills to seek income and thus exploit the people . . . In order to implement the policies of the Center [Party leadership], we must clearly distinguish the different types [of staff], by mobilising them to study the Center's policy documents. If some of these staff are good, we should allow them to continue studying documents about the characteristics of revolutionary health workers (*phet pativat*), so that they can change their political thinking and use their technical skills once again for the service of the people . . . under strict Party leadership.[138]

A separate but parallel process was the integration of the Village Health Program network. The coalition government reiterated the need for integration, and so in 1974 the goal of the Village Health Program was amended to: "helping the PGNU [Provisional Government of National Union] provide medical care to refugees and rural areas. Provide medical facilities and training and integrate them into the PGNU Medical Service."[139] The anti-USAID demonstrations of May 1975, in the wake of the fall of Phnom Penh and Saigon the previous month, brought the "premature, abrupt, unplanned turnover of all health facilities" to the coalition government. All international personnel of USAID and Operation Brotherhood were required to depart Laos before 30 June—a hurried departure for the international assistance agencies and staff who had assisted the Lao health sector for almost two decades.[140]

The political situation changed rapidly. Minister of Health Khamphaï did not return to Vientiane from a WHO meeting in Geneva in May 1975, and was granted political asylum in France.[141] Dr Tiao Jaisvasd, former Director of the Royal School of Medicine and the Department of Hospital Services, replaced him as minister. He recalls hoping that Lao health professionals of all political persuasions would find a way of working together. However, from 29 September 1975 he was confined with Crown Prince Vong Savang to the former USAID compound, and was presumably unable to perform his role as minister.[142] Fearing possible consignment to a re-education camp, Dr Tiao Jaisvasd fled to Thailand four days after the establishment of the Lao PDR in December 1975, and resettled in France as a refugee.[143]

Concluding Remarks

Independence from France presented Laos with the potential to shape a health service managed and delivered by Lao nationals, which focused on the needs of the Lao population rather than colonial policy imperatives centered on Hanoi or a more distant Paris. However, the 25 years from the initial handover of the colonial health service to the Lao government until the establishment of the Lao PDR in 1975 resulted in the fragmentation of the colonial health service into a variety of foreign-influenced, foreign-supported health services.

Ultimately, the Lao health sector was caught in the political and military struggle aggravated and supported by Cold War rivalries. The consolidation of the sector was jeopardized by the geographic and administrative division of Laos into two territorial zones, the introduction of foreign aid to both political factions, and the prosecution of the Second Indochina War, which included heavy bombing of large areas of the country for a period of nine years (1964–73). The long-running political conflict between the Royal Lao Government and the NLHX, fueled by the geopolitical interests of their respective allies and supporters, created divisions in the technical expertise and financial resources available for health sector development, and fragmented the considerable development efforts that took place during this period.

National independence did not remove the colonial-era problems of geographical, political and cultural marginality or afford Laos much control over its own destiny. Instead, the newly independent nation plunged into decades of armed conflict, divided along political and territorial lines but which also influenced the development of technical skills and services, which in turn consolidated its dependence on external assistance. While foreign aid boosted budgets available for health development, especially in the Royal Lao Government zone, the strength and coherence of the health sector was severely constrained by its high degree of fragmentation.

All three civilian health services made important achievements during this period. The number of health facilities more than doubled, the number of Lao health staff increased more than tenfold, and the first Lao became fully-qualified medical doctors, pharmacists, registered nurses and midwives. International assistance supported the implementation of a number of specific projects: the provision of medical care, yaws and malaria eradication, maternal and child healthcare, as well as nursing and medical education. The range of healthcare services broadened, and was supplemented by an emerging private sector.

The quality of healthcare continued to struggle, however, because it relied on the availability and equitable distribution of limited trained staff, equipment and supplies. The Royal Lao Government recruited the most highly qualified staff of the three services, but faced difficulties with staff distribution. In contrast the USAID-funded Village Health Program and NLHX services had no choice but to adopt more flexible recruitment and training standards, and consequently their staff were more likely to remain in rural areas. All three services struggled to provide basic equipment, supplies and utilities to health facilities, especially in rural areas. Weak budgets and supply chains, compounded by poor roads and expensive air access, resulted in gaps in the supply of pharmaceuticals and basic medical supplies, and health staff. Equipment was difficult to maintain, and utilities such as electricity and piped water were often absent. Such limitations were characteristic of Laos' international marginality as a geographically remote, extremely poor, war-torn country caught up in the Cold War. In the words of a United States project proposal from 1974: "Laos compares unfavorably with most of the developing countries by almost any yardstick of national development."[144]

Lao health sector development was not only limited by Laos' poverty, but also, paradoxically, by its dependence on foreign aid. Aid donors had their own interests in mind, a point picked up by the revolutionaries. The NLHX criticized the Royal Lao Government for accepting foreign aid, and the political expectations attached to it, from capitalist nations who they saw as meddling in the domestic political affairs of Laos. The revolutionaries contrasted their own receipt of aid from fraternal socialist nations as no-strings-attached assistance to a just cause.

The diversity of international donors, and their political motivations, resulted in a jumble of technical advice, scholarships and training, as well as medical equipment and supplies which were not necessarily complementary or interchangeable. The cultural and technical uniformity of the French colonial period was gone. The professional classifications and training curricula used by the various health services of the Royal Lao Government and Liberated Zones did not correspond, and health professionals working in the various services did not share a common technical approach, nor a common language of training.

Finally, a large portion of Laos' limited human and financial resources, and the potential opportunities of foreign aid, had been channeled into a civil war fueled by the regional and international Cold War, rather than into national development, including the development of the health sector. This is the legacy of the Lao health sector.

NOTES

1. Perry Stieglitz, *In a Little Kingdom* (Armonk, NY: M.E. Sharpe, 1990), pp. 202–3.
2. Responsibility for the government health service was handed over by the Commissioner of the French Republic in Laos to the semi-autonomous Royal Lao Government in April 1950, in line with the Franco-Lao Treaty of July 1949 and the practical agreements of February 1950. See *Laos Mil neuf cent cinquante. Le Royaume du Laos, ses institutions et son organisation générale* (Pathet Lao, 1950. Rabiabkane Pok-khong lae Kanechattang Thoua-pay) (no publication details, no

date), p. 108; Katay Don Sasorith, *Le Laos. Son évolution politique. Sa place dans l'Union française* (Paris: Éditions Berger-Levrault, 1953), pp. 72–3; and ANOM, RSL, Box 12: "Rapport annuel de 1950," [Annual Report, 1950] p. 15.

3. I refer to the two zones as the Royal Lao Government zone (pejoratively referred to by the current regime as the Vientiane zone); and the Liberated Zone, administered by the revolutionary *Neo Lao Hak Xat.*

4. Khammeung Volachit, *Nang Phet Pativat. Xivit tit-phanh kab Hongmoh 101 vilaxon* [Revolutionary Female Nurses. Life and the Heroic Hospital 101] (Vientiane: Manthatoulath Press, 2012); Chanpheng Thongphimpha, "Botbanhtheuk: Xivit kanekheuanvay pakobsouan het kanepativat nay vongkanephet khong Pa Chanpheng Thongphimpha tae pii 1953 theung pii 2000" [The Revolutionary Contribution of Aunt Chanpheng Thongphimpha to the Health Sector from 1953 to 2000] (Vientiane: self-published, 2013); Anonymous, *60 pii heng kane-teub-nyay khong lao-hob Senahak, 1.11.1954–1.11.2014* [60 Years of Development of the Military Health Service, 1.11.1954–1.11.2014] (Vientiane: Lao People's Army, 2014); Keo Phimphachanh, unpublished draft manuscript of memoirs (Vientiane, 2020).

5. Staff at the University of Health Sciences in Vientiane, Lao PDR, expressly advised me not to research the military health services.

6. In 1950 the Ministry of Health was referred to as the Department of Health [Direction générale de la Santé publique] and the Health Service [Assistance médicale laotienne or the Phanek Satharanasouk]. For the sake of simplicity, I use the term "Ministry of Health" throughout this chapter to refer to both the administrative health department and the technical health service, as well as the government health services at central, provincial and district levels.

7. Judith Cousins and Alfred W. McCoy, "Living it up in Laos. Congressional Testimony on US aid to Laos in the 1950s," in *Laos: War and Revolution,* ed. Nina S. Adams and Alfred W. McCoy (New York: Harper and Row, 1970), p. 340.

8. WHO, WPR/RC2, 18–21 September 1951, p. 14 and p. 79; and WHO, WPR/RC3, 25–30 September 1952, p. 13.

9. Despite its rhetoric of neutrality, the WHO assisted South Vietnam rather than North Vietnam, and Taiwan rather than the People's Republic of China during this period.

10. RSL, Box 12: "Rapport annuel de 1950," p. 7.

11. RSL, Box 12: "Rapport annuel de 1950," p. 7, insert between p. 6 and p. 7; LNAD, RLG/MOH, 211-004: "Rapport statistique de l'Assistance médicale, Anneé 1966," Table L/1, and 211-024: "Rapport annuel de l'Assistance médicale, Année 1973," p. 23.

12. Thomas A. Dooley, *Dr Tom Dooley's Three Great Books: Deliver Us from Evil, The Edge of Tomorrow [and] The Night They Burned the Mountain* (New York: Farrar, Straus and Cudahy, 1960), p. 234.

13. RSL, Box 12: "Rapport annuel de 1950," p. 18; and LNAD, RLG/MOH, 211-024: "Rapport annuel de l'Assistance médicale, Anneé 1973," p. 24.

14. USAID, "Foreign Assistance to Laos" (Vientiane: USAID, 1969), p. 7.

15. USAID, "Report of Audit of Maternal and Child Health Project No. 439-11-570-081, 31 March 1969 to 31 March 1971" (Laos Program), p. 2.

16. Martin Stuart-Fox, *A History of Laos* (Cambridge: Cambridge University Press, 1997), p. 154.

17. A Lao national, Dr Oudom Souvannavong, graduated with a degree in medicine from the University of Paris in 1949, and was licensed to practice medicine in France as well as the French colonies.

18. Lao nationals who had graduated with a lesser medical degree from the colonial medical school in Hanoi, and were licensed to practice medicine only within Indochina.

19. ANOM, RSL, Box 12: "Rapport annuel de 1950," p. 7. However, the annual report of the Lao Health Service for 1950 indicates a greater number of Lao staff than the Lao government publication, *Laos Mille Neuf Cent Cinquante*.

20. LNAD, RLG/MOH, 211-004: "Rapport statistique de l'Assistance médicale, Anneé 1966," Table P/8; and Khamphao Phonekeo, "Les recherches sur la géographie du Laos," in *Les Recherches en Sciences Humaines sur le Laos, Actes de la conférence international organiseé à Vientiane, 7–10 décembre 1993*, ed. Pierre-Bernard Lafont (Paris: Publications du Centre d'Histoire et Civilisations de la Peninsule Indochinoise, 1994), p. 29.

21. LNAD, RLG/MOH, 211-004: "Rapport statistique de l'Assistance médicale, Anneé 1966," Table P/8.

22. Anonymous, *Mil neuf cent cinquante. Le Royaume du Laos, ses institutions et son organisation générale* [Laos 1950. The Kingdom of Laos, its Institutions and its General Organization], no publication details, no date, p. 100.

23. The Ministry of Health and the University of Health Sciences (UHS) celebrated the 55th anniversary of the medical school in November 2013, despite Khamsone Sassady and WHO stating the school opened in 1957. It is unclear how the Ministry and UHS selected the date of the celebrations. One response I received suggested that management took a consensus decision, rather than consulting historical sources. See Khamsone Sassady, "Contribution à l'étude de la médecine laotienne," Thesis, Doctorat en médecine, University of Paris, 1962, p. 113; WHO, WP/RC16/5, 1965, p. 57; and the University of Health Sciences' pamphlet, "Saleum salong khop hob 55 pii khong kane-sangtang hong hian phet" [55th Anniversary Celebrations of the Establishment of the Medical School] (Vientiane: UHS, 2013).

24. L. Mathurin and R. Fontan, "La médecine au Laos," *Médecine tropicale* 33, 6 (November–December 1973): 647.

25. WHO, WPR/RC21/4, 1970, p. 55; and Manivanh Souphanthong, "Kane seuksa phetsard thi mahavitthayalay vitthayasat soukhaphapsard vivatthanakane 55 pii pheua pitouphoum khong bouangxon lao" [Medical Education at the University of Health Sciences, 55 Years of Service to the Lao People], in *Peumbotkhatyo*

botthopthouan vixakane Kongpaxoum vitthayasard saleum salong van-sang-tang honghianphed khob-hob 55 pii [Abstracts for the Scientific Conference to cele-brate the 55th Anniversary of the Establishment of the Medical School], 30 October 2013, p. 140.

26.   Anonymous, "Hang lay-ngane saphab viak-ngan sathalanasouk you kongpasoum-ngay khang thi I tae 1 ha 12 toula 1979" [Draft Report on the Health Situation for the First Conference of Health from 1–12 October 1979] (Vientiane: Ministry of Health, 1979), p. 4.

27.   Bruce Lockhart, "Education in Laos in Historical Perspective," unpublished paper, 2001, p. 9.

28.   USAID, "Termination Report. USAID Laos" (Washington, DC: USAID, 1976), p. 162.

29.   NARA, RG 286, Box 2: "Draft GAO Report. Medical section," November 1971, chapter 1, p. 3.

30.   Joel M. Halpern, *Laotian Health Problems*, Laos project paper 20 (Amherst, MA: University of Massachusetts, 1961), p. 25.

31.   Khamsone Sassady, "Contribution à l'étude de la médecine laotienne," pp. 122–3.

32.   LNAD, RLG/MOH, 211-024: "Rapport annuel de l'Assistance médicale, Anneé 1973," p. 11.

33.   USAID, "Foreign Assistance to Laos" (Vientiane: USAID, 1969), p. 10, and Mervyn Brown, *At War in Shangri-La: A Memoir of Civil War in Laos* (London and New York: Radcliffe Press, 2001), pp. 34, 93–4, 123.

34.   NARA, RG 59, Box 2560: "Bi-weekly economic review for Laos, No. 6 (March 11–24), 28 March 1960"; and LNAD, RLG/MOH, 211-024: "Rapport annuel de l'Assistance médicale, Anneé 1973," p. 11.

35.   LNAD, RLG/MOH, 211-024: "Rapport annuel de l'Assistance médicale, Anneé 1973," p. 11.

36.   USAID, "Foreign Assistance to Laos" (Vientiane: USAID, 1969), p. 13.

37.   LNAD, RLG/MOH, 211-017: "Rapport annuel des statistiques sanitaires, 1970," Table P/9.

38.   LNAD, RLG/MOH, 211-024: "Rapport annuel de l'Assistance médicale, Anneé 1973," p. 4.

39.   RSL, Box 12: "Rapport annuel de 1950," p. 6; and NARA, RG 59, Box 4601: "Health: Lao Government Hospital and Medical Personnel Facilities [sic] in Laos as of June 30, 1959," 13 August 1959.

40.   RSL, Box 12: "Rapport annuel de 1950," p. 6; and LNAD, RLG/MOH, 211-024: "Rapport annuel de l'Assistance médicale, Anneé 1973," p. 4. No reports for the years 1974 or 1975, during the period of the Provisional Government of National Union, were available for consultation.

41.   Yaws, or endemic treponematosis (*pian* in French; *khi moh* in Lao) is: "a chronic infection that affects mainly skin, bone and cartilage. It is caused by a bacterium related to the one that causes venereal syphilis. However, yaws is an infection

transmitted mainly through skin contact with an infected person. It is rarely encountered in Laos anymore, due to the successful eradication program of the 1950s. See WHO, *50 Years Working for Health in the Lao People's Democratic Republic, 1962–2012* (Manila: WHO, 2013), p. 5.

42.   WHO, WPR/RC10/2, 1959, p. 40.

43.   WHO, WPR/RC16/5, 1965, p. 86.

44.   RSL, Box 12: "Rapport annuel de 1950," p. 29; Frank LeBar and Adrienne Suddard, ed., *Laos. Its People, Its Society, Its Culture* (New Haven: HRAF Press, 1967 revised edition [1960]), p. 179, and Laura Watson, "Lao Malaria Review," unpublished paper, 1999.

45.   RLG/MOH, *Bulletin statistique du Laos*, No. 4, 1958, p. 82, cited in Joel M. Halpern, *Laotian Health Statistics*, Laos project paper 10 (Amherst, MA: University of Massachusetts, 1961), p. 4.

46.   Halpern, *Laotian Health Problems*, p. 24.

47.   Watson, "Lao Malaria Review," unpublished paper, 1999, p. 17.

48.   WHO, *50 Years Working for Health in the Lao People's Democratic Republic, 1962–2012*, p. 12.

49.   USAID, "Termination Report," pp. 167–8.

50.   WHO, WPR/RC21/4, 1970, p. 90.

51.   WHO, WPR/RC11/3, 1959, p. 100; and WHO, WPR/RC21/4, 1970, p. 91.

52.   LNAD, RLG/MOH, 211-027: Service national de PMI, "Rapport annuel 1969," p. 7.

53.   WHO, WPR/RC13/2, 1962, p. 14.

54.   See Richard Pottier, *Santé et Société au Laos (1973–1978)* (Paris: Comité pour la Coopération avec le Laos, 2004).

55.   WHO, WPR/RC15/3, 1964, p. 11.

56.   *Journal Officiel du Royaume du Laos* (JORL), 1957–1958.

57.   Khamsone Sassady, "Contribution à l'étude de la médecine laotienne," p. 111.

58.   LNAD, RLG/MOH, 211-024: "Rapport annuel de l'Assistance médicale, Anneé 1973," p. 30.

59.   NARA, RG 59, Box 4598: "Chinese Business Concerns in Vientiane, Laos," 19 February 1959.

60.   Khamsone Sassady, "Contribution à l'étude de la médecine laotienne," p. 121.

61.   USAID, "Termination Report," p. 162.

62.   LNAD, RLG/MOH, 211-024: "Rapport annuel de l'Assistance médicale, Anneé 1973," p. 7.

63.   USAID, "Termination Report," p. 165.

64.   Charles Weldon, *Tragedy in Paradise. A Country Doctor at War in Laos* (Bangkok: Asia Books, 1999). Weldon was Chief of USAID's Public Health Division in Laos from 1963 to 1974.

65.   I refer to Operation Brotherhood by its full name throughout this chapter in an effort to minimize the use of acronyms, while acknowledging that the organization was commonly referred to in Laos as OB.

66. The cover of Miguel A. Bernad, *Filipinos in Laos, with "Postscripts" by J "Pete" Fuentecila* (New York: Mekong Circle International, 2004), describes Operation Brotherhood's work in Laos as an "Asian People Partnership."

67. NARA, RG 286, Box 2: "Draft Government Accountability Office Report. Medical section," November 1971, chapter 4, p. 2.

68. Timothy N. Castle, *At War in the Shadow of Vietnam. US military aid to the Royal Lao Government, 1955–1975* (New York: Columbia University Press, 1993), pp. 59, 99.

69. For Operation Brotherhood's work from 1956 to 1960, see Miguel A. Bernad, *Filipinos in Laos, with "Postscripts" by J "Pete" Fuentecila*. The NGOs work from 1963 to 1975 is discussed in Charles Weldon, *Tragedy in Paradise: A Country Doctor at War in Laos*, pp. 42–50.

70. See USAID, "US Economic Assistance to the Royal Lao Government, 1962–1972," Vientiane, December 1972, p. 10; LNAD, RLG/MOH, 211-004: "Rapport statistique de l'Assistance médicale, Anneé 1973," Table L/1; and 211-024: "Rapport annuel de l'Assistance médicale, Anneé 1973," p. 23.

71. USAID, "Termination Report," pp. 158, 162, 166.

72. USAID, "American Aid to Laos" (Vientiane: USAID, 1964), p. 9.

73. USAID, "Termination Report," pp. 158–9, 166.

74. Ms Bounthanh Oudom, retired Operation Brotherhood and Lao PR nurse, interviewed in Vientiane, 3 February 2012.

75. Several Filipino staff of Operation Brotherhood who worked in Laos for many years spoke Lao very well.

76. See Miguel A. Bernad, *Filipinos in Laos, with "Postscripts" by J "Pete" Fuentecila*, p. 5; and USAID, "Project Appraisal Report for National Health Development Project—Operation Brotherhood," FY74, p. 3.

77. Dr Joe Westermeyer, former USAID doctor, interviewed by email, 13 June 2013.

78. NARA, RG 286, Box 4: "USAID Local Staffing—Refugee Relief," 30 July 1973.

79. The Mekong Circle International pamphlet "Those Were the Days" (produced in 2004) states Operation Brotherhood trained 130 practical nurses between 1963 and 1969, but the year-on-year total from figures in the same pamphlet is 148.

80. USAID, "Termination Report," p. 159.

81. USAID, Project Appraisal Report, Public Health Development—VHP, OBI, 12 July 1973–20 July 1975.

82. NARA, RG 286, Box 2: "Draft Village Health Program report. Medical section," chapter 2, November 1971, p. 6.

83. NARA, RG 286, Box 1: "The Civilian Health and War Casualty Program in Laos. Report to the Sub-committee to Investigate Problems with Refugees and Escapees Committee on the Judiciary," US Senate, 25 November 1970, p. 20; and USAID, "Termination Report," p. 161.

84. NARA, RG 286, Box 2: "Draft Government Accountability Office report, November 1971," chapter 4, p. 4.

85. LNAD, RLG/MOH, 211-017: "Rapport annuel des statistiques sanitaires, 1970," Table 7; 211-018: "Rapport annuel des statistiques sanitaires, 1971," Table 39.
86. USAID, "Termination Report," p. 161.
87. USAID, "Termination Report," p. 164.
88. NARA, RG 286, Box 2: "Draft Government Accountability Office Report. Medical section," chapter 2, p. 3.
89. NARA, RG 286, Box 2: "Draft Government Accountability Office Report. Medical section," chapter 2, p. 8.
90. NARA, RG 286, Box 2: "Draft Government Accountability Office Report. Medical section," chapter 2, p. 12.
91. USAID, "Termination Report," p. 163.
92. Ms Syphanom Viravong, former Operation Brotherhood nurse, interviewed in Sydney, Australia, 25 July 2012.
93. USAID, "Termination Report," pp. 164–5.
94. Chanpheng Thongphimpha, "The revolutionary contribution of Aunt Chanpheng Thongphimpha to the Health Sector from 1953–2000." See also, Anonymous, *60 Years of Growth of the Military Health Service, 1.11.1954–1.11.2014* [60 Pii heng kane teub-nyay khong lao-hob Senahak, 1.11.1954–1.11.2014] (Vientiane: Lao People's Army, 2014), p. 11.
95. The official history of the military health service is supported by an undated NLHX report (presumably from 1970). Both sources state the civilian health service separated from the military service in 1965. See Anonymous, *60 Years of Growth of the Military Health Service*, p. 28 and NLHX/CHC, 01/02/425: "Lay-ngane saloup kane-patibat viak-ngane sathalanasouk nay 3 p. ii (1967–1970)" [Report of the Implementation of Health Work for the Past Three Years (1967–1970)], undated.
96. Xam Neua province was renamed Houaphan province by the Lao PDR authorities.
97. Anonymous, "Draft Report on the Health Situation for the First Conference of Health from 1–12 October 1979," p. 6.
98. Donald P. Whitaker et al., *Laos: A Country Study* (Washington, DC: Foreign Areas Studies, The American University, 1985 [1971]), p. 68.
99. LNAD, NLHX/CHC, 01/02/426: Handwritten note attached to "Sathiti viak-ngane sathalanasouk thi day patibath nay laya 3 pii thi phane mah" [Statistics of Health Work Implemented in the Past 3 Years], 14 March 1971.
100. Nguyen Tien Dinh, "Ten Years of Providing Healthcare for Leaders of the Lao Patriotic Front in the Anti-American Resistance (1966–1975)," in *History of Vietnam-Laos, Laos-Vietnam Special Relationship 1930–2007*, ed. Vietnamese and Lao Compilatory Steering Committees (Hanoi: National Political Publishing House, 2012), pp. 531–8.
101. LNAD, NLHX/CHC, 01/02/423: "Bantheuk kong-paxoum khong khana-satha-sounkang kio kap kane pap-poung sap-xone khana-satha" [Minutes of the Central Health Committee meeting to improve and reorganise the Health Committee], 15 March 1970.

102. Julie Feinsilver, "Fifty Years of Cuba's Medical Diplomacy: From Idealism to Pragmatism," *Cuban Studies* 41 (2010): 85.
103. Anonymous, "Draft Report on the Health Situation for the First Conference of Health from 1–12 October 1979," p. 6.
104. Chanpheng Thongphimpha, "Memoirs of Aunt Chanpheng Thongphimpha's contribution to the revolution in the medical sector, from 1953–2000," p. 11.
105. LNAD, NLHX/CHC, 01/02/425: "Lay-ngane saloup kane-patibat viak-ngane sathalanasouk nay 3 pii (1967–1970)" [Report of the implementation of health work for the past three years (1967–1970)], undated, unpaginated.
106. LNAD, NLHX/CHC, 23-05: "Saloup saphap sathalanasouk 1974" [Summary of the Health Situation, 1974], 25 February 1974, p. 3.
107. RSL, Box 12: "Rapport annuel de 1950," pp. 19–21.
108. Bounheng Banxalith, "Special Relationship between Laos and Vietnam in Military Medicine," in *History of Vietnam-Laos, Laos-Vietnam Special Relationship (1930–2007). Memoirs—Volume II*, ed. Vietnamese and Lao Compilatory Steering Committees (Hanoi: National Political Publishing House, 2012), p. 193.
109. See photos V.2041-/V.2055 in KPL archives.
110. See Khammeung Volachit, *Revolutionary Female Nurses.*
111. Paul F. Langer and Joseph J. Zasloff, *North Vietnam and the Pathet Lao. Partners in the Struggle for Laos* (Cambridge, MA: Harvard University Press, 1970), p. 158.
112. Interview with Bounlap, published in the Lao neutralist newspaper, *Sai Kang* 97 (March 1964): 10–11.
113. Nguyen Phuong Thoan, "The Lao Twins Saved and Brought Up by the Truong Son Military Medical Corps—Then and Now," in *History of Vietnam-Laos, Laos-Vietnam Special Relationship (1930–2007). Memoirs—Volume II*, ed. Vietnamese and Lao Compilatory Steering Committees (Hanoi: National Political Publishing House, 2012), p. 632.
114. Anonymous, *60 Years of Development of the Military Health Service*, pp. 17, 27.
115. LNAD, NLHX/CHC, 01/02/426: "Samlouad tilahkha khong kanexouay-leua lae phouaphanh lavang lao lae Vietnam" [An Evaluation of the Assistance and Liaison between Laos and Vietnam], 18 July 1971.
116. Personal discussions with former NLHX and retired Lao PDR doctor (anonymous), in Vientiane, Lao PDR, November 2012 and August 2013.
117. LNAD, NLHX/CHC, 01/02/423: "Khamsang—theung bandah phanek-kane, hong-kane, hong-ngane, samnak-gnane ome-khang sounkang" [Order—To All Departments, Offices, Factories and Offices Surrounding the Centre], 20 October 1969.
118. Anonymous, "Draft Report on the Health Situation for the First Conference of Health from 1–12 October 1979," p. 6. It is unclear if this is the same hospital that Oliver Tappe refers to as the Lao-Cuban Friendship Hospital. See Oliver Tappe, "National *Lieu de Mémoire* vs. Multivocal Memories: The Case of

Viengxay, Lao PDR," in *Interactions with a Violent Past. Reading Post-Conflict Landscapes in Cambodia, Laos and Vietnam*, ed. Vatthana Pholsena and Oliver Tappe (Singapore: NUS Press, 2013), p. 55.

119. LNAD, NLHX/CHC, 01/02/424: "Assessment of the 1967–1970 plan for health" (Kouad-ka phene-kane pii tae 1967–1970 khong sathalanasouk), undated, unpaginated.

120. Chanpheng Thongphimpha, "The revolutionary contribution of Aunt Chanpheng Thongphimpha to the Health Sector from 1953–2000," p. 2.

121. Vatthana Pholsena, "La production d'hommes et de femmes socialistes nouveaux. Expériences de l'éducation communiste au Laos révolutionnaire," in *Laos. Sociétés et pouvoirs*, ed. Vanina Bouté and Vatthana Pholsena (Bangkok: IRASEC, 2012), pp. 45–67.

122. Bui Van Y, "Public Health Support for Lao Friends During the Resistance Against French Colonialists," in *History of Vietnam-Laos, Laos-Vietnam Special Relationship 1930–2007*, ed. Vietnamese and Lao Compilatory Steering Committees (Hanoi: National Political Publishing House, 2012), pp. 243–8.

123. LNAD, NLHX/CHC, 01/02/426: "Samlouad tilahkha khong kanexouay-leua lae phouaphanh lavang lao lae Vietnam" [An Evaluation of the Assistance and Liaison between Laos and Vietnam], 18 July 1971.

124. LNAD, NLHX/CHC, 01/02/424: "Kouad-ka phene-kane pii tae 1967–1970 khong sathalanasouk" [Assessment of the 1967–1970 Plan for Health], undated, unpaginated.

125. Bui Van Y, "Public Health Support for Lao Friends During the Resistance Against French Colonialists," p. 244.

126. Bui Van Y, "Public Health Support for Lao Friends During the Resistance Against French Colonialists," p. 246.

127. *Sai Kang* 97 (March 1964): 10–11.

128. Chanpheng Thongphimpha, "The revolutionary contribution of Aunt Chanpheng Thongphimpha to the Health Sector from 1953–2000," pp. 8–9.

129. LNAD, NLHX/CHC, 23-05: "Lay-ngane saloup viak-ngane sathalanasouk nay 6 deuane ton pii 1973" [Summary Report of Health Work for the First 6 Months of 1973], 1 July 1973, p. 10.

130. Bounthan Bandavong, "Vietnam-Laos Special Solidarity in Military Medicine," in *History of Vietnam-Laos, Laos-Vietnam Special Relationship (1930–2007). Memoirs Volume II*, ed. Vietnamese and Lao Compilatory Steering Committees (Hanoi: National Political Publishing House, 2012), p. 508.

131. Anonymous, "Draft Report on the Health Situation for the First Conference of Health from 1–12 October 1979," pp. 8–9. Information about the number of cohorts is provided by the KPL photographic archives collection in captions to photographs TK 7158–7160.

132. Bounheng Banxalith, "Special Relationship between Laos and Vietnam in Military Medicine," pp. 193–4.

133. Anonymous, "Draft Report on the Health Situation for the First Conference of Health from 1–12 October 1979," p. 6.

134. Former NLHX nurse, quoted in Fred Branfman, *Voices from the Plain of Jars. Life under an Air War* (New York: Harper Colophon Books, 1972), p. 51.

135. LNAD, NLHX/CHC, 23-05: "Summary of the Health Situation 1974" (Saloup saphap sathalanasouk 1974), p. 2.

136. LNAD, PGNU/MOH, AF-03: "Bantheuk kane-paxoum khanakamakane phicha-lana kane-pin-poua kharaxakane thi bo sia kha thang mot" [Minutes of the Committee Meeting to Consider Free Medical Treatment of Staff], No. 72/KS-TB, 2 July 1975.

137. LNAD, NLHX/CHC, 23-03: "Phenekane khong sathalanasouk sapho nay khet yeud amnat kanebok-khong nay khet beuang nanh" [Plan for Health Work Only in the Seized (RLG) Zone Administered by That Side], No. 551, 13 July 1975.

138. LNAD, NLHX/CHC, 23-03: "Plan for health work only in the Seized [RLG] Zone administered by that side," No. 551, 13 July 1975.

139. USAID, "Project Appraisal Report, VHP, 12 July 1973 to 20 July 1975," p. 3.

140. USAID, "Termination Report," p. 10.

141. Dr Khamphaï Abhay, former RLG Minister of Health, interviewed by email, 10 October 2012.

142. Dr Tiao Jaisvasd's curriculum vitae, kindly provided at interview in Torcy, France, 2 December 2012.

143. Dr Tiao Jaisvasd, interviewed in Torcy, France, 2 December 2012.

144. USAID, Laos: "Maternal and Child Health/Family Planning Prop" (FY 75–79) (USAID, 1974), p. 17.

CHAPTER 4

More Eastern than Traditional: The Making of *Đông y* in the Republic of Vietnam during the Cold War

Nara Oda[1]

Introduction

This chapter considers the complex modern history of traditional Vietnamese medicine vis-à-vis Chinese medicine during the Cold War with a focus on South Vietnam (Việt Nam Cộng hòa, Republic of Vietnam, 1954–75). It examines how the governments of South Vietnam institutionalized *Đông y* (Eastern medicine), or traditional medicine, in their medical system. Specifically, this chapter argues that South Vietnam promoted traditional medicine and legally integrated it into the public healthcare system, parallel to North Vietnam. This process revealed that, unlike North Vietnam, the South found it difficult to define the daily practice of traditional medicine as a "Vietnamese tradition" due to a greater influence of the Chinese population than in the North.

In 1954, Vietnam was divided into North and South territories by the Geneva Accords. During this territorial division, the concepts of Eastern medicine (*Y học Đông phương* or *Đông y*) and family medicine (*Y học gia truyền*) coexisted in both North and South Vietnam. There was no unified usage of these three terms. However, the South Vietnamese government used the term *Đông y* to promote it along with Western medicine in the institutionalized medical system.

Practices of *Đông y* comprise two forms of medicinal herbs or treatments—*Thuốc Nam*, which means "medicine (thuốc) of the South (Nam)" and *Thuốc*

119

Bắc, meaning "medicine of the North." The distinction between "South" and "North," in this context, is a geographic distinction, relative to China, hence, *Thuốc Nam* means Vietnamese herbal medicine.

The term, *Thuốc Nam*, is believed to have originated around the 14th century during *Đại Việt's* rivalry with the politically and culturally dominant China. During the independence movement of the late 1940s and 1950s, it received considerable attention, especially in North Vietnam, as the national and original Vietnamese medicine.

The momentum toward adopting traditional Vietnamese medical practices became increasingly urgent during Vietnam's independence movements, particularly in North Vietnam.[2] Therefore, the distinction between *Thuốc Nam* and *Thuốc Bắc* is both geographic and pharmacological and a reflection of Vietnam's growing independence from Chinese influence in contemporary history. Researchers have shown that North Vietnam treated Eastern medicine, *Đông y*, and *Thuốc Nam* as distinguished medicine to rival Western medicine.[3]

Despite some studies examining the history of Vietnamese traditional medicine, the situation in South Vietnam has not been sufficiently considered.[4] This is partly because Vietnamese historiography has long been described through the perspective of North Vietnam, which became the foundation for the establishment of contemporary Vietnam. For instance, Lê Trần Đức's work on the history of traditional medicine in Vietnam is written to be compatible with the national historiography, which follows the North Vietnamese/Communist Party's authorized political view.[5] In addition, prior research describes that *Đông y*, Eastern medicine, was to be restricted or even suppressed in the South as the state was supported by the West. Did South Vietnam genuinely restrict the role of *Đông y* and its practitioners? If yes, why and how did the government execute this plan?

This chapter traces the endeavors of South Vietnamese governments to institutionalize *Đông y*, that is to simultaneously valorize it and bring it under governmental control. This process consisted of the standardization of practice and education of *Đông y* in South Vietnam's medical system, and thus reveals the characteristics of *Đông y* in the South. While the term *Đông y* was understood in the North as a medical practice, using a combination of *Thuốc Nam* and *Thuốc Bắc*, *Đông y* in South Vietnam witnessed a greater Chinese influence and less influence of *Thuốc Nam*.

I first summarize the current scholarship on the contemporary history of *Đông y* in North Vietnam. The second part chronologically describes the situation in South Vietnam, based on my archival research of official documents (for example, from the Ministry of Health (MOH) and the Prime Minister's

Office), articles in newspapers and magazines from this period, and oral interviews. Specifically, legal analysis of the medical policy shows its transition from the colonial regime, or the decolonization process of medical policy making, and the Chinese impact on *Đông y* in South Vietnam. The final section examines to what extent such political and social changes affected official medical education that had begun during the French colonial period.

Traditional Medicine in North Vietnam

In 1955, Hồ Chí Minh of North Vietnam (*Việt Nam Dân chủ Cộng hòa*, the Democratic Republic of Vietnam) urged medical practitioners to thoroughly study traditional medicine:

> [We] must build our own medicine . . . our ancestors had rich experience [concerning] treatment [that uses] local medicines and those of the North [China]. To inaugurate medicine, one should focus on researching medicine of the East and the West as well as [the] integration of the two.[6]

After this letter was publicized, the MOH began to standardize traditional medical practices and permit traditional local doctors to practice for the first time.[7]

Even before Hồ Chí Minh's letter, however, North Vietnam had begun promoting traditional medicine. In 1946 the Ministry of Interior in North Vietnam gave permission to establish a research committee for *Thuốc Nam* medicine. However, by 1954, this committee could not achieve any specific results.

The Research Committee for *Đông y*, established under the MOH in 1949, was the first to officially research both *Thuốc Nam* and *Thuốc Bắc*. The committee published a list of Southern and Northern medicines in their investigation of effective medicinal plants; however, this work and the committee itself did not have any further accomplishments. Instead, the MOH announced their policy to "scientize *Đông y*"; that is, they attempted to eliminate the superstitious elements of local traditional medicine from the practice and knowledge of *Đông y*.[8] In addition, the MOH aimed to promote Southern plant-based medicine, *Thuốc Nam*, at health stations in rural areas. Finally, they set the goal of integrating Eastern and Western medicine (*Tây y*) in North Vietnam.

In 1957, the MOH promoted its initiative to institutionalize *Đông y* by establishing a *Đông y* research institute and practitioner's association. Interestingly, the majority of the research center staff were doctors and pharmacists of Western medicine who had been educated at the Hanoi Medical School during the French Indochina period. This situation did not change significantly even after a few years. While the research center collected materials and information from local *Đông y* practitioners, the MOH dispatched a research group from the institution to China. Among the four members of the group, three were practitioners of Western medicine.

Under the leadership of Western medicine practitioners, in the newly established institution, the MOH decided to form an association for the local *Đông y* practitioners and let each individual register as a member. Unsurprisingly, this garnered criticism from the local practitioners. One complaint, for example, showed mistrust as the association was led by Western medical staff in the MOH. Another pointed out the differences in the ability or performance of the *Đông y* practitioners, demanding that more capable practitioners must be differentiated. Their opinion was that while *Đông y* discipline was traditionally researched by Confucian practitioners and was originally written in Chinese characters, new *Đông y* practitioners only knew *quốc ngữ*, the romanized Vietnamese script, and could not reference the original manuscripts.[9] Some practitioners insisted on studying the written traditional texts as scientizing *Đông y* might eliminate its core ideas.[10] These varied opinions indicate the challenges faced by the practitioners attempting to scientize *Đông y*. Despite dissent, the Association of *Đông y* practitioners eventually spread all over North Vietnam. Meanwhile, the MOH performed its initiative to institutionalize *Đông y* by reorganizing practitioners into one institution.

Traditional Medicine in South Vietnam

Given the influence of the overseas Chinese on the southern part of Vietnam and the fact that laws in the Republic of Vietnam authorized only the Vietnamese *Đông y* with the title of practitioner, it is worth considering the historical background of the South Vietnam–China relationship and the conditions of Chinese residents in South Vietnam.

Geographically, the southern part of Vietnam is distant from China; however, the size of the Chinese-origin population there was much higher than in the northern part of Vietnam. At the same time, compared to the northern part, the southern part had only recently become Vietnamese territory. Understanding the history of South Vietnam's integration into Vietnam, focusing on the settlement of Chinese immigrants in the region, is important.

The *Việt* (*Kinh*) political forces began a southward advance (*Nam tiến*) around the 15th century. This expansion, which consisted of over 3,000 asylum seekers from China's Ming Dynasty (*Minh Hương*), continued until after the latter half of the 17th century when several political powers dominated *Đại Việt*, including the Nguyễn lords.[11]

From the late 17th century to the 18th century, the Chinese developed communities in southern *Đại Việt*, with permission from the Nguyễn lords of *Đàng Trong*, which was ruled by the *Việt* (*Kinh*). As they spread their roots, they mixed with the local Khmer and Vietnamese people. Today, these immigrants enjoy Vietnamese nationality, speak Vietnamese, and are legally registered as "Vietnamese." However, their descendants who maintain this identity continue to be called *Minh Hương*.

The area stretching from the present territory of Cambodia to the southern tip of Vietnam was inhabited by people who spoke Khmer; however, it was exploited by people of Chinese descent, especially in Bien Hoa, along with areas in the Mekong Delta, such as Ha Tien.[12]

Modern immigration from China to Vietnam began toward the end of the 19th century, particularly from southern China (for example, Guangdong and Fujian) to Cochinchina. The population of overseas Chinese in Cochinchina increased by approximately 13,000 between 1879 and 1889, which resulted in 57,000 Chinese residing in Cochinchina. Following this, the outbreak of the Sino-Japanese War increased immigration. In 1906, the Governor General's order concerning immigration control was issued, which made it difficult for new overseas Chinese to migrate and, temporarily, slowed the Chinese population growth rate. Yet, as of 1943, 396,000 overseas Chinese lived in Cochinchina.[13]

The distribution map[14] of overseas Chinese in 1931 shows that more than 10 percent of the total population of overseas Chinese were living in Cochinchina, in the southern part of Indochina, particularly in Saigon, and the area stretching from Phnom Penh to the coast of Cochinchina. In contrast, in Tonkin, northern Indochina, only 5–10 percent of the Chinese population was concentrated in the Hai Phong area near the ports. Therefore, it is assumed that a majority of the overseas Chinese population lived in Cochinchina because they were either merchants or engaged in the rice trade. Cochinchina was considered a highly advantageous location because it was suitable for rice production and convenient for river transportation. Another reason for the increased immigration rate was its low population density compared to the north in the Red River Delta.[15]

According to the 1928 statistics, before the Indochina War, half of the Saigon population consisted of overseas Chinese, which totaled approximately 319,000 people.[16] Many ethnic Chinese had settled in the Cholon district, a large southern commercial district. Since the French colonial period, the rice trade has been monopolized by the overseas Chinese.[17] The first and second Indochina Wars influenced economic transactions, which affected the Chinese merchants in Cochinchina.[18] However, during the conflict they still had the distribution power and influence in the rice polishing industry. After the mid-1950s, it is estimated that the Chinese in South Vietnam accounted for nearly 90 percent of non-European capital.[19] In the early 1970s, the overseas Chinese population in South Vietnam was approximately 1.5 million.[20] This large population had a significant impact on South Vietnam's culture.

Due to a completely different historical formation process, in comparison with the North, the South developed a complex social structure. From the perspective of Vietnam as a whole, it was a newly developed area, where various ethnic groups were distributed and/or mixed. Specifically, the Chinese held considerable status and importance in South Vietnam's society.

Decolonizing the Regulation of *Đông y*

In 1955, in South Vietnam, Prime Minister Ngô Đình Diệm became the first Vietnamese president with the support of the United States. After Ngô Đình Diệm refused to hold a general election, which had been scheduled to be held within two years of the Geneva Agreement, Vietnam became two opposing states on opposite sides of the Cold War.

Diệm was a Catholic from Hue who had once served in the Nguyễn Dynasty. The process of establishing his regime and autocratic style, with the involvement of his family, resulted in him being regarded as a puppet of the United States. His regime was appraised as a powerful attempt to reflect Vietnam's traditional Confucian values in politics.[21] However, recent studies suggest that Diệm sought to build a modern Vietnam during the Cold War period, which would not be affected by either Western or communist influences,[22] and establish a new cultural infrastructure.[23]

In 1958, a report published in North Vietnam, submitted to the MOH, described how Ngô Đình Diệm's regime in South Vietnam had not been utilizing traditional medicine as it did not have the appropriate authorization. The report concluded that the Diệm government did not intend to develop healthcare in its territory as it wanted to receive medical assistance from the United States.[24] Hence, North Vietnam strongly criticized Diệm's government for not promoting traditional medicine.

It must be noted that the North Vietnam MOH may have published the report to display its efforts in comparison with South Vietnam; however, similar narratives continued to appear post-Cold War. Previous research concluded that, while Hồ Chí Minh urged the "harmonization" of Eastern and Western medicinal remedies in North Vietnam, the government in the South extolled Western medicine and attempted to restrict the role and status of traditional practitioners.[25]

This section of the chapter examines the South Vietnamese government's legislative attempts to institutionalize *Đông y*. It compares the two rival states and demonstrates the decolonization process during nation-building amidst the Cold War. While North Vietnam took measures to institutionalize traditional/local practices independently, South Vietnam inherited colonial legal measures, since the regulations placed on traditional medicine by the French colonial government were still in effect at the beginning of the Diệm regime. The South Vietnamese government considered amending the former regulations when discussing the practices of *Đông y*.

The French colonial government legally recognized traditional medicine as "Sino-Indochinese" medicine by the "regulation of the Sino-Indochinese pharmacopeia" in 1942 after discriminatory legislative projects.[26] In 1943, another decree, called the *Arrete du 17 juillet 1943*, was enacted under Governor General Decoux.[27] The decree further regulated the import and practice of Sino-Vietnamese medicine in French Indochina. On 23 August of the same year, the government proclaimed a list of acceptable medicinal products to prohibit the sale of "toxic medicines." These medicinal ingredients included 13 minerals (nine types, if classified by their Latin names), 36 plants (37 types, if classified by their Latin names) and two animals (three types, if classified by their Latin names) used by traditional practitioners, such as cannabis, belladonna or mylabris.[28]

Although Decoux's decree was not necessarily known to all medical practitioners, as it was written in French, these continued restrictions provoked antipathy in *Đông y* practitioners.[29] As discussed later, in 1958, one of the associations for medical practitioners demanded the abolition of the Decoux decree. Decoux's resolution was an obstacle for *Đông y* practitioners hoping to revive traditional medicine.

Imposed Hardships in Practicing *Đông y*

As of 1957, in South Vietnam there were four medical associations for *Đông y* practitioners.[30] These were the *Đông y dược* Union (Eastern medicine and pharmacopeia union), the *Việt y sĩ* Medical Association (the Vietnam Medical Association), the *Việt Nam Y Dược* association (the Vietnamese medical and medicinal association), and the Northern Migrants' Medical Association.[31]

Among these, the *Đông y dược* Union in Cholon, known for being the largest mercantile center with a Chinese population in Saigon, published a journal called "*Đông y dược*." They expressed concern that "Western medicine has an advantage over Eastern medicine" and asked their readers, "will *Đông y* regain its value in Vietnam? Can *Đông y* restore its vital duty to protect the health of the Vietnamese?"[32]

Before issuing these statements, the *Đông y dược* Union had suggested the promotion of traditional medicine through government cooperation. "*Đông y dược*" had previously claimed that Vietnamese traditional medicine was considered a "unique science for the Vietnamese"[33] and had expressed their opposition to Decoux's decree. "The decree on July 17, 1943, by the Decoux colonial government will be abolished and replaced by the new condition for Eastern medicine in the Republic of Vietnam . . . this can be done when people engaging in Eastern medicine unite together with the government."[34]

By 1958, the practitioners in the union claimed that "everybody had been united to repeal Decoux's decree. Everyone in the organization of Eastern medicine wants to reconstruct the knowledge of *Đông y*."[35]

Along with legislative issues, there was another practical concern for the union—the stagnation of the distribution of medicine due to the country's division into Northern and Southern territories. In an article published in April 1957, they argued that it had become increasingly difficult to obtain medicine from the Northern part of Vietnam and China.[36]

> In recent years, the northern part (North Vietnam and China) has been an opponent to our nation. Commerce with Communist countries has ceased, and it is becoming very difficult to obtain materials . . . (Therefore, we must seek the cooperation of the government and create a good environment for Eastern medicine "*Y học Đông dương*").[37]

Despite the *Đông y* practitioners' complaints about the shortage of medicinal materials and the regulations of the colonial government, the new South Vietnamese government did not take any measures to deal with the issues. On 10 January 1958, the government set regulations to limit the number of *Đông y* pharmacists in each province[38] and, from 1958 to 1960, the government drew up a list of prescriptions.[39] It can be assumed that the aim was to differentiate trustable *Đông y* practitioners from other local practitioners by making a list of reliable prescriptions.

According to the official records, some people misused Western medicinal tools for diagnosis and treatment, disguised under the title of *Đông y sĩ* (*Đông y* practitioners), and advertised false information about the medicines. To solve this issue, the authorities established a committee to inspect medicine and medical product advertisements in 1962.[40] Based on their inspection, some clinics were forced to temporarily close, while some were prohibited from using the names of *Đông y sĩ* and *Đông dược sĩ* (*Đông y* pharmacists).

Following the coup d'état on 1 November 1963, and the collapse of the Ngô Đình Diệm government, these practitioners reopened their businesses and called themselves *Đông y sĩ* and *Đông dược sĩ*.[41]

Incorporating *Đông y* in Institutionalized Medicine

The new government of South Vietnam launched a full-fledged effort to introduce traditional medicine into the healthcare system by amending Decoux's decree. On 23 January 1964, the MOH proposed that the government revise Decoux's decree. The minister of health submitted the second revised version on 7 February. It stated that "the most important thing is to increase the value of the *Đông y*" and the aim was to "rationalize" the regulations for traditional medicine to suit the current situation.[42]

The draft consisted of the following chapters:

- Chapter 1 defined traditional medicines.
- Chapter 2 defined the conditions, such as business licenses and sales by practitioners.
- Chapter 3 listed the necessary conditions for operating as practitioners.
- Chapter 4 set out the conditions for importing drugs.
- Chapter 5 established the Vietnamese versions of the names of drugs containing toxic elements and specified the conditions under which they could be used.
- Chapter 6 described the transitional measures that enabled the treatment of those who did not meet the conditions for *Đông y* practitioners.[43]

According to the instructions sent by the MOH to the Prime Minister's Office, practitioners were required to obtain government permission to practice medicine; however, the number of people permitted to practice per province was no longer limited. Additionally, those who had received a medical education within their family tradition (*gia truyền*) could become qualified practitioners.[44]

These instructions permitted the use of Western medical tools and techniques for the advancement of *Đông y*. Simultaneously, the draft stated that severe penalties would be imposed for the abuse of Western medicinal techniques or deception involving medical materials containing poison.[45]

The documents attached to the draft indicate two major reasons for the revision of Decoux's decree. First, the MOH pointed out language issues. Most *Đông y* practitioners did not know the regulations or only vaguely understood the laws and regulations related to their profession since they were Confucian scholars who had not received a French-language education.[46] In addition, the majority of the public, including local herbal practitioners, did not recognize the precise content of the decree and the punishment for a violator was insufficient. The latter limitation urged the MOH to amend the Decoux decree in Vietnamese with their definition of *Đông y*.

Second, the MOH noted that the Decoux decree prohibited "chemical, synthetic substances, or tablets," thus practitioners were only able to legally use raw medicinal materials and could not prescribe Western medicines, such as aspirin. To be precise, any medical products in the form of tablets and capsules were prohibited for *Đông y* practitioners under the Decoux decree.[47]

Due to the limitations of the historical records, it is difficult to evaluate the inconvenience faced by the practitioners due to the prohibition on prescribing Western medicines. However, it is evident that they may have found themselves at a disadvantage in improving medical knowledge or technology, such as manufacturing tablets. Moreover, they could have been dissatisfied with the limited range of medicines that they could prescribe in spite of being recognized as medical practitioners. A second draft to organize *Đông y*, as mentioned above, was issued against this backdrop.

The draft led to the passing of a new statute in the National Assembly on 29 April. The new statute, named statute number 9 of 1964 (hereinafter, 9/64 Statute), aimed to increase the value of *Đông y* by expanding the range of treatments available to medical practitioners, whilst offering better means of differentiating the skilled doctors from the unskilled ones.

This statute defined the qualifications for practicing *Đông y*. In addition, it defined the provisions for practicing traditional medicine and allowed practitioners to use medicine with toxic elements for two days per patient. As a result, all medicinal materials prohibited by Decoux's decree remained on the list after the 1964 revision. However, it became possible for *Đông y* practitioners to administer such medicines to a patient only for two days with the patient's acknowledgment that they accepted the treatment voluntarily.[48]

Differentiating State *Đông y* from the West

The 9/64 Statute defined *Đông y* as traditional medicine[49] that "includes any products in their natural state or processed by traditional methods made of minerals, plants, or animals," whereas "purified water, serum drugs, vaccines, drugs processed by filling glass bottles or tubes for injection" were banned from being used.[50] In addition, they were prohibited from performing dental or midwifery surgery and using instruments used in Western medicine, for both diagnosis and treatment. Specifically, "stethoscopes, anesthetics, electricity (X-ray, infrared, ultraviolet and electrothermal treatments), vaccine therapy, chemobiological or microbiological component analysis, and serotherapy" were banned.[51]

While this distanced *Đông y* practitioners from Western medical tools, the definition of *Đông y* in the statute did not exclude all new instruments. The practitioners could use products, such as camphor, peppermint oil, white tree oil or fennel oil, manufactured by machines if they were processed in "traditional ways."[52] Additionally, the statute allowed the use of a machine to crush and refine the medicine or round it into a pill. Traditional methods, such as acupuncture and moxibustion, were officially recognized as *Đông y*.[53]

Although the law allowed *Đông y* practitioners to introduce machines and devices to support the production of traditional medicine, they were still unable to prescribe or use Western medicine and instruments. These changes were an attempt to maintain the differentiation between *Đông y* practitioners and Western doctors.

As science-based biomedicine and related technologies spread in South Vietnam, especially in those cities largely under the influence of, and receiving medical aid from, the West during the Cold War, the MOH faced the problem of maintaining and redefining *Đông y* along with new pharmaceutical knowledge. Hence, the 9/64 Statue must be understood not only as an amendment or denial of Decoux's decree, but also as a process of decolonization by identifying indigenous medicine against Western medicine under the Vietnamese regime.

Another significant change brought about by the statute was the categorization of *Đông y* practitioners. The statute defined two types of *Đông y* practitioners. *Đông y sĩ* was defined as a practitioner "who learned the medical theory of *Đông y* through Chinese or translated books and obtained the authorization from the Ministry of Health," or "a person who graduated from a public or foreign *Đông y* medical school and had a license equivalent to that of the Ministry of Health."[54] *Gia truyền* practitioners, literally meaning "family-transmitted" practitioners, could only provide particular medical prescriptions that had been passed on by their family and who were registered with the MOH. While *gia truyền* practitioners did not necessarily have the knowledge of medical theory, their prescriptions were limited to a small number of ancestral remedies.[55]

Those who engaged in buying and selling *Đông y* medicine were defined in three categories. *Đông dược sĩ* could prepare raw materials for a pack of medicines for the patients. *Thực dược viên* were the vendors within the country.[56] Hence, theoretically, *Đông dược sĩ* bought materials from *Thực dược viên* and sold them to the patients. *Sinh dược viên* were those who could engage in trading *Đông y* medicines. When importing such prescriptions, *Sinh dược viên* would be registered drug importers with the Ministry of Economy and the MOH. Hence, *Sinh dược viên* could import *Thuốc Bắc* from overseas and sell raw materials in South Vietnam. Setting each category as an authorized profession, especially the professionalization of trade, reflected the development of the commercial medicinal market in the South.

A crucial factor that must be considered is that a person's nationality determined whether or not they could obtain these positions in *Đông y*. Except for *gia truyền* practitioners, all the types of *Đông y* practitioners mentioned above (*Đông y sĩ*, *Sinh dược viên*, *Thực dược viên* and *Đông dược sĩ*) were required to have Vietnamese nationality and be above 25 years of age. They were required to graduate from a public or overseas *Đông y* medical school, which provided a license equivalent to that of the MOH.[57]

In South Vietnam, individuals who wished to study *Đông y* overseas would have to study either in Hong Kong or Taiwan, as these two places were allies of South Vietnam during the Cold War. However, there may have been senior practitioners who studied in mainland China before 1949 and the establishment of the People's Republic of China.

However, the education rules were not strictly applied. For example, *Đông y* practitioner L, who was of Chinese ethnicity and resided in Hồ Chí Minh City, told the author that his father never received a medical school degree, but rather studied traditional medicine intermittently in his youth in mainland China. L's father was born in 1928 in Fujian and moved to Beijing and Nanjing after joining Chiang Kai Shek's army. Eventually, he moved to Saigon from mainland China in 1952. He taught mathematics, physics and chemistry at a British school before starting his career as a *Đông y sĩ* in Saigon. It is not clear when he obtained Vietnamese nationality; however, he was practicing *Đông y* as an authorized *Đông y sĩ* in 1960.[58]

Regarding medicinal sales, those who sold *Đông y* medicine at local markets without obtaining a certain title were required to be over 21 years, able to read Vietnamese or Chinese characters and understand each ingredient in the medicine.[59] Unlike *Đông y* practitioners, local merchants selling *Đông y* medicine were not necessarily required to have Vietnamese nationality. Hence, the merchants involved in *Đông y* medicine in local markets and family (*gia truyền*) practitioners could be non-Vietnamese nationals, allowing people of Chinese origin, who could read Chinese characters, to practice.

For example, Mr C was born in 1945. He lived in Bien Hoa, Dong Nai, where his father ran a Chinese herbal medicine (*Thuốc Bắc*) store before 1975. His whole family, including his father, obtained Vietnamese citizenship in

1956/1957. Mr C did not remember the specific kind of *Đông y* medicine his father practiced; however, he remembered his father taking a pulse before prescribing medicines. Nevertheless, his father was not a practitioner but a medicine seller.[60] The case of Mr C indicates that merchants involved in medicinal product sales or family-run medical practices could be non-Vietnamese.

Moreover, the new statue did not exclude Chinese medicinal products. It did not have a particular regulation for the use of *Thuốc Bắc* nor for the endorsement of *Thuốc Nam*. Instead, it provided a supplementary list of *Đông y* prescriptions permitted to be imported from overseas. This list included 22 kinds of prescriptions, namely, oil medicines, preparations and pills and powders with particular names, such as *Bao anh đơn*, *Hải cầu hoàn* or *Ngưu hoàng hoàn*.[61] As these medical products are still imported from overseas, it can be suggested that South Vietnamese got these medicines from Hong Kong or Taiwan.

The government approved and defined authentic *Đông y* practitioners by categorizing practitioners and setting a restriction on nationality. This meant that ethnic Chinese practitioners could no longer practice advanced medical care without Vietnamese nationality. South Vietnam's Vietnamization and the assimilation of the Chinese went in tandem, as explained later. The ethnic Chinese population was likely targeted by these standards of professionalization. The government attempted to institutionalize *Đông y* primarily by professionalizing practitioners and differentiating Vietnamese practitioners from other nationalities.

Đông y and the Chinese in South Vietnam

The regulation of nationality regarding *Đông y* practitioners in the 9/64 Statute can be understood in the light of China–South Vietnam tensions, namely, the government's suspicion towards the Chinese-origin population. Since the Chinese population was dominant in *Đông y*, both culturally and economically, the South Vietnamese government was keen to eliminate Chinese influences when establishing *Đông y* in the official medical system.

Although there are few reliable statistics about the Chinese population from the beginning of South Vietnam, the available information shows that *Đông y* in the South could not be practiced without Chinese-origin people. During the French colonial rule, one of the major goods imported from China was medicine.[62] In the Republic of Vietnam, the Chinese population remained engaged in retail trade businesses, selling goods and medicine. The Chinese had enormous economic power in the *Đông y* industry in South Vietnam.[63]

Yet in 1955, Diệm, a nationalist, on becoming the first president of South Vietnam, implemented harsh policies and restrictions, which negatively impacted the Chinese residents in Vietnam. Residents were forced to adopt Vietnamese nationality. Those who refused had to face various restrictions on their freedom of occupation. In Resolution No. 48 of 21 August 1956, it was decided to grant Vietnamese nationality to the overseas Chinese born in Vietnam so that the government could impose tax and military service.[64] In other words, it forced the overseas Chinese to become ethnic Chinese with Vietnamese nationality.

In contrast, the overseas Chinese without Vietnamese nationality had to renew their residence permits as "foreigners."[65] This could be problematic for Chinese residents, since, in 1957, the government issued Decision No. 53, which stipulated that only Vietnamese nationals could engage in 11 occupations which were dominated by Chinese residents,[66] causing confusion among the overseas Chinese.

Furthermore, in February 1963, the government implemented a strict investment law for the overseas Chinese. The law forbade the diversion of profits earned by the overseas Chinese and ethnic Chinese in commerce outside South Vietnam. In addition, the stores or offices were to be owned by the state after 15 years of operation.[67] Even after the collapse of Diệm's administration, these harsh regulations continued.

Even in 1974, the Chinese held a large proportion of the South Vietnamese capital. It is believed that the Chinese capital investment accounted for 16 percent of the total investment that funded a total of 11,747 business establishments and stores. Among these, 500 business establishments of Chinese origin involved Chinese herbal medicines with an investment of $730,000 in *Đông y*. These establishments of Chinese origin accounted for about 80 percent of the total investment in Eastern medicine.[68]

While these statistics do not include the profits from individual or small-scale commercial activities, Chinese herbal medicines accounted for most of the commercial profits of Chinese residents. For example, in Hue, before 1975, traditional Chinese physicians would obtain herbal drugs from Hong Kong through an agent in Cholon, Saigon.[69] In Bien Hoa in Dong Nai prefecture, medicine was imported from Hong Kong via Saigon. At the time, when Mr C's father was running a herbal medicinal (*Thuốc Bắc*) store, there were more than ten *Thuốc Bắc* stores in the same market.[70] *Đông y* practitioners near Cholon would buy medicinal herbs from these markets.[71] These examples indicate that Chinese residents were at the center of the drug trade network.

As explained, the South Vietnamese government suppressed Chinese residents, urging them to be more Vietnamese in South Vietnam and hoping to exclude the influence of overseas Chinese people. At this time China was being controlled by the communists and was called the People's Republic of China. Moreover, Diệm and his brother, Ngô Đình Nhu, had their eyes on the Emergency in Malaya, where communists, who drew heavily from the Chinese community, were challenging the British colonial rule and the Federation of Malaya.[72] The Diệm administration's mindset continued to be evident in the next government, which ruled that all medical practitioners had to have Vietnamese nationality.

The greater numbers of overseas Chinese in South Vietnam, compared to the North, and the southern government's strict policies towards its Chinese residents is reflected in the institutionalization process of *Đông y* in South Vietnam.

Second Amendment: Qualifying in the "Western" Way

The 9/64 Statute focused on categorizing professions regarding *Đông y* according to age and nationality; however, it lacked precise protocols. Soon after Nguyễn Văn Thiệu became the president in 1967, controversy on *Đông y* professions arose in the National Assembly. This time, as South Vietnam became politically stable after the coup, discussions continued for a few years. This led to the second amendment of Decoux's decree with more attention paid to physicians of Western medicine.

In 1967, a South Vietnamese Senate, Trần Thế Minh, announced in the Diet that *Đông y* practitioners in Saigon should be regulated in a similar way as the Western physicians. At that time, the Diet was divided into two groups concerning issues regarding the qualifications of *Đông y* practitioners.[73] Minh argued that it was necessary to set an independent clause regarding the qualifications of *Đông y* doctors. He stated, "they [*Đông y* practitioners] have helped us from rural to urban areas for several thousand years. Therefore, to develop *Đông y*, which has been ostracized by French Medicine [or French doctors] during the French colonial period, the independence [from French-influenced medicine] is necessary."[74]

Congressman Nguyễn Văn Chuẩn argued: "We need an [medical] examination, which balances French medicine and *Đông y* . . . there is no need for a provision concerning the qualifications of independent *Đông y* practitioners."[75] However, Minh opposed this idea, stating: "I think that medical care in the past has never supported *Đông y* and it seems now somebody is willing to put more negative pressure on *Đông y* than in the colonial period."[76] As a result of the Diet's vote, a clause was added that stipulated the need for an independent qualification, an established method for the protection of *Đông y* practitioners, which was similar to that required by Western medical doctors.

On 6 January 1970, the Diet's Committee of Health and Hygiene (*Ủy ban Y tế*) and the House of Representatives proposed the "Draft of Regulation on Eastern Medical Occupations." It was submitted in 1969 and consisted of two drafts.[77] Based on a draft drawn up by 12 senators in March 1969 and a draft composed by six members of the House of Representatives, the Diet's Committee of Health and Hygiene prepared a new draft. Opinions from four organizations engaged in *Tây y* (Western medicine), two organizations related to *Đông y* and the deans of medical/pharmaceutical universities were taken into consideration in the drafting process.[78]

The requirements specified in the submitted draft were as follows. First, one must "restore the skills of the lost *Đông y.*" Second, one must "form a reliable medical organization [. . .] [for the] scientization of *Đông y* (like Western medicine)." It must be noted that the scientization of *Đông y* should be understood as making *Đông y* a non-religious and non-superstitious medical practice. The discussion assumed *Đông y* as a medicine that did not include rituals or religious revelation, as noted by the MOH in 1964 as a problem of the Decoux decree, which did not forbid treatment by oracle.[79]

The draft urged the formation of a research institute, specializing in *Đông y*, and a professional association, claiming that "cooperation between Eastern medicine and Western medicine" is needed.[80] Furthermore, it proposed to permit the use of tools used by Western physicians "for an accurate diagnosis."[81]

Practitioners of Western medicine saw the draft as a threat as it allowed *Đông y* to practice with *Tây y* skills. As the House of Representatives began debating the bill, lawmakers' opinions were divided. On 23 May, the House voted for the first time on the bill. However, only 46 of the 76 members of the House were present and the bill did not acquire the minimum number of affirmative votes.

The House was divided concerning the preparation of medicines.[82] Some thought that *Đông y* medicine should be prepared in a traditional way and should remain in its natural state. Supporters advocated that it was dangerous to change the preparations by adding newly discovered treatments. By contrast, some saw this as an opportunity to reform *Đông y* and insisted that the new treatments of Western medicine should be adopted.[83] Others pointed out that some of the *Tây y* doctors in cities used *Đông y* treatments and medicine, hence it would be fair to allow *Đông y* practitioners to use *Tây y* medicine and enhance the authority of *Đông y* practitioners.[84] This group of people emphasized that "*Đông y* and *Tây y* (Western medicine) are one medicine and the patient's perspective should be considered first."

The arguments were not clear. They expressed their opinions rather than negotiating to conclude a certain agreement. All of the three opinions on *Đông y* were intended to position it in comparison with the *Tây y*. In the end, some argued that the *Đông y sĩ* and *Đông dược sĩ* professions should be defined in more detail, while others argued that *Đông y* medicinal products should be defined first. The argument diffused and these points were not reflected in the new bill.

Ultimately, after the vote on 1 June 1970, in the Senate,[85] the bill was sent to the House of Representatives on 19 July 1972, and was finally passed on 22 July.[86] Unlike previous legislation, this bill required the government to administer qualification tests for *Đông y* practitioners and establish specialized research institutions.[87] The bill stated:

> within two years of the enforcement of this Law, the Ministry of Health aims to establish a qualification test for doctors, pharmacists, and traders of *Đông y* in Association of each professional. At the latest, one year after the enforcement, the Ministry of Health and the Ministry of Education will establish the Research center of *Đông y* and Educational Institution in cooperation.[88]

It became clear that the MOH intended to manage *Đông y* practitioners and standardize education, medical treatment and *Đông y* treatment. These measures were similar to Western medical practices.

Another Discussion on *Đông y*, *Tây y* and Science

Along with the discussion in the Diet, some opinions on *Đông y* reform appeared in a newspaper, arguing for the modernization of *Đông y*. As a term, "scientization" first appeared in the 1969 draft. A doctor named Trần Văn Thích raised the question whether it was possible for *Đông y* to become scientific and gain people's trust, adding that unless practitioners modernized their medicine, *Đông y* would be absorbed by Western medicine.[89]

This question received negative feedback. Thích wrote an article, "Concrete suggestions to modernize *Đông y*"; however, unlike the title, he only introduced a revival movement of traditional medicine in the People's Republic of China and Japan and advocated the establishment of a research center and educational institution for *Đông y*.

Another physician, Nguyễn Hữu Phiểm, maintained that it was impossible to modernize *Đông y* and to educate the practitioners in a modern form, as he understood that such a process was an attempt to reform *Đông y* theory by introducing Western science into it. In his article, he criticized the whole idea of the modernization or scientization of *Đông y* in the amended bill as being unrealistic. According to him, Western medicine was progressing every day "based on science"; however, *Đông y* is based on the theory of yin-yang and the five elements, which is "not based on science." Moreover, he insisted that *Đông y* was not as easy to "scientize" as Western medicine and doubted if *Đông y* practitioners, without higher education, could undertake medicine "based on science."[90]

Discussion in the Diet and physicians' argument around 1967–72 show that each side had different concerns. As already pointed out, the discussion concerning the bill amendment continued on the premise that institutionalized *Đông y* should not be superstitious, while pre-modern *Đông y* possibly contained such practice. Among lawmakers, the aim was to differentiate *Đông y* professions from Western medicine by employing the medical institutionalized system of Western medicine.

Physicians' arguments in the newspapers showed that they understood institutionalizing *Đông y* as modernization using Western notions of science. Whether possible or not, it seems that physicians' opinions were more realistic. Nevertheless, because of the difficulties pointed out by the physicians, the bill passed in 1972 had the minimum regulations that could be offered.

Making Institutionalized *Đông y* Medical Education

As mentioned above, South Vietnam set a goal to standardize education programs on *Đông y* in 1972. In South Vietnam, a medical education could be obtained at the University of Saigon Medical School and at the University of Hue Medical School. After 1966, US medical assistance played a major role and US educational assistance continued until 1974 through the Office of Education, as part of the United States Agency for International Development (USAID), a division of the US Department of State in Saigon.[91] From 1963 to 1966, funding for the construction of a new medical school at the University of Saigon was shared between the Vietnamese government and the United States.[92] At this point, there was no institutionalized education for *Đông y* practice at the medical schools in South Vietnam.

According to recollections from this period, the primary language of the lectures was French; however, gradually the textbooks supported by the United States were used by the US physicians for teaching the students in English.[93] Classes began to be conducted in Vietnamese around 1970, yet the Saigon University School of Medicine did not include *Đông y* in their curriculum.[94]

Before 1963, at the Hue Medical School, classes were taught by German and French teachers in English and French. After the Diệm administration ended, the nationalities of the teaching staff ranged from Canadian to North American to French.[95] Thus, Western medicine remained the foundation of the medical education curriculum at the university.

However, efforts to improve the system did yield some results. In 1968, the president of Hue Medical School, Bùi Duy Tâm, and others on the university committee, began to consider the introduction of elements of traditional medicine in their graduation ceremony.[96] The university committee discussed studying the "education of traditional medicine in accordance with modern medical and scientific methods for the medical students."[97]

A report to the American health workers on traditional medical care in Saigon provides some information on traditional medicine in institutionalized medical education. According to the report, traditional medicine had become a part of the university curriculum by 1974 in the South.[98] It was presented by an American officer from the US Information Agency, Chester A. Bain, who conducted four surveys after 1958.[99]

According to his report, the *Đông y* practitioner community was thriving in South Vietnam. For example, in 1969, at a meeting in Saigon to honor Lãn Ông, one of the most prominent figures in the history of traditional medicine in Vietnam,[100] the Vietnamese Academy of Medicine announced its plan to develop "traditional Oriental medicine" and contribute to the culture of the country.[101] Bain presented folk therapists' medical treatments in Vietnam in his report, including treatments that primarily involved magic in rural areas.

Then, as of 1974, lectures on acupuncture and moxibustion began at the Saigon University School of Medicine.[102] *Đông y* techniques were voluntarily introduced in institutionalized medical education. It can be suggested that medical doctors were seeking for "new" and simple medical formulas as the Vietnam War intensified in the South. Compared to North Vietnam, there is scant information on the institutionalization of traditional medicine in South Vietnam. However, despite the 1964 policy change, the integration of *Đông y* into South Vietnam's public health system did not make significant progress.[103]

Conclusion

Attempts to institutionalize *Đông y* in South Vietnam reveal its characteristics there. In the South, it underwent a greater Chinese influence and was exposed to lesser *Thuốc Nam* (Southern Vietnamese medicine) influence than in the North. Thus, *Đông y* in South Vietnam reflected mixed medical and social practices of Chinese and Vietnamese elements.

Although *Đông y* in the South was different compared to that in the North, and despite the political competition of the Cold War, both states eventually set a goal of institutionalizing *Đông y* in each of their medical systems. Moreover, both states were eager to establish *Đông y* along with its nation-building process. This chapter thus has offered mainly two perspectives to understand institutionalized *Đông y* in South Vietnam.

The first element is the difference of *Đông y* with respect to Chinese influences between the two states. In North Vietnam, Western medical and pharmaceutical practitioners took the initiative to institutionalize Eastern medicine, hailing the case of the People's Republic of China as a model. In contrast, in South Vietnam, the institutionalization of *Đông y* was achieved by differentiating *Đông y* practitioners from Chinese and Western influences under the political rivalry of communist states and the inflow of Western medical knowledge.

The second point is how South Vietnam defined its own *Đông y*. Later, after restricting *Đông y* practitioners to Vietnamese nationals in South Vietnam, the discussion on *Đông y* concentrated on how to differentiate it from Western medical practice. This was done by tracing the formula of Western medical institutions, such as their educational system. While government and lawmakers understood this institutionalizing process as showing a state's authenticity and a process of making *Đông y* practical, some understood it as a matter of modernization. Physicians saw such modernization as the scientization of *Đông y*, with an image of renewal and improvement in a contemporary Western context. Such understandings at least shared a common understanding of *Đông y* as not being superstitious.

South Vietnam's case of institutionalizing *Đông y* was a struggle to create one's own image against competition from North Vietnam and supporting states. It was not only an attempt to make *Đông y* more Vietnamese than Chinese but was representative of South Vietnam's decolonizing process. It was a process of defining self in contrast to Western medicine and the political and social influence of the West in the Cold War.

NOTES

1. Acknowledgments: This chapter was partly supported by JSPS KAKENHI Grant numbers JP16H03310 and JP19K20523. I am particularly grateful for insightful comments and helpful suggestions on my manuscript from the editorial team, Dr Michitake Aso, Dr Michele C. Thompson and Dr Kathryn Sweet. I also appreciate the feedback offered by anonymous reviewers.
2. See C. Michele Thompson, "Medicine, Nationalism, and Revolution in Vietnam: The Roots of a Medical Collaboration to 1945," *East Asian Science, Technology &*

Medicine 21 (2003): 114–48, and C. Michele Thompson, *Vietnamese Traditional Medicine: A Social History* (Singapore: NUS Press, 2015).

3. See David Craig, *Familiar Medicine: Everyday Health Knowledge and Practice in Today's Vietnam* (Honolulu: University of Hawai'i Press, 2002); Thompson, "Medicine, Nationalism, and Revolution in Vietnam"; Nara Oda, "Betonamu Kingendaishi ni okeru Dento-igaku: Minzoku igaku no tanjo ['Traditional Medicine' in the Modern History of Vietnam: Invention of 'National Medicine'] [In Japanese]," *Tonan Ajia* [Southeast Asia: History and Culture] 40 (2010): 126–44; Oda, *Dentou Igakuga Tsukurareru Toki: Betonamu Iryo-seisaku-shi* [The Making of 'Traditional Medicine': A History of Vietnam's Medical Policies] [In Japanese] (Kyoto: Kyoto University Press, 2022); Ayo Wahlberg, "Revolutionary Movement to Bring Traditional Medicine Back to the Grassroots Level: On the Biopolitization of Herbal Medicine in Vietnam," in *Global Movements, Local Concerns: Medicine and Health in Southeast Asia*, ed. Laurence Monnais and Harold J. Cook (Singapore: NUS Press, 2014), pp. 207–25.

4. For instance, *Sơ Thảo Lịch Sử Y Học Cổ Truyền Việt Nam* written by Lê Trần Đức does not even mention how traditional medicine was treated in South Vietnam.

5. See Lê Trần Đức, *Sơ Thảo Lịch Sử Y Học Cổ Truyền Việt Nam* (Hà Nội: NXB Y Học, 1995); Hoang Bao Chau, ed., *Vietnamese Traditional Medicine* (2nd edn) (Hanoi: The Gioi Publishers, 1999); and Hoang Bao Chau, "The Revival and Development of Vietnamese Traditional Medicine: Towards Keeping the Nation in Good Health," in *Southern Medicine for Southern People: Vietnamese Medicine in the Making*, ed. Laurence Monnais, C. Michele Thompson and Ayo Wahlberg (Newcastle upon Tyne: Cambridge Scholars, 2012), pp. 113–52.

6. Trung ương Hội Đông Y Việt Nam 2011, pp. 1–2. The original document was displayed at Vietnam National Archive No. 3 on 27 February 2018. The copy of the letter can be read in the newspaper article reporting the exhibition (Available at: https://dangcongsan.vn/thoi-su/trao-tang-bo-y-te-ban-sao-thu-cua-chu-tich-ho-chi-minh-gui-hoi-nghi-can-bo-y-te-dau-nam-1955-474649.html [accessed on 8 September 2021]).

7. Craig, *Familiar Medicine*, pp. 1–60.

8. Trung tâm Lưu trữ quốc gia 1 [National Archives of Vietnam No. 1, hereafter TTLT1], TTLT1, file BYT (Bộ Y tế, Ministry of Health) 8509, Nghị quyết "Đoàn kết đông tây y" tại Hội nghị quân dân y Nam Bộ năm 1954.

9. TTLT1, file BYT 8525, Báo cáo của Vụ Đông y—Bộ Y tế về tình hình Đông y trước cách mạng tháng 8 đến năm 1958.

10. TTLT1, file BYT 8525, Báo cáo của Vụ Đông y.

11. Li Tana, *Nguyễn Cochinchina: Southern Vietnam in the Seventeenth and Eighteenth Centuries* (Ithaca, NY: Cornell University Press, 1998), pp. 12–16.

12. Khanh Tran, *The Ethnic Chinese and Economic Development in Vietnam* (Singapore: Institute of Southeast Asian Studies, 1993), pp. 15–16.

13. Thomas Engelbert, "Vietnamese- Chinese Relations in Southern Vietnam during the First Indochina Conflict," *Journal of Vietnamese Studies* 3, 3 (2008): 197.

14. Mantetsu East Asia Economic Survey (満鉄調査局), *Futsuryo-Indoshina ni okeru Kakyo* (Chinese in French Indochina) [In Japanese] (Tokyo: The East Asiatic Economic Investigation Bureau, 1939), p. 55.

15. Pacific Association（太平洋調査会）ed., *Futsuryo-Indoshina (French Indochina)* [In Japanese] (Tokyo: Kawade-shobo, 1940), pp. 418–32.

16. Engelbert, "Vietnamese- Chinese Relations in Southern Vietnam during the First Indochina Conflict," p. 193; Li Tana, "In Search of the History of the Chinese in South Vietnam, 1945–75," in *The Chinese/ Vietnamese Diaspora*, ed. Yuk Wah Chan (New York: Routledge, 2011), p. 53.

17. Shigeo Itsumi, *Futsuryo-Indoshina-Kenkyu* (Research on French Indochina) [In Japanese] (Tokyo: Nihon-Hyoron-sha, 1942), p. 79.

18. See Li, "In Search of the History of the Chinese in South Vietnam."

19. Tran, *The Ethnic Chinese*, p. 23.

20. Tran, *The Ethnic Chinese*, p. 23.

21. Edward Miller, *Misalliance: Ngo Dinh Diem, the United States, and the Fate of South Vietnam* (Cambridge, MA: Harvard University Press, 2013), pp. 14–15.

22. Miller, *Misalliance,* pp. 15–16.

23. Duy Lap Nguyen, *The Unimagined Community: Imperialism and Culture in South Vietnam* (Manchester: Manchester University Press, 2020).

24. Trung tâm Lưu trữ quốc gia 3 (National Archives of Vietnam No. 3, hereafter TTLT3), file BYT 8531.

25. David Marr, *Vietnamese Tradition on Trial, 1920–1945* (Berkeley: University of California Press, 1987), p. 183.

26. Laurence Monnais, *The Colonial Life of Pharmaceuticals: Medicines and Modernity in Vietnam* (Cambridge: Cambridge University Press, 2019), pp. 243–4.

27. TTLT 3, BYT 8531. Báo cáo tình hình đông y miền nam năm 1957–1958 của Vụ Quan hệ Bắc Nam, Ban Thống nhất Trung ương.

28. Phạm Huy Lục, *Luật mới về nghề làm thuốc Bắc thuốc Nam* (Hà Nội: Imprimerie de Hanoi, 1943).

29. Trung tâm Lưu trữ quốc gia 2 (National Archives of Vietnam No. 2, hereafter TTLT2), file Phủ thủ tướng, PTT29.316. Arrêté du 17 Juillet 1943, Nghị định 17/7/1943.

30. TTLTI 2, file PTT 29.316, Sặc Luật số 9/64 ngày 29.4.1964 Ấn Định Thể Lệ Hành Nghề Đông y Dược (1964). On 4 November 1963, right after the coup d'état, the first draft of Decoux's revised order was submitted to the Ministry of Health.

31. In South Vietnam, *Đông y* practitioners were called *Đông y sĩ* or *Việt y sĩ*. See Đoàn Văn Quýnh, "Y Miếu Huế," *Nghiên Cứu Huế* 7 (2010): 443–6. Following the division of North and South, up to 90,0000–100,0000 people, including wealthy people such as pro-French forces, landlords and Catholics, moved from North Vietnam to South Vietnam. See Gerald Hickey, *Free in the Forest:*

Ethnohistory of the Vietnamese Central Highlands, 1954–1976 (New Haven, CT: Yale University Press, 1982), p. 16. The Northern Migrants' Medical Association can be considered as a group of *Đông y* practitioners consisting of those who migrated from the North.

32. Đông y Dược [*Đông y Dược,* Eastern Medicine and Pharmacopeia Union. Hereafter Đông y Dược], April 1957.

33. Đông y Dược, September 1956.

34. Đông y Dược, February 1957.

35. Đông y Dược, later than August 1958.

36. Đông y Dược, April 1957.

37. Đông y Dược, April 1957.

38. TTLT 2, Sặc Luật số 9/64 ngày 29.4.1964 Ấn Định Thể Lệ Hành Nghề Đông Y Dược (1964).

39. Công Báo Việt Nam Cộng Hòa [Official Daily Gazette of Democratic Vietnam, hereafter CBVN) 1971: 73.

40. CBVN 1962: 1936.

41. TTLT2, file PTT 29.316, Tờ Trình Thủ Tướng Chánh Phủ Lâm Thời ngày 23 tháng 1 năm 1964 (1964).

42. TTLT2, file PTT 29.316, Tờ Trình Thủ Tướng Chánh Phủ Lâm Thời (1964).

43. TTLT2, file PTT 29.316, Sặc Luật số 9/64 ngày 29.4.1964 Ấn Định Thể Lệ Hành Nghề Đông Y Dược (1964).

44. TTLT2, file PTT 29.316, Sặc Luật số 9/64 (1964).

45. TTLT2, file PTT 29.316, Sặc Luật số 9/64 (1964).

46. TTLT2, file PTT 29.316, Tờ Trình Thủ Tướng Chánh Phủ Lâm Thời (1964).

47. TTLT2, file PTT 29.316, Trình Bày Lý Do về việc Dự Thảo Sặc Luật Ấn Định Lại Quy chế Hành Nghề Đông Y Dược (1964).

48. According to the current encyclopedia of medicinal material for traditional medicine, materials vary in terms of toxicity. Not all of them are recognized as traditional medicine today. See Đỗ Tất Lợi, *Những Cây Thuốc và Vị Thuốc Việt Nam* (Hà Nội: NXB Khoa Học và Kỹ Thuật, 2009).

49. TTLT2, file PTT29.316, Sặc Luật số 9/64 ngày 29.4.1964 Ấn Định Thể Lệ Hành Nghề Đông Y Dược (1964).

50. TTLT2, file PTT29.316, Sặc Luật số 9/64 (1964).

51. TTLT2, file PTT29.316, Sặc Luật số 9/64 (1964).

52. TTLT2, file PTT29.316, Sặc Luật số 9/64 (1964).

53. TTLT2, file PTT29.316, Sặc Luật số 9/64 (1964).

54. TTLT2, file PTT29.316, Sặc Luật số 9/64 (1964).

55. TTLT2, file PTT29.316, Sặc Luật số 9/64 (1964).

56. TTLT2, file PTT29.316, Sặc Luật số 9/64 (1964).

57. TTLT2, file PTT29.316, Sặc Luật số 9/64 (1964).

58. Interview with *Đông y* practitioner L in Hồ Chí Minh City conducted on 15 March 2016.

59. TTLT2, file PTT29.316, Sắc Luật số 9/64 ngày 29.4.1964 Ấn Định Thể Lệ Hành Nghề Đông Y Dược (1964).
60. Interview with Mr C, a descendant of Chinese migrants in Dong Nai, on 8 August 2016.
61. TTLT2, file PTT 29.316, Danh Sách Các Cao Đôn Hoàn Tán Được Phép Nhập Cảng theo Chương IV Điều 22 (1964).
62. Mantetsu East Asia Economic Survey, *Futsuryo-Indoshina ni okeru Kakyo* [Chinese in French Indochina], p. 116.
63. Joann Schrock et al., *Minority Groups in the Republic of Vietnam* (Washington, DC: American University Cultural Information Analysis Center, 1966), p. 990.
64. Schrock, *Minority Groups in the Republic of Vietnam*, p. 986.
65. Tran, *The Ethnic Chinese*, p. 28
66. Tran, *The Ethnic Chinese*, p. 29. See also Luong Nhi Ky, "The Chinese in Vietnam: a Study of Vietnamese-Chinese Relations with Special Attention to the Period 1862–1961" (Doctoral Thesis, University of Michigan, 1963), p. 183 and Xiaorong Han, "Spoiled Guests or Dedicated Patriots? The Chinese in North Vietnam," *International Journal of Asian Studies* 6, 1 (2009): 11.
67. Tran, *The Ethnic Chinese*, pp. 41–3.
68. Tran, *The Ethnic Chinese*, p. 43.
69. Interview with Lê Hữu Mạch, *Đông y* practitioner, in Hue on 25 December 2014.
70. Interview with Mr C, a descendant of Chinese migrants in Dong Nai, on 8 August 2016.
71. Interview with *Đông y* practitioner L on 15 March 2016.
72. Miller, *Misalliance*, p. 232.
73. *Chính Luận*, 15 December 1967.
74. *Chính Luận*, 15 December 1967.
75. *Chính Luận*, 15 December 1967.
76. *Chính Luận*, 15 December 1967.
77. TTLT 2, file PTT 30.952, Việc về Dự Luật Quy Chế Đông Y của ba Nghị Sĩ Phạm Nam Sách, Trần Thế Minh và Nguyễn Văn Ngãi (1969).
78. TTLT 2, file PTT 30.952, Việc về Dự Luật Quy Chế Đông Y của ba Nghị Sĩ Phạm Nam Sách (1969).
79. TTLT2, file PTT 29.316, Trình Bày Lý Do về việc Dự Thảo Sắc Luật Ấn Định Lại Quy chế Hành Nghề Đông Y Dược (1964).
80. TTLT 2, file 30.952, Về Dự Thảo Luật Ấn Định Qui Chế Hành Nghề Y Dược Đông Phương (1970).
81. *Chính Luận*, 21 May 1970.
82. *Chính Luận*, 24–25 May 1970.
83. *Chính Luận*, 24–25 May 1970.
84. *Chính Luận*, 24–25 May 1970.
85. CBVN 1971: 183.

86. TTLT 2, file PTT30.952, Dự Án Luật "Hàng Nghề Đông-Y- Dược" đã được Thượng-Viện biểu quyết ngày 19.7.1972 (1972).
87. TTLT 2, file PTT30.952, Việc về Dự Luật Quy Chế Đông Y của ba Nghị Sĩ Phạm Nam Sách, Trần Thế Minh và Nguyễn Văn Ngãi (1969).
88. TTLT 2, file PTT30.952, Dự Án Luật "Hàng Nghề Đông-Y- Dược" đã được Thượng-Viện biểu quyết ngày 19.7.1972 (1972).
89. For example, a doctor, Trần Văn Thích, criticized *Đông y* itself and the way North Vietnam was institutionalizing traditional medicine around that time (*Chính Luận*, 11–12 January 1970). Also, a citizen, Quan Chánh Quản, wrote his opinion from patients' points of view on *Đông y* and *Tây y* in *Chính Luận* newspaper from 8 January 1970 for two days (*Chính Luận*, 8–9 January 1970).
90. *Chính Luận*, 21–23 May 1970.
91. For an overview of the medical assistance of the US, see the policy report written by Alister Brass, "The Importance of Foreign Medical Aid for South Vietnam," *The Australian Quarterly* 39, 2 (1967): 45–55 (Available at: https://doi.org/10.2307/20634128 [accessed 19 May 2023]).
92. Hien V. Ho, "I Went to Medical School," in *The Vietnamese Mayflowers of 1975*, ed. Chat V Dang, Hien V. Ho, Nghia M. Vo and Anne R. Capdeville (Scotts Valley, CA: Create Space, 2010), pp. 178–81.
93. Hien V. Ho, "I Went to Medical School."
94. An interview with Đoàn Văn Quýnh in Hue on 21 December 2014. He obtained a PhD in Medicine in 1971.
95. An interview with Đoàn Văn Quýnh and Trần Thị Như Mai (PhD in Pharmacology) in Hue on 13 December 2014.
96. *Chính Luận*, 9 August 1968.
97. *Chính Luận*, 9 August 1968.
98. Chester A. Bain, "The Persistence of Tradition in Modern Vietnamese Medicine," *Southeast Asia: An International Quarterly* 3, 1 (1974): 618.
99. For Bain's personal background and his work, see Geoffrey Fairbairn, review, "*Vietnam: The Roots of Conflict*. By Chester A. Bain," *Journal of Southeast Asian History* 9, 2 (1968): 362 (doi:10.1017/S0217781100004828).
100. For two prominent Vietnamese medical practitioner/scholars recognized nowadays, see C. Michele Thompson, "Tuệ Tĩnh Vietnamese Monk-Physician at the Ming Court," in *The Illustrated History of Chinese Medicine and Healing*, ed. T.J. Heinrichs and Linda L. Barnes (Cambridge: Harvard University Press, 2013), pp. 134–5 and Thompson, *Vietnamese Traditional Medicine: A Social History*.
101. Bain, "The Persistence of Tradition in Modern Vietnamese Medicine," p. 618.
102. Bain, "The Persistence of Tradition in Modern Vietnamese Medicine," p. 618.
103. However, as a life history of the practitioner in *Tiger's Apprentice*, directed by Trinh M. Nguyen and produced by Trinh M. Nguyen (Royal Anthropological Institute, 1998), illustrates, traditional medical practices have been handed

down through the generations through unofficial channels of *gia truyền*. For details, see https://raifilm.org.uk/films/tigers-apprentice/ [accessed 19 May 2023]. For the unofficial medical education including esoteric practice, see Quang Van Nguyen and Majorie Pivar, *Fourth Uncle in the Mountain: The Remarkable Legacy of a Buddhist Itinerant Doctor in Vietnam* (New York: St. Martin's Griffin, 2006).

CHAPTER 5

Building a "Socialist Health System": Soviet Assistance in Malaria Control in the Democratic Republic of Vietnam during the Cold War

Annick Guénel[1]

In January 1956, the North Vietnam Ministry of Health welcomed a team of Soviet specialists in zoology and parasitology. Composed of eight members, six of them women, its ten-month mission was described through four key actions:

1. the study of ticks and fleas in North Vietnam;
2. the study of small mammals on which these parasites fed;
3. the study of interaction between parasites and their hosts, and an investigation of the environmental conditions which potentially allowed contact with humans; and
4. finally, determining the epidemiological value of the above studies, and defining subsequent lines of research.

An essential task of the Soviet visit, it was added, was training the "Vietnamese comrades" both in entomo-parasitological working methods in the field, and in experimental work from the collected material in the lab. According to the Soviet scientists who conducted the program, although those wild animals likely to become reservoirs of diseases were numerous in Vietnam, the medical education provided by the French had been inadequate.

Moreover, many cases of illness had been probably incorrectly registered, such as influenza or malaria, without laboratory tests.[2]

The request for Soviet assistance from the Vice-Minister of Health, Phạm Ngọc Thạch, relied upon the Soviet scientific expertise in the study of "the natural foci of communicable diseases." This referred to a theory developed by a Russian biologist, E.N. Pavlovsky, which had provided a study method to the Soviet scientists, who carried out significant research on a wide range of parasitic diseases throughout the USSR territory and its variety of climates.[3]

Actually, it was not the first mission of Soviet parasitology experts to visit the Democratic Republic of Vietnam (DRV). In October 1955, 12 Soviet malaria specialists had already been sent to the DRV. Among other infectious diseases, malaria was by far the most serious concern for the North Vietnamese government since its return to Hanoi following the Geneva Agreement. The year 1955 was also when the World Health Organization (WHO) launched its program of global malaria eradication. The use of DDT, a long-lasting and relatively inexpensive insecticide, synthetized at the beginning of World War II, gave hope that malaria control could be extended over a large part of the world. However, when the WHO had been officially established in 1948, the world had already begun to enter into the Cold War. There were disagreements among health officials about integration of disease control and broader development programs. Furthermore, as a UN agency, the WHO was very quickly dominated by the United States, which reduced the funding available to the Soviet bloc countries. In response to this restricted medical help, the Soviet Union left the WHO in 1949, and returned only in 1957. Followed by several countries of the socialist bloc, they built their own system of health cooperation.[4]

As the program detailed above shows, Soviet assistance to the DRV in the control of malaria, and more generally in the control of parasitic diseases, was not a mere material assistance, but included training, research and participation in health activities. Furthermore, in 1959, Leonard J. Bruce-Chwatt made a detailed account of Soviet scientific work in malariology, and noted that "the general strategy of malaria eradication in the USSR has many technical, administrative and economic and social features not seen elsewhere."[5] Much more recently, Michitake Aso also pointed out that, in the 1950s in Vietnam, the production of malaria knowledge entered a new phase, or "a postcolonial rationality," which led to a change of strategy developed with Soviet aid.[6]

The present chapter aims to extend the debate on this issue, and to question the Soviet legacy. While the borrowing of Soviet model by the Vietnamese political leaders was widely investigated,[7] there is relatively little research on the scientific transfer to the DRV, especially in the biomedical field. Yet, several teams of specialists in parasitology and malariology from the Soviet Union were sent to the DRV over the period 1955–63, during which time a program of malaria eradication was set up. The Soviet assistance continued thereafter and during the American war, with mass shipments of equipment, medicines and DDT.

This chapter draws on materials held in the Center of National Archives in Hanoi, as well as published books and articles. When the North Vietnamese authorities called for Soviet assistance, they responded to a difficult health situation combined with a lack of material and human resources, two factors which shall be taken into account. From 1955, understanding of, and control strategies for, malaria developed by the Vietnamese in cooperation with Soviet experts focused on the environmental features of specific areas. That leads us to address the question of state-induced transformation of spaces and the role played by scientific practices and public health policies. As Matthias Braun noticed in a paper concerning the anti-malaria policy in Soviet Azerbaijan, at an early time of the USSR, "state-induced spatial practices [was] a picture very common to and best studies in states 'in becoming'."[8] Moreover, during this period of state-building, maintaining the legitimacy and authority of the DRV government over the entire territory was all the more crucial as Vietnam had been divided into two parts following the Geneva Agreements in 1954.

South of the 17th parallel, in the Republic of Vietnam (RVN) under US control, public health efforts were also undertaken. The RVN was included in a malaria eradication program launched in 1958, which covered the entire Western Pacific region, and was supervised by the WHO Regional Office.[9] The South Vietnam government received particularly important financial and material aid as well as expert assistance from the United States International Cooperation Administration (ICA). However, DDT spraying experiments had been conducted as soon as 1951 under the WHO auspices with the assistance of the American Economic mission. Interestingly, Marcos Cueto, regarding the US efforts to eradicate malaria in Latin America, pointed out that DDT was called the "atomic bomb" of insecticides by US scientists, and emphasized how these efforts served the policy of communism containment by expanding its influence around the world.[10]

Prior to 1954

Malaria distribution in Vietnam was closely tied to human settlements and ethnicity.[11] With a few exceptions, it also divided the territory between lowlands, where malaria was non- or hypoendemic, and the hyper-endemic uplands, where minorities lived. As a consequence, the economic agricultural development policy of the latter, pursued by the French from the beginning of the 20th century, acted as a spur to conduct research on malaria. Aso analysed the successive stages of knowledge production about malaria from the 1920s, marked by the development of rubber plantations on "red lands" in the south of Vietnam. He notably discussed several factors which were driving a new interest in rural conditions of life and their impact on malaria during the interwar period. Among them was the pressure of the League of Nations Health Organisation (LNHO) which argued that malaria control could not succeed without rural economic development.[12]

The international organization collapsed in 1946, and the little improvements in the rural areas were wiped out during World War II.[13] From the onset of the first Indochinese War, 1946–54, which immediately followed, the North and the South faced different challenges.[14] The war turned the central highlands into strategic areas and their inhabitants into potential allies of the French forces, which rekindled malaria research there.[15] Meanwhile, in the northern uplands, or Việt Bắc, where Ho Chi Minh's government had escaped, the sparseness of means gave an incentive to find innovative means of malaria treatment and prevention.

In the early years of the first Indochinese War, the shortage of antimalarial drugs incited Vietnamese doctors to look for local folk remedies. The plant Thường sơn (*Dichroa febrifuga*), from which the army laboratory prepared tablets, was particularly prized. However, up to 30 tablets per day were sometimes necessary to stop a malaria crisis. Later on, the laboratory succeeded in producing the active compounds from the plant, which were more efficient in a shorter time.[16] It was only after the victory by Mao Zedong's troops in 1949 that the North Vietnamese could receive the first supplies of the latest antimalarial drugs from China and the Soviet Union.

Health campaigns were another aspect of the war period. Prevention education was first conducted among the army units, which, in turn, had to spread simple messages in the local villages. They were in the form of slogans, like "tidy up the house," "sleep under the net," "smoke out the mosquitoes," or "wear long clothing in the evening," and later viewed as having played an important role in malaria control at that time.[17] In any event, this mass propaganda, which was a first step in the setting up of a health network, also contributed to the general policy of local population rallying the Việt Minh.

The war period also prevented the Vietnamese medical doctors who had joined the Việt Minh from obtaining the latest scientific knowledge and practices in malaria control. DDT, available since the end of the 1930s, and new

antimalarial drugs were first trialled only from 1948 in the Central High pla-
teaux, which was occupied by the French.[18] Moreover, among the Vietnamese
trained at the French Medical School of Hanoi, very few had acquired any competence in malariology. Hoàng Tích Trí, appointed Minister of Health in 1946,
should be mentioned as he had conducted malaria surveys with the Pasteur
Institute of Hanoi before the war.[19] However, the only Vietnamese physician
trained in parasitology at the Hanoi school was Đặng Văn Ngữ. Like Tôn Thất
Tùng, he was one of the very few Vietnamese to specialize at the faculty after
completing his medical thesis.[20] In 1937, he became Henri Galliard's assistant in
the department of parasitology, where he remained until 1941, when he left to
study mycology in Japan. He was only able to return to Vietnam clandestinely
in 1947, when he joined the resistance. There, he was responsible for teaching
parasitology at the medical university set up at Chiêm Hoá (Tuyên Quang
Province in the northeast of Vietnam) during the war.[21]

The Soviet Program of Staff Training

The scale of population movement following the Geneva Agreements in 1954
and the consequences of the war itself were major causes of the spread of malaria. This was worsened by natural disasters, such as the floods of 1955, and
by the continuing population displacement due to the rapid implementation of
the "new economic zones" in the uplands, dictated by the Party.[22]

The first response was to establish a basic laboratory for the study of malaria within the premises of the Microbiology Institute, set up by the maquis
during the war, rather than at the Pasteur Institute of Hanoi, which had the
prerogative of malaria studies until 1945.[23] The laboratory team comprised
15 members—half of them had a medical education—of various origins:
civilian and seconded military cadres, from the North and from the South, as
well as some former members of the Pasteur Institute. It conducted preliminary studies on parasites as well as on vectors in the surrounding areas of Hanoi.
But, facing up to inexperienced staff, its main function seems to have been to
prepare for the arrival of Soviet experts.[24]

The first Soviet antimalarial mission (1955) was supervised by Professor Pravikov. He was one of the Soviet malariologists who had participated in
the national program of malaria eradication in the USSR, launched in 1951.[25]
A steering committee, composed of two medical physicians and one epidemiologist from Pravikov's team, was set up in Thái Nguyên, capital of the province
of the same name. Located in a region of medium altitude of the Việt Bắc, Thái
Nguyên was one of the most malaria-affected provinces in the country.
The other Soviet members of the mission formed mobile teams, joined by

the Vietnamese staff sent by the Ministry of Health and the Army Medical Department.

The mobile teams conducted inquiries not only in many Thái Nguyên communes, but also in other provinces. They visited villages as well as industrial zones, such as the apatite mines in Lào Cai province in the northwest, or farms of the Nghệ An and Ninh Bình provinces in the south of the DRV. At every place, the prevalence of splenomegaly as well as blood parasites among the population was reported. This was combined by mosquito collections and evaluation of their density. The distribution of medicines, and gaining the trust of the local people, was another task of the mobile teams.[26] The assessment of treatments with antimalarial drugs provided by the Soviets could be carried out at the local hospitals, where most patients were the *cán bộ* (public officers) and their families, the great majority of which were Kinh.[27] During the Pravikov mission, 48 million tablets were supplied to the DRV by the Soviets, in addition to 13 tons of DDT.[28]

It was already clear that the pre-war data was not only incomplete but also obsolete due to environmental changes and population displacements. The inquiries conducted during the first two years of Soviet collaboration provided updated information, notably on the intensity of malaria transmission and the distribution of the *plasmodia* species depending on the season and the region. This confirmed the predominance of *P. falciparum*, especially in the north and northwest of the country, as French scientists had already stated, while it was observed that *P. vivax* prevailed over *P. falciparum* during the winter and spring in some regions of Central Vietnam.[29] In-depth entomological observations also allowed the teams to specify the role of some Anopheles species as parasite vectors.[30]

Last but not least, these inquiries provided the opportunity to educate the Vietnamese in malaria theory and Soviet data collection methods. And being in charge of propaganda campaigns for disease prevention, like those started during the war, meant that the development of mobile teams was strongly encouraged by the Vietnamese Ministry of Health. For their part, the Soviet experts organized training on malaria for nurses, students and health propagandists in the areas they were surveying. The training of local teams was later noted as one of the most important points by A. Ya. Lysenko, who succeeded Pravikov as malariology expert in North Vietnam. He stressed "that during the detachment of Soviet malariologists to the DRV [1955–57], numerous local cadres were trained among the malariologist-medical specialists, entomologists, and laboratory workers with whose cooperation it was possible to perform later (in 1957–59) a series of studies on the epidemiology of malaria and the efficiency of antimalarial measures."[31]

"Topographical—Malariological Zoning," Applied to the Program of Malaria Eradication in the DRV

Throughout the first Soviet mission, the malaria situation remained very serious. Among the most affected regions were the provinces of Thái Nguyên and Tuyên Quang, and the Thái-Mèo region, where the percentage of malaria cases in the hospitals was 41.5, 47 and 24 percent, respectively. At the end of 1956 and the beginning of 1957, the situation was getting worse. Epidemics broke out on building sites in particular, and in industrial and agricultural enterprises located in endemic areas, impacting production.[32]

It was under these health conditions that Lysenko, who had previously led the malaria eradication campaign in Tajikistan, was appointed as a new expert in North Vietnam in 1957.[33] In August of that year, the Malaria Research Institute, *Viện nghiên cứu sốt rét*, was officially created, as had been recommended during the first Soviet mission. The Institute brought together the Vietnamese malaria specialists in the country at that time.[34] In the early stages, the staff was composed of 70 cadres, including Đặng Văn Ngữ, who was appointed director. With 27 physicians (including only five medical doctors and two military doctors), 21 nurses and eight microscopists, the specialist capacity was still limited, as was the technical equipment.[35] However, the setting up of a command post rapidly allowed the development and implementation of a malaria control program throughout North Vietnam.

The DRV government and the Party decreed that the malaria eradication program should run over an eight-year period (1958–65), with a preparation phase scheduled from 1958 to 1960. It is noteworthy that the Republic of Vietnam, on the other side of the 17th parallel, started its malaria eradication program at the same time as the DRV. On both sides, proceeding along a stepwise approach with four phases was the same: preparation, attack, consolidation and maintenance.

To draw up the control plan, Lysenko proposed a mapping of malaria with the method of "topographical—malariological zoning," which had been successfully used in Soviet Tajikistan before. The method comprised six steps:

1. Using a topographical map, choosing routes to be investigated with coverage of the whole variety of oro-hydrographical conditions;
2. carrying out a complex exploration of the places and populations along the chosen routes;
3. typing of the malarial foci in inhabited sites;
4. sorting by using topographical maps and, by analogy, with identified types of malarial foci of all other inhabited sites of the locality and grouping together similar types of breeding grounds;

5.   reappraisal of the situation in sections whose classification is doubtful (that is, zonal boundaries);
6.   characterizing the zones using the sum of all data available (demographic, economic . . .).[36]

The Ministry of Health and the Administrative Committee of the Việt Bắc designated Thái Nguyên province as the pilot area for the first experimentation of this method. The province was highly diversified in terms of epidemiology, with different patterns of malaria transmission, including high transmission all year round, and severe cases. It was also a multi-ethnic province, and the most important zone of industrial development in the region. Therefore, the choice of Thái Nguyên spotlighted the policy towards the minorities (*chính sách dân tộc*), and "the priority given by the Party and the government to the economic and cultural development of the mountainous regions" (*ưu tiên phát triển kinh tế, văn hóa miền núi của Đảng và Chính phủ ta*).[37]

During the exploration of the Thái Nguyên province, in October and November 1957, entomological and epidemiological data were collected in 116 inhabited sites, the spleens of 8,292 people were examined, thick blood tests were performed in 7,609 people, and 461 Anopheles mosquitoes were caught and examined. Other factors were considered, such as the population's way of life, types of dwelling, quantity of livestock, water bodies and the migration of people. In all, 948 sites were studied.[38]

Thirteen species of Anopheles mosquitoes were collected during the investigation, *A. vagus* accounting for the largest share, but *A. minimus* being the most important vector. Following the method described above, and according to the collected data, the province was classified into four zones: endemic-malaria mountain-river zone, low mountain-river zone, hilly-river zone, and non-endemic sparsely populated high-mountain zone. This classification served as a basis for developing appropriate and economic malaria control programs or, in a malariologist's words, for developing "tailor-made plans for both cure and prevention activities."[39]

Experimentation continued with a Malaria Institute team, based in Thái Nguyên, responsible for following up DDT spraying operations and medical treatments on 14 sites determined by the Soviet experts. Several dozen teams of spraying workers had been trained at the launch of the study, and a DDT amount supplied to cover at least 1 million square meters during the first two months. More than 2.5 million antimalarial tablets had also been provided.[40] It should be noted that chemotherapy played at least as an important role as residual insecticide in the Soviet program of malaria control.[41] From the end of the war, the Soviets provided North Vietnam mostly with Plasmocide (similar to rhodoquine), synthetized as early as 1931 in the USSR, and Acriquine (mepacrine type), synthetized in 1933. They also provided Bigumal (proguanil), synthetized in 1947. The more recent Quinocide (4-amino-quinoleine), synthetized by the Institute of Malariology and Parasitology in Moscow, was also tested against *Plasmodium vivax* in some areas, in association with DDT spraying.[42]

Between 1957 and 1960, in Thái Nguyên province, the malaria prevalence rate fell from 9.2 percent to 0.3 percent, and nearly all the vectors were declared as having disappeared. This first achievement, which was planned to be extended to the rest of the country, could not be realized without training an important number of people. At least until 1960, the significant Soviet participation in parasitology training was fully recognized. It was notably reported that, from 1958 to 1959, 179 chief district doctors were educated in malaria control measures. Through mass health education, and the decentralized health system progressively implemented by the Vietnamese government from 1955, community involvement in malaria prevention resulted in lower levels.[43]

In July and October 1958, the Lysenko method was applied to the huge autonomous region of Thái Mèo. The special attention paid to the periodic migration of the people was one of the major factors of this study, supervised by Đặng Văn Ngữ and Nguyễn Tiến Bửu.[44] Notably, it led to understanding the reasons for the high infestation among Mèo adults living at an altitude above 1,200 meters, which could be considered as hypoendemic.

The Transformation of Rural Areas

Agrarian reform, actually started during the First Indochina War, was a broad modernization project pursued by the DRV in rural areas.[45] Often named "cooperativization," it inspired Đặng Văn Ngữ to propose a change to the malaria control strategy. He argued that the cooperative movement, which was "revolutionizing" the mode of production and agricultural techniques, had a direct impact on the Anopheles. As examples, he described the new method of densely transplanting rice, which removed the larvae from the surface of the paddy fields, or, in the mountains, the construction of dams by the cooperative peasants to retain running water in the streams, a favorite breeding place for *A. minimus*. Extolling the virtues of socialism, Ngữ even considered that the improvement of rural livelihoods accompanying these transformations was happening at a much faster rate than in European countries where it had taken several centuries.

These environmental changes, as he wrote in a letter addressed to Sergiev, head of the plan for malaria elimination in the USSR,[46] were able to shorten the length of the program, without massive DDT spraying, and would be at a lower cost for the country. According to Ngữ, the use of DDT should be limited to the construction sites, factories or other public enterprises located in endemic areas. In rural areas, besides health education, he encouraged the use of simple traditional means to eradicate larvae and adult mosquitoes, such as larvivorous fish, destruction by fire, fumigation and the use of local plants.[47]

In his answer, one month later, Sergiev agreed with Ngữ's plan in many respects. Control measures complying with the national economy, adaptation to environmental changes by the experts, as well as the likelihood of the successful acceptance and participation by the population, were in accordance, as he said, with "the malaria control experience in the Soviet Union." However, he expressed serious doubts regarding the possibility of a spontaneous malaria regression in the climatic conditions prevailing in Vietnam, which were conducive for malaria. Moreover, providing substantial evidence from his malariologist experience on Soviet territory, Sergiev raised strong reservations about the level of larvicide efficiency and the sustainability of agricultural methods described by Ngữ. As for the extermination of the adult insects by traditional means, he was also not very positive. Why spend the strength of the population on inefficient and scarcely long-lasting measures, such as fumigation and mosquito swatting, Sergiev asked, when there was a highly effective and safe insecticide, such as DDT. His conclusion was that "given the current malaria situation in the world, when all the countries have set the target of eradicating malaria in a very short time, the principles set out in [Ngữ's] letter cannot guarantee malaria eradication in [the] country, even more within the time allowed by the other tropical countries."[48]

Studies of "alternative" means to DDT, against both larvae and adult mosquitoes, were pursued at the Malaria Institute, at the behest of the Vietnamese Ministry of Health, beyond 1960.[49] Therapeutic trials, such as splenomegaly treatment by acupuncture, and use of well-known medicinal plants, were also performed. Nevertheless, all these studies were conducted only at the level of a few villages, while massive DDT spraying was experimented with in new regions. As soon as December 1959, in Ngọc Lạc district (Thanh Hóa province), and in Hoà Bình province, a team led by Vũ Phi Hùng conducted a pilot experiment similar to that conducted in Thái Nguyên, this time with the assistance of four Romanian experts. DDT spraying combined with mass treatment of people affected by or suspected of having malaria led to a 75 percent decline of its prevalence in one year.[50]

Therefore, in 1958, indoor DDT spraying was conducted in an area of about 11,000 sq km, in 1959 in an area of about 16,000 sq km, and in 1960 in an area of more than 48,000 sq km. Over three years, 2.5 million people had been protected and the decrease of malaria incidence in sprayed areas was dramatic.[51] This encouraging result made it possible to move into the attack phase. Moreover, the Soviet government allocated 20 million rubles of non-reimbursable aid in the form of insecticide and other equipment.[52]

Besides material assistance, at the beginning of 1962 the Soviets sent a five-member team, led by the epidemiologist Kompantsev, to assist the Institute during the attack phase. He reported that, during that year, the population living in malaria areas (that is 5.3 million people) was protected by DDT. As the number of malaria patients dropped by 32 percent between 1961 and 1962, and the mortality dropped by 50 percent, only 2 million received antimalarial medicines. According to Kompantsev, the incidence of malaria continued to fall. Until 1963, a dozen Soviet experts still participated in the deployment of spraying operations and surveillance in the DRV.[53]

Propaganda

As already mentioned, propaganda (*tuyên truyền*) was a substantial component of the malaria eradication program. Propagandists (*cán bộ tuyên truyền*) were recruited among local authorities and governmental mass organizations (like the Youth Union and the Women's Union) and were trained as the beginning of the first malaria mission. They were generally also responsible for collecting data from the villages in the endemic areas. Their visits to remote villages were reportedly the first time the inhabitants had met Party and government representatives.[54]

After enumerating the problems caused by malaria, and stressing the role of mosquitoes as vectors of the disease, medical propaganda strove to explain contemporary ways of eradication, including DDT, the importance of compliance with drugs delivered by health workers, and other hygiene and preventive measures.[55] The malaria eradication committee required the use of all available media. For example in the Thái-Mèo region, the following were proposed: text and illustrated books (*Tìm hiểu về bệnh sốt rét* [Learning about malaria], *Chống bệnh sốt rét* [Fighting malaria]), including copies in Vietnamese as well as in Thái languages, talks, exhibitions, as well as radio broadcasts by the Propaganda and Education Committee, relating to eradication work carried out in the region.[56]

Propaganda was targeted primarily toward ethnic minorities. The "obscurantist policies of the former feudal regime" were accused of having left these populations in the lurch, and the latter were often presented as falling prey to superstitions and fatalism about the disease. Besides the fact there was a common vision of people living in peripheral regions in several modern nations, one could find other similarities with the medical propaganda in Soviet Kazakhstan, launched three decades earlier, as depicted by Paula A. Michaels.[57] A similar emphasis on the link between economic, social and cultural environments and hygiene issues was given in propaganda reports in both cases.[58] Providing populations with basic scientific knowledge about health and disease and introducing them to new habits was expected to lead to a major transformation of these regions.[59] At the outset of the eradication program throughout North Vietnam, the Minister of Culture, responsible for propaganda, stated that the program was not only aimed at protecting human health, but also at developing the local economy, army and culture in minority regions.

Ultimately, the health program participated in the "building of a socialist society," which also meant a society based on national unity, with the minority acceding to a new culture.[60] Enhanced solidarity amongst the fraternal countries was also put forward. However, still more important since the beginning of the 1960s was the "great political impact" of the malaria eradication plan, "which reaches our compatriots in the South as well as neighboring countries like Laos."[61]

Interestingly, a 2014 publication dedicated to Đặng Văn Ngữ reproduced a radio message he himself delivered to his compatriots in the South on 15 October 1960. In his discourse, after a harsh judgment of the colonial scientific institutions for their lack of concern about the Vietnamese population suffering from malaria, he continued with the epic tale of malaria control in the North since the anti-French Resistance. He pointed out the inquiries conducted by the malaria teams "from the top of the mountains to the delta, from the streams to the rivers," and the distribution of medicines. He especially focused on the last three years with the number of health staff, the people protected by DDT, and on the decline in the incidence of malaria. The end of the message was probably the most important part, as it was in support of the struggle against Ngô Đình Diệm's government and the United States. Despite a lot of money spent to fight malaria in the South, the main objective, he said, was to control the population. The program was used as a means of propaganda and espionage purposes, he argued, mentioning the major general at the head of malaria control and commandos disguised as health agents, searching the houses to track down patriots.[62]

Readiness before the War?

According to some data, by 1964 there was a drastic reduction in the number of Soviet and East European technicians in the DRV, which could be due to high tensions between Moscow and Hanoi at this time.[63] We do not know when exactly the last Soviet health experts left the DRV, nor the cause of their departure. In any event, in 1964 the Institute report noted intense activity.

There was some new entomological research, not only on malaria vectors, but also on vectors of other parasitic diseases. Indeed, through the Soviet training in parasitology and entomology, the Institute had expanded its field of research. In 1961, it had been renamed *Viện Sốt rét, Ký sinh trùng và Côn trùng* (Institute of Malariology, Parasitology and Entomology – IMPE). In 1964, studies were notably undertaken on filariasis and encephalitis, and on their vectors.

Training activities continued to be among the most important roles of the Institute. They were addressed to all levels: local malaria teams, responsible for the detection and treatment of the sick, province and district chiefs, assistant doctors, and administrators. Additional training on malaria was even given to *Cán bộ* belonging to the Ministry of Transport, as well as to members of the army. In 1964, the Institute also moved towards further decentralization, by progressively creating provincial stations responsible for health service organization. The provincial stations also allowed more rapid processing of epidemiological, parasitological and entomological data, and thus participated in malaria surveillance.

At the end of 1964, all the regions had already moved to the attack phase and many regions could move to the maintenance phase, although caution was advised for others. However, some "unusual phenomena" also happened, such as epidemics in the delta, which could be explained and then solved thanks to spraying measures.[64] Malaria resurgence after the end of DDT spraying, especially in Thái Nguyên province, was more alarming. Did this involve *A. minimus* resistance to DDT, and/or mosquito change of habits? In any event, in 1964, right on the eve of the first American bombings of North Vietnam, the overall malaria prevalence had fallen to 0.28 percent, as compared to 5.64 percent in 1958 (20 times less). In the mountainous regions, the decrease in prevalence was of course strongest (40 times less).[65]

Conclusion

With the assistance of Soviet and Romanian experts in malaria research and control, the DRV built a health system modeled along the same lines as the USSR's: centralized health planning and supervision combined with the development of a wide health network, reaching the smallest administrative units. This structure allowed the teams to conduct comprehensive epidemiology and environmental surveys, based on the Soviet scientific expertise in malariology, and the deployment of a large-scale anti-malaria program.

Launching an eradication program at the same time as the land collectivization process and the development of new economic zones was taking
place met both public health and political-economic concerns. Priority was
given to some provinces, depending not only on their malaria situation, but also
on government economic projects of construction of "state spaces."[66] Introducing health services and hygiene rules through active propaganda, and fighting
"backwardness" in peripheral areas, such as those occupied by ethnic minorities, helped in this construction. It also aimed to reinforce the unity of the nation
and to promote the formation of a "socialist society."

Regardless of the Soviet part in malaria control, the Vietnamese health
authorities had their own agenda. Phạm Ngọc Thạch, the DRV Minister of
Health from 1958 to 1968, had set up specific guidelines, adapted to the
low-level resources of the country. They included "mass mobilization and
self-reliance," "optimal use of local medication and pharmacopeia" and the re-
course to both "modern and traditional care," clearly put into practice in
the new strategy of malaria control proposed by Đặng Văn Ngữ in 1959.[67]
Was he really confident in an alternative strategy? It is, of course, impossible
to answer.[68] In any case, and although in some places there was a large population participation in control measures, no alternative means of that time
appears to have successfully reduced the use of DDT.

Until the eve of the first American bombings, in 1965, major progress was
made in disease control, and despite some early signs of DDT resistance, several regions achieved the stage of near-eradication. The spraying operations
even increased in the North during the Vietnamese–American war, which led
the Institute to change its strategy and focus more on the battle zones. Malaria
became a major policy challenge, which led Phạm Ngọc Thạch to declare: "Malaria eradication is a strategic task, a struggle against the American enemy."[69]

The war period hindered malaria control in South Vietnam even more.
Despite very important support from the ICA, the program had to face many
obstacles. Among them, exophilic vectors and important population movements, in particular in hyperendemic areas, were the most permanent obstacles.
In addition, the difficulty of coordination among the different actors of the
program, and the lack of general organization, slowed down the process.
The more and more difficult recruitment of malaria agents, and above all
the growing "insecurity," due to "Vietcong" incursion in the villages during
the war, finally put a stop to the program.[70]

Progressively the "liberated zones" in the South were occupied by malaria control teams from the North, and, in 1973, the assistance was under the
responsibility of the DRV Prime Minister.[71] Despite the numerous doctors,

technicians and equipment sent to the South, the basis and the strategy from which a program could be conducted were lacking. Moreover, the malaria situation had deteriorated in the North, and new challenges had appeared: exophilic vectors and parasite chemoresistance. In this year, a Soviet team of three members arrived in Hanoi. During its visit, a 12-year assistance program (1973–85) was developed, focusing first on the North, but opening the door for aid directed to the South and neighboring countries.[72]

Further research would allow us to know more about the development of this project. In any event, after 1975, from the Institute of Malariology, Parasitology and Entomology, which could be considered as the heritage of the Soviet assistance period, two branches were created, one in Hồ Chí Minh City, the second one in Quy Nhơn. As for the WHO, it was not until the beginning of the 1980s that experts made first contact with the Hanoi authorities.

NOTES

1. Many thanks to all the staff members at the Vietnamese National Archives no. 3, especially for helping me in ordering documents. I am very grateful to Jovan Latinovic for not only his help in reading Russian documents, but also in collecting information on Soviet experts' careers. Dr Phạm Huy Tiên, who was an early player in the malaria control in Vietnam, helped me a lot with his experience and his scientific knowledge and contacts in my research. His warm welcome during my visits to Hanoi was also a source of encouragement in my work.

2. National Archives of Vietnam, Centre no. 3, Hanoi (NAV3), Bộ Y Tế 5466: Báo cáo hoạt đông của Đoàn chuyên gia Liên Xô chông sốt rét tại VN năm 1956 [Report on the Soviet Union malaria control activities in Vietnam in 1956]. For an overview of public health in colonial Vietnam, see for example: H. Meyer, *Public Health in Indochina* (prepared for the Health Research Unit of the League of Nations), (Washington, DC, December 1944, WHO Archives: 8A/43045/21641 (R. 6141).

3. VIu Litvin and E.I. Korenberg, "Natural Foci of Diseases: The Development of the Concept at the Close of the Century" (in Russian), *Parazitologiia* 33, 3 (1999): 179–91; Yu. S. Balashov, "Academician E. N. Pavlovskiĭ's Parasitology School in the Zoological Institute RAS" (in Russian), *Parazitologiia* 37, 4 (2003): 249–58; L.N. Pavlovskyĭ, "Outstanding Soviet Zoologist and Parasitologist E.N. Pavlovsky—the Creator of the Theory of Natural Foci of Disease" (in Ukrainian), *Lik Sprava* 5–6 (2011): 142–9.

4. Randall M. Packard, "'Roll Back Malaria, Roll in Development'? Reassessing Burden of Malaria," *Population and Development Review* 35, 1 (2009): 53–87; Socrates Litsios, "Malaria Control, the Cold War, and the Reorganization of International Assistance," *Medical Anthropology: Cross-Cultural Studies in*

Health and Illness 17, 3 (1997): 255–78; Anne-Emmanuelle Birn and Nikolai Krementsov, "'Socialising' Primary Health Care? The Soviet Union, WHO and the 1978 Alma-Ata Conference," *BMJ Global Health* 3 (2018). Available at: http://dx.doi.org/10.1136/bmjgh-2018-000992 [accessed 19 May 2023].

5.   Leonard J. Bruce-Chwatt, "Malaria Research and Eradication in the USSR: A Review of Soviet Achievements in the Field of Malariology," *Bulletin of the World Health Organization* 21 (1959): 737–72. Marcus Klingberg, who was trained as epidemiologist in the USSR, also provided a possible explanation for the difference of "tradition" with Western epidemiology: Alfredo, Morabia, "'East Side Story': On Being an Epidemiologist in the Former USSR: An Interview with Marcus Klingberg," *Epidemiology* 17, 1 (2006): 115–19.

6.   Michitake Aso, *Rubber and the making of Vietnam: An Ecological History 1897–1975* (Chapel Hill: The University of North Carolina Press, 2018), pp. 217–23.

7.   Among other publications: Buu Hoan, "Soviet Economic Aid to Vietnam," *Contemporary Southeast Asia* 12, 4 (1991): 360–76; Melanie Beresford and Phong Đặng, *Economic Transition in Vietnam: Trade and Aid in the Demise of a Centrally Planned Economy* (Northampton: Edward Elgar, 2000); George C. Herring, "The Cold War and Vietnam," *OAH Magazine of History* 18, 5 (2004): 18–21.

8.   Matthias Braun, "From Landscapes to Labscapes: Malaria Research and Anti-Malaria Policy in Soviet Azerbaijan, 1920–41," *Jahrbücher für Geschichte Osteuropas* 61 (2013): 514.

9.   Western Pacific Regional Organization (WPRO). When it was founded in 1951, the region was composed of Australia, New Zealand, Japan, Korea, the Philippines, Vietnam, Laos, Cambodia, Burma, Thailand and the Federation of Malaya. The regional office was established in Manila.

10.   Marcos Cueto, "Appropriation and Resistance: Local Responses to Malaria Eradication in Mexico, 1955–1970," *Journal of Latin American Studies* 37, 3 (2005): 533–59.

11.   Annick Guénel, "Malaria Control, Land Occupation and Scientific Developments in Vietnam in the XXth Century" (1999). Available at: https://halshs.archives-ouvertes.fr/halshs-00137031 [accessed 19 May 2023].

12.   Michitake Aso, "Patriotic Hygiene: Tracing New Places of Knowledge Production about Malaria in Vietnam, 1919–75," *Journal of Southeast Asian Studies* 44, 3 (2013): 423–43. Malaria was a major topic at the international conference on rural hygiene in Java, organized by the LNHO in 1937.

13.   About the control of malaria before and after the war, Socrates Litsios published several articles; René J. Dubos and Fred L. Soper, "Their Contrasting Views on Vector and Disease Eradication," *Perspectives in Biology and Medicine* (Autumn 1997): 138–49; "Arnoldo Gabalon's Independent Path for Malaria Control and Public Health in the Tropics: A Lost 'Paradigm' for WHO," *Parassitologia* 40 (1998): 231–8 (see also note 3).

14. We could note that research work respectively conducted in the northern and central highlands by French scientists had, already, generally followed separate agendas, depending on the current colonial purposes.

15. Archives du Service de Santé, Institut de médecine tropicale (Le Pharo), Marseille: Territoire des populations montagnardes du Sud-Indochinois, 1948–50, dossier 168.

16. Bộ Y Tế, *Lịch sử Viện sốt sét ký sinh trùng và côn trùng (1957–1997)* [History of the Institute of Malariology, Parasitology and Entomology (1957–1997)] (Hà Nội: Nhà Xuất Bản Chính Trị Quốc Gia, 1998), p. 24; Đặng Văn Ngữ, "Mười lăm năm ngành ký sinh trùng học ở nước Việt Nam Dân Chủ Cộng Hòa [Fifteen Years of Parasitology in Democratic Republic of Vietnam]," in Bộ Y Tế, *Đặng Văn Ngữ. Một Trí Thức Lớn, Một Nhân Cách Lớn* [Dang Van Ngu: A Great Intellectual, a Great Man] (Hà Nội: Nhà Xuất Bản Y Học, 2010), p. 180.

17. Some other slogans have been often quoted in stories of Vietnamese resistance, such as the "3 clean" (eat clean, drink clean, live clean) and the "4 killers" (flies, mosquitoes, mice, lice).

18. M.E. Farinaud, *Rapport sur le paludisme dans le Sud Viet-Nam et sur les activités de l'équipe antimalarienne de l'OMS* (Geneva: WHO, Project Files VNR/MRD/001, 1952).

19. *Hoàng Tích Trí* remained Minister of Health until his death in 1958.

20. Michitake Aso and Annick Guénel, "The Itinerary of a North Vietnamese Surgeon: Medical Science and Politics during the Cold War," *Science, Technology and Society* 18, 3 (2013): 291–306.

21. "Tự Thuật của Giáo Đặng Văn Ngữ từ nhỏ đến khi về nước tham gia kháng chiến (1910–1949) [Dang Van Ngu's Autobiography since Childhood until the Return to the Home Country to Join the Resistance (1910–1949)]," in *Đặng Văn Ngữ*, 2010, pp. 49–79.

22. At this date, officially called "Worker's Party of Vietnam" as the Communist Party of Vietnam was dissolved in 1951. Merging with the People's Revolutionary Party of South Vietnam, it reverted to "Communist Party of Vietnam" in 1976.

23. The unsuccessful negotiations between the DRV government and the Pasteur Institute of Paris resulted in the departure of the last French scientists working in the Institute of Hanoi, in 1957, and the merging of the latter with the Institute of Microbiology, then renamed "National Institute of Hygiene and Epidemiology": Annick Guénel, "The Pasteur Institutes in Vietnam: A Long History," in *History of Science in the Multiculture: Proceedings of the Tenth International Conference on the History of Science in East Asia*, ed. Jiang Xiaoyuan (Shanghai: Jiao Tong University Press, 2005), pp. 161–72.

24. *Lịch sử Viện sốt sét*, p. 29.

25. Based on his role in the Soviet Union's malaria program, likewise his colleagues. He was awarded the Stalin Prize: G.A. Pravikov, "The Stalin Prize for the Elaboration and Application of Measures in Malarial Liquidation," *Izvest. Akad. NauklurVmen SSR, Ashkhabad* 4 (1952): 90–1.

26. NAV3, UBHC KHU TT Tây Bac 7314: Kế hoạch, báo cáo các đợt chống sốt rét cơn của khu tự trị Thái Mèo [Programme and Report on the Stages of Malaria Control in the Autonomous Region of Thái Mèo].

27. NAV3, UBHC LK3, 2128: Báo cáo tổng kết kinh nghiểm về điều trị các bệnh sốt rét thương hàn của các bệnh viện Hà Nam—Hòa Bình, 1956 [Summary Report on Malaria and Typhoid Treatments at Hospitals of Hà Nam—Hòa Bình, 1956].

28. *Lịch sử Viện sốt sét*, pp. 30–4; *Đặng Văn Ngữ*, 2010, p. 183.

29. Vũ Thị Phan, *Epidémiologie du paludisme et lutte antipaludique au Vietnam* (Hanoi: Editions Médicales Vietnam, 1998), p. 31.

30. See: L.I. Zalutskaya, "Comparative Data on the Biology of *Anopheles minimus* and *A. vagus* at Tay-Nguyen [Democratic Republic of Vietnam]," *Meditsinskaya Parazitologiya i Parazitarnyye Bolezni* 28 (1959): 548–53.

31. A. Ya. Lysenko, Đặng Văn Ngữ, Hồ Văn Hưu and Đặng Tùng Thổ, "Studies in Malaria Epidemiology in North Vietnam. 1. Topographical Malariological Exploration of Thai-Nguyen Province," *Med Parazitol (Moskva)* 30 (Nov. 1961): 293–8. Available at: https://apps.dtic.mil/sti/pdfs/AD0671272.pdf [accessed 19 May 2023].

32. *Lịch sử Viện sốt sét*, pp. 34, 45. The percentage of deaths from malaria in the three regions was respectively: 22, 41 and 21 percent.

33. Andreï Yakolevich Lysenko [Лысенко, Андреї Ыаковлевич] had been at the head of the Health Department of Tajikistan. In 1957, he was at the head of the Epidemiology and Tropical Disease Prevention Department in the Institute of Medical Parasitology and Tropical Medicine. Later on, in 1962, he was appointed as a parasitology expert at the WHO. In 1974, he was nominated chief parasitologist at the Ministry of Health of the USSR, and later the Russian Federation (dic.academic.ru).

34. Since 1955 and before this date, three different institutions dealt with malaria research and prevention: the Parasitology Department of the Faculty of Medicine and Pharmacy (Đặng Văn Ngư, dir.), the malaria laboratory of the Institute of Microbiology (Hoàng Tích Trí, dir.) and the Army Malariology Department headed by Nguyễn Sĩ Quốc.

35. *Lịch sử Viện sốt sét*, p. 41.

36. Lysenko, 1961, note 31. See also: A.Y. Lysenko and I.N. Semashko, *Geography of Malaria* (Moscow, 1968). Available at: https://endmalaria.org/sites/default /files/lysenko.pdf [accessed 19 May 2023].

37. *Lịch sử Viện sốt sét*, p. 60.

38. Lysenko, 1961, note 31.

39. Lysenko and Semashko, *Geography of Malaria*, p. 27.

40. *Lịch sử Viện sốt sét*, p. 61.

41. Bruce-Chwatt, "Malaria Research and Eradication in the USSR," p. 753.

42. *Đặng Văn Ngữ*, 2010, p. 180.

43. *Lịch sử Viện sốt sét*, pp. 49–51. About the role of DRV political regime at this time, and its health system in the prevention of infectious diseases, see: John Bryant, "Communism, Poverty, and Demographic Change in North Vietnam," *Population and Development Review* 24, 2 (1998): 235–69.

44. A. Ya. Lysenko and Nguyễn Tiến Bửu, "Studies in Malaria Epidemiology in North Viet Nam. 2. Topographical Malariological Exploration of the Thái Mèo Autonomous Region," *Med Parazitol (Moskva)* 30 (Nov–Dec 1961): 643–51. Available at: https://apps.dtic.mil/sti/pdfs/AD0671273.pdf [accessed 19 May 2023].

45. About the process of agricultural reform conducted in DRV, see: Alexander Woodside, "Decolonization and Agricultural Reform in Northern Vietnam," *Asian Survey* 10, 8 (1970): 705–23. For a comparison with China: Benedict J. Tria Kerkvliet and Mark Selden, "Agrarian Transformations in China and Vietnam," *The China Journal* 40 (1998): 37–58.

46. Pyotr Grigorievich Sergiev [Пётр Григорьевич Сéргиев], 1893–1973, was parasitologist and epidemiologist, member of the Academy of Medical Sciences of the USSR (1944) and hero of Socialist Labour (1963). He led the plan for malaria elimination in the USSR (dic.academic.ru).

47. NAVN3, Bộ Y Tế 5585, Công văn, kế hoạch, đề án nghiên cứu bệnh mặt hột, sốt rét ở Việt nam của Bộ Y tế Liên Xô, năm 1959 [Official Correspondence, Plan, and Project of Research on Trachoma and Malaria in Vietnam by the Soviet Ministry of Health, 1959]: Letter Đặng Văn Ngữ–Sergiev, 14 August 1959. This file contains the correspondence in French between the two men (probably their only common language), but translations exist in Vietnamese as well as in Russian, which are also kept in other files of the National Archives.

48. NAVN3, Bộ Y Tế 5585, Công văn, kế hoạch, đề án nghiên cứu [Official Correspondence, Plan, and Project of Research].

49. *Đặng văn Ngữ*, 2010, p. 185. Several larvicide methods were studied: larvivorous fish (*Tilapia Mossambica*), green manure . . . In every district of DRV, there was one pilot commune designated to apply these methods.

50. Romania, one of the southern-most countries of the Soviet sphere, had developed a wide network of malaria control after WWII, and achieved very effective results in eradicating the disease: M. Ciucă, "Le paludisme en Roumanie de 1949 à 1955," *Bulletin of the World Health Organization* 15 (1956): 725–51. Pr Mihai Ciucă, of the Cantacuzene Institute in Bucarest, was the most eminent Romanian malaria expert. He undertook several research visits in Asia, but we do not know whether he took part in the mission cited above.

51. NAVN3, Bộ Y Tế 718, Đề án, Báo cáo tổng kết công tác Y tế năm 1958–1960 và 1960 của viện sốt rét thuộc Bộ Y tế [Plan and Summary Report on Work of the Malaria Institute (Ministry of Health) in 1958–1960 and 1960]. In the Thái Nguyên province, the malaria incidence was 33 times lower, in the Hoà Bình province 180 times lower.

52. *Lịch sử Viện sốt sét*, p. 66.

53. N.F. Kompantsev, "Кампания ликвидации малярии в Северном Вьетнаме и помощь Советского Союза" [Malaria Eradication Campaign in Northern Vietnam, and Assistance Given by the USSR] *Медицинская паразитология и паразитарные болезни* [Medical Parasitology and Parasitic Diseases] 32, 6 (1963): 752–3.

54. *Lịch sử Viện sốt sét*, pp. 58–60.

55. NAVN3, Bộ Văn Hóa 3187: Thông tri của Bộ Văn Hóa về công tác văn hóa phục vụ công tác tiêu diệt sốt rét trên toàn miền Bắc năm 1961, Hanoi 30/9/1961 [Ministry of Culture Circular Concerning Cultural Work Serving Malaria Eradication in the North in 1961].

56. NAVN3, UBHC Khu Tự Trị Tây Bắc 7357: Thông tri của UBHC Tự Trị Thái Méo về hướng dẫn cộng tác tuyên truyền phục vụụ kế hoạạch tiêu diệt bệnh sốt rét năm 1961 [Thái Mèo Autonomous Committee Circular Providing Propaganda Guidelines for Malaria Eradication Plan in 1961].

57. Paula A. Michaels, "Medical Propaganda and Cultural Revolution in Soviet Kazakhstan, 1928–41," *The Russian Review* 59, 2 (2000): 159–78.

58. NAVN3, UBHC KHU TT Tây Bắc 7314: Kế hoạch, báo cáo các đợt chống sốt rét cơn của khu tự trị Thái Mèo [Malaria Report and Control Plan in the Autonomous Region Thái Mèo].

59. Medical propaganda focused on other common transmissible diseases as well. For a more general view of "hygiene education" in the North Vietnam countryside after 1954, see: Shaun Kingsley Malarney, "Germ Theory, Hygiene and the Transcendence of 'Backwardness' in Revolutionary Vietnam (1954–60)," in *Southern Medicine for Southern People: Vietnamese Medicine in the Making*, ed. L. Monnais, C.M. Thompson and A. Wahlberg (Newcastle Upon Tyne, UK: Cambridge Scholars, 2012), pp. 107–32.

60. About the Vietnamese State policy toward ethnic minorities since 1954, see: Céline Marangé, *Le communisme vietnamien* (Paris: Presse de Science Po, 2012), pp. 467–86. See also: Patricia Pelley, "'Barbarians' and 'Younger Brothers': The Remaking of Race in Postcolonial Vietnam," *Journal of Southeast Asian Studies* 29, 2 (1998): 374–91.

61. NAVN3, UBHC Khu Tự Trị Tây Bắc 7357: "hoạch này . . . còn có một ý nghĩa chính trị rộng lớn gây ảnh hưởng tốt tới đồng bào miền Nam và các nước lành giềng với ta như Lào. . . ."

62. "Công Tác Chống Sốt Rét Ở Miền Nam. Bài của Giáo sư Đặng Văn Ngữ, phát trong 'Buổi phát thanh dành cho đồng bào' Nam 22 giờ 30, ngày 15-10-1960, *Đài Tiếng nói Việt Nam*" [Malaria Control in the South. Pr Dang Van Ngu's Speech, Broadcasted in 'Program for the Compatriots' 10:30 pm, 15-10-1960, on the Radio *Vietnam Voice*], in *Đặng Văn Ngữ Một Trí Tuệ Việt Nam* [Dang Van Ngu, a Vietnamese Intellectual], ed. Trường Đại Học Y Hà Nội (Hà Nội: Nhà Xuất Bản Chính Trị Quốc Gia - Sự Thật, 2014), pp. 74–80.

63. Marangé, *Le communisme vietnamien*, pp. 314–15. The main ideological and strategical conflict dealt with the continuation of armed struggle in the South versus "peaceful coexistence," advocated by Moscow. This also resulted in a new rapprochement with Beijing. However, relations with Moscow recovered before the end of 1964.

64. Dr Phạm Huy Tiến was in charge of studying this problem, which was due to mosquitoes transporting on boats from high regions to the delta. In this study, besides *A. minimus*, which was the main vector responsible for epidemics in the delta, he could identify two new Anopheles species there (several interviews).

65. *Lịch sử Viện sốt sét*, pp. 88–91.

66. According to Eric D. Carter, "in the 'integral' sense, which refers to State projects that target specific locations for development and public investment": "State Visions, Landscape, and Disease: Discovering Malaria in Argentina, 1890–1920," *Geoforum* 39 (2008): 280.

67. Vu Man Loi, "Le système sanitaire et la protection de la santé," in *Population et développement au Viêt-nam*, ed. Patrick Gubry (Paris: Karthala/CEPED, 2000), pp. 140–1.

68. Đặng Văn Ngữ was certainly a fervent patriot, but he was above all a high-level scientist (see several articles in *Đặng Văn Ngữ Một Trí Tuệ Việt Nam*). Although he had himself joined the Vietnamese Party, according to a former member of the Malariology Institute, he was always seconded by a member of the Political Bureau during the meetings with the Soviet experts. In any case, the Soviet assistance did not prevent Ngữ from pursuing his own agenda. He was killed in April 1967 by an American bomb, on the South side of the 17th parallel, where he tried to develop a vaccine against malaria. The Soviet influence in Vietnamese policy has also been challenged, although in other areas of expertise, in: Vladimir Mazyrin and Adam Fforde, "Soviet Influence on Vietnamese Development Policy—Some Myths," in *Mythbusting Vietnam, Facts, Fictions, Fantasies*, ed. Catherine Earl (Copenhagen: NIAS Press, 2018), pp. 99–129.

69. *Phạm Ngọc Thạch*, February 1966: "Phải coi nhiệm vụ tiêu diệt sốt rét là nhiệm vụ chiến lược, phải coi công tác tiêu diệt sốt rét như diệt giặc Mỹ," in *Lịch sử Viện sốt sét*, p. 105.

70. WHO Archives, Geneva, Project Files, VNR/MRD/001, no. 1: Programme for malaria eradication in Vietnam; VTN-MPD-001, n°2: Malaria Control. Republic of Vietnam. General.

71. *Lịch sử Viện sốt sét*, pp. 143–60.

72. NAVN3, Phủ Thủ Tướng 9195: Báo cáo. Hoạt động của Đoàn Chuyên gia sốt rét Liên xô từ 24/2 đến 10/3/1973 [Activity of the Soviet Specialists in Malaria from 24/2 to AO/3/1973]; 18401: Biên bản làm việc của đoàn chuyên viên sốt rét Bộ Y tế nước Việt Nam Dân chủ Cộng hòa và đoàn chuyên viên sốt rét Bộ Y tế Liên xô [Working Minutes of the Delegation of Malaria Experts from the Ministry of Health of the Democratic Republic of Vietnam and the Delegation of Malaria

Experts from the Ministry of Health of the Soviet Union]. The soviet team comprised an epidemiologist, Robert Kouznetsov, an assistant physician, Serguei Litvinov, and an entomologist, Vera Anoufrieva. On the Vietnamese side, two IMPE members, including the director, Mrs Vũ Thị Phan, and Nguyễn Tiến Bửu, epidemiologist, as well as Hô Như Vinh, also an epidemiologist from the Health Ministry, were responsible for preparing a new project.

CHAPTER 6

Mobilizing Applied Medical Knowledge in Indonesia: Soekarnoist Science and Asian–African Solidarity in the 1950s

Vivek Neelakantan

Introduction

On 8 August 1958, at the closing reception of the First Indonesian Science Conference in Malang, President Soekarno highlighted the significance of applied sciences to nation-building.

> Life has not taken me to any house of science but has destined me to go to villages, cities, markets, to get in touch with farmers and workers. Science has always been revolutionary. Science is always searching whereas religion is based on belief.[1]

For Soekarno, science was an instrument to realize the objective of the Indonesian Revolution (1945–49), of a just and prosperous society ("masjarakat jang adil dan makmur"). At the conference, the president exhorted Indonesians to rethink whether the application of science in the country was congruent with the revolutionary objective. To this end, Soekarno suggested a reappraisal of science that would not only be confined to Indonesia's national orbit but would also embrace humankind. This vignette highlights the simultaneity of science as universal phenomenon and local effect, a discerning feature of Soekarno-era science (1945–67).

This chapter explicates the historical circumstances that led to the mobilization of applied sciences, especially medicine, in nation-building in post-colonial

Indonesia.[2] In 1943, at the height of the Japanese occupation of the Indonesian archipelago, Soekarno had, for the first time, articulated the symbolic role physicians would play in future Indonesia in terms of nurturing a strong and healthy population ("rakjat jang sehat dan kuat").[3] As the Indonesian novelist Pramoedya Ananta Toer put it succinctly in *Jejak Langkah* (Footsteps), "A doctor must not only cure the disease of the body, he must also awaken the spirit of his people anesthetized by their own ignorance."[4]

Physicians dominated the first generation of nationalist leaders in the Dutch East Indies (present-day Indonesia) and the Philippines under American colonialism (1898–1946). For the nationalist physicians of both colonies, decolonization was yoked to the tropes of scientific progress. Physicians from the Dutch East Indies and the Philippines under American control deployed organic metaphors derived from their medical training to diagnose ills of the proto-national body politic.[5] This chapter contends that subsequent to the transfer of political sovereignty to Indonesia (1949), the legacy of nationalist physicians in shaping the trajectory of scientific thinking continued in terms of symbolically aligning medical research with national exigencies, arising partially in response to the Cold War.

The early 1950s coincided with decolonization in Southeast Asia. The US was apprehensive about the spread of communism and sought to purchase the loyalties of leaders of newly independent nations of Asia through technical assistance, channeled through UN agencies such as the The World Health Organization (WHO). By portraying poverty and disease as the breeding grounds of communism, the US sought to assist disease eradication, especially the anti-malaria campaigns in Indonesia. Indonesian leaders were aware of the political ramifications of participating in disease eradication programs led by the US.[6] President Soekarno sought to achieve a delicate equilibrium between maintaining Indonesia's political sovereignty on one hand, with increased receptiveness to technical assistance from the US and the Soviet Union, on the other.

This chapter outlines a notion of Soekarnoist science. The argument has three strands. First, Soekarnoist science was packaged as a comprehensive program of delivery intended to address the basic needs of the people. Second, Soekarno understood science functionally, in terms of relating it to national needs; and strategically, in terms of nurturing Indonesia's Cold War ambitions as leader of the Non-Aligned Movement resulting from the Asian–African Conference convened in Bandung (1955). Third, physicians occupied a prominent niche in the evolution of post-colonial science. The prosopographies of three physicians—Sardjito, Sarwono Prawirohardjo and Soedjono Djoened Poesponegoro—collectively illustrate science was both central to the autobiography of the Indonesian nation and a nation-building project (*pembangunan*). This chapter does not focus on specific disease eradication campaigns in Indonesia during the 1950s. Rather, it examines the specific meanings attributed to disease by President Soekarno and Indonesian physicians in the context of nation-building. Medical sciences such as nutrition and pediatrics—which physicians strategically related to the nationalist objective of economic self-sufficiency—shaped the trajectory of Soekarnoist science.

Qualifying the "post-colonial" in Soekarnoist science is problematic. Post-colonial has been taken to signify a time period after colonialism; a critique of the legacy of colonialism; an ideological backing for newly independent states; a demonstration of the complicity of Western knowledge with colonial projects; or an argument that colonial engagements can reveal the ambivalence, anxiety and instability deep within Western thought and practice.[7] Post-colonial theory has worked to destabilize or challenge the notion that Western knowledge is objective, authoritative and universally applicable. Post-colonial science as a field of enquiry crosses geopolitical boundaries as it tracks flows, circuits of scientists, knowledges, machines and techniques.[8] Post-colonial science— that focuses on contact zones of clashing knowledges—is dangerously incomplete unless it is firmly situated in political and institutional contexts.[9] Science is central to the forging of the post-colonial state. As a result, it exists simultaneously as history, myth, political slogan, as technology and as an instrument of change.[10] In the Indonesian context, post-colonial science existed simultaneously as history, myth and political slogan—as reflected in Soekarno's speeches—and as an instrument of change indicating the confidence in Indonesia's ancient and modern scientific credentials and the commanding role of the state in nation-building.[11]

Soekarno's Authorial Voice in Science

Given his antecedents as a civil engineer and president of Indonesia, Soekarno lent his authorial voice to science, as was evident in his speeches and writings. Soekarnoist science was packaged as a comprehensive program of socio-economic change, intended to transform the prevalent mindset of the Indonesians. While inspiring national pride in Indonesia's past accomplishments, science was also a negotiation tool in Indonesia's international relations with both the USSR and the US.[12]

While laying the foundation stone of the Faculty of Agriculture at Bogor in 1952, Soekarno observed that the problem of food scarcity was one of the most pressing problems for Indonesia.[13] He noted that the population of Indonesia was growing at a rate of 800,000 per annum during the early 1950s, whereas the rice deficit was estimated at 700,000 tonnes.[14] He cited the estimates of the Food and Agriculture Organization to indicate that the per capita intake of the average Indonesian was only 1,700 calories as opposed to 2,121 calories for India, 2,348 calories for Burma, 2,918 calories for Cuba and 2,127 calories for Indochina.[15]

For Soekarno, increasing the daily caloric intake of the average Indonesian was congruent with his vision of a strong and healthy nation.[16] For increasing the caloric intake of the average Indonesian, Soekarno noted that the country had either to increase the production of rice, or had to turn to locally available sources of carbohydrate such as corn or cassava. Widespread hunger, attributed to a scarcity of rice, had resulted, in Soekarno's words, in a "want-to-live" or "want-to-die" situation ("mau hidup ataukah mau mati").[17] The importation of rice had drained Indonesia of millions of dollars' worth of foreign exchange. To alleviate the situation, Soekarno recommended the intensive cultivation of paddy fields, the opening up of new lands for cultivation in the Outer Islands (especially in Sumatra and Kalimantan), and changing the dietary habits of the people by increasing the intake of animal protein.[18] By the late 1950s, the Soviet Union had offered the results of its rice research to Indonesia, but Soekarno was dissatisfied. He stressed that the research into high-yielding varieties of rice needed to be undertaken in Indonesia itself.

For Soekarno, industrialization was Indonesia's solution to alleviating the excessive pressure of population on land and harnessing the country's natural resources. Industrialization was contingent on nurturing the technical skills of the population. At a public lecture delivered to students at Universitas Gadjah Mada in Yogyakarta (1962), Soekarno asserted that unlike Mahatma Gandhi—who had a distrust of industrialization and labeled machines the "world of the devil"—Indonesian planners would apply mechanized production to achieve the equitable distribution of essential commodities.[19] For Soekarnoist science, technology was the means to develop the foundations of a socialist society.

The president situated science in the autobiography of the Indonesian nation. He observed that in the 17th century, the country had a self-supporting textile industry, but by the 19th century Indonesia depended on imported textiles from the Netherlands.[20] With the industrial revolution in Europe in the 19th century, demand for raw materials, sugarcane and tobacco replaced rice as the staple crops on the island of Java. Soekarno blamed the colonial legacy for Java's rice shortages and poverty. Soekarno maintained that due to Dutch colonialism, Indonesia was reduced to "Een volk van koelies een koelie onder de naties" (A nation among coolies and a coolie among nations).[21] Science provided Indonesia with a means of redemption from economic dependence on foreign countries and a revived national glory.[22]

Soekarno sought to gain respectability for Indonesian science on the world stage. He noted that subsequent to the transfer of political sovereignty, the Indonesian Revolution was transformed into a struggle to conquer nature, given the challenges of natural disasters such as floods, volcanoes and earthquakes.[23] His exemplar was the 11th-century King Airlangga (which literally means Water Gulper) who tamed the wild Brantas river—notorious for its devastating floods—and established an irrigation system.[24] Soekarno pointed out that as Indonesians were heirs to a glorious past, they could not be considered a weak nation ("satu bangsa tempe").[25] By the ninth century, Indonesia had built grand monuments such as Borobudur and Prambanan. By presenting these two examples from history, Soekarno lent credibility to the notion that Indonesian knowledge was useful to the world of science.[26]

Salient features of Soekarnoist science included Indonesia-centeredness and self-sufficiency in economic affairs. In positing science as central to the autobiography of the Indonesian nation, Soekarno's reading of Indonesian history portrayed a glorious past, loss of economic independence under Dutch colonialism and challenges associated with nation-building in the 1950s.

The Bandung Moment, Medicine and Cold War Propaganda in Indonesia

The economic self-sufficiency of newly independent nations in Asia and Africa was a defining feature of the Bandung Conference (1955). The immediate outcome of the conference was the communique, which spelt out the urgency of promoting economic development in Asia and Africa, cultural cooperation and world peace. The notion of the "Third World," which has gained currency since the Bandung Conference, refers to a political alternative to the communist and capitalist worldviews.[27] Although raising the health standards of people in Asia and Africa was not directly mentioned in the communique, Soekarno mentioned this goal in his opening address.

In addition to Soekarno, the Bandung Conference hosted delegates of various ideological persuasions, particularly Jawaharlal Nehru from India, Gamel Abdul Nasser from Egypt, Zhou-en-Lai from China, U Nu from Burma and Hồ Chí Minh from North Vietnam. Delegates looked beyond ideological disagreements among capitalism, communism and pan-Islamism and focused instead on repudiation of colonialism, of relations of dependency, war, racism and questions associated with poverty. Domestically, Soekarno aspired to promote such solidarity, partly to address ethnic and ideological differences extant in Indonesia between 1950 and 1955.

Soekarno's view of development was shaped by a need to balance contending political forces such as nationalism, communism and Islam. He tried to unify the contending forces through a shared project of *pembangunan*. *Pembangunan* was embodied in projects such as a massive national telecommunications network across the Indonesian archipelago, a high-rise hotel and numerous monuments across Jakarta. These lighthouse projects fulfilled a symbolic function as they signalled to Indonesia and the rest of the world that the country was capable of pursuing its own path to modernity, independent of the US or the USSR.[28]

Between 1950 and 1957, Indonesia witnessed the rise and fall of no less than seven cabinets in quick succession and no government could constitute an absolute majority. A number of political parties, led by the Islamist Masjumi, sought to forge closer ties with the US while weakening communism at home, in contrast to the Partai Nasional Indonesia (PNI) that espoused a more radical foreign policy.[29] During the Soekiman Cabinet (1951–52), dominated by the Masjumi politicians, Indonesia's Foreign Minister Subardjo secretly signed an agreement committing Indonesia to technical and economic assistance from the US. Not surprisingly, disclosure of the agreement led to the fall of Soekiman's Cabinet in 1952 due to the fear of compromising the country's hard-won political sovereignty. The fall of Wilopo's Cabinet in 1953 was due to the weak coalition between the PNI and Masjumi.

Between 1950 and 1955, Indonesia faced two sets of economic problems: (a) political instability made it difficult for the government to execute austerity measures; and (b) Indonesian dependence on a narrow range of export commodities such as rubber, petroleum and tin.[30] In 1951, riding on the high prices of export commodities brought about by the Korean War, Indonesia recorded a budgetary surplus of 1,200 million rupiah. In contrast, in the following year, the country recorded a 4,300 million rupiah deficit.[31] Indonesia's economic troubles created disillusionments with US aid promises.

The Bandung Conference of 1955 coincided with a need to improve the image of the PNI prior to the country's first general elections. The outgoing PNI's poor record regarding its economic policies attracted criticism from the Masjumi. The country attracted international criticism for failing to liberate West Irian by peaceful means. The conference generated considerable political capital for Prime Minister Ali Sastroamidjojo of the PNI as it established Indonesia's credentials as a leader of the Third World.[32]

The Bandung Conference resolved to promote the economic development of the Asian and African nations.[33] First, the conference advocated cooperation between countries based on mutual interest and respect for national sovereignty. Second, participating countries agreed to provide technical assistance to one another. Third, the conference delegates recommended collective action be taken to stabilize the prices and demand for primary commodities through bilateral and multilateral agencies and working together for that purpose with international agencies. Although the Bandung Conference delegates welcomed international aid—especially in the field of capital investments, both through bilateral arrangements and through such institutions as the International Bank—they emphasized that such aid should not interfere with national sovereignty.[34] The Bandung Conference left several questions pertaining to economic development unanswered. For example, how would newly independent countries secure technical and managerial knowhow suitable for their conditions? The conference alluded to mutual aid and cooperation between Asian and African nations but did not specify the fields, for example the sharing of technical expertise in agriculture and medicine, in which such cooperation could materialize.

In his opening address delivered at the Bandung Conference on 18 April 1955, in an effort to nurture solidarity amongst Asian and African nations of disparate political leanings, Soekarno denounced imperialism and racism:

> The twentieth century has been a period of terrific dynamism. Perhaps the last fifty years have seen more developments and more material progress than the previous five hundred years. Man has learned to control many of the scourges which once threatened him. He has learned to overcome distance. He has learned to project his voice across oceans and continents. He has probed deep into the secrets of nature and learned how to make the deserts bloom and the plants of the earth increase their bounty. He has learned how to release the immense forces locked in the smallest particles of matter.[35]

The underlining concern of Soekarno's opening address was world peace. Soekarno noted that war was the consequence of human fears, such as the fear of the hydrogen bomb and fear of ideologies.[36] He urged delegates to the Bandung Conference to mobilize the spiritual and political strength of Asia and Africa in the cause of peace.

During the early and mid-1950s, in its efforts to contain the spread of communist ideology, the US policy in Indonesia was based on strengthening the anti-communist forces, such as the Masjumi Party, in order to wean Soekarno from the Partai Komunis Indonesia (PKI). But, given the losses sustained by the Masjumi in the 1955 election, and the fear of losing Indonesia to the

Soviet orbit, the US loaned Indonesia $6 million per annum for developmental assistance, mainly directed at malaria control.[37]

In a 1955 speech, President Dwight D. Eisenhower noted that improved health stymied poverty and misery, well-known breeding grounds of disorder (and consequently communism):

> Of all diseases, malaria, which attacked 200 million people last year and killed two million is probably the world's worst remaining source of poverty and misery. We are now to undertake, in cooperation with the World Health Organization and the countries affected, a project to abolish malaria once and for all from the face of the earth. We are willing to cooperate with Soviet Russia and Communist China in this work of peace, if they will agree.[38]

The above speech highlighted the Eisenhower administration's Cold War propaganda to differentiate the purpose of the US aid program that was based on raising the standards of the people in Asia and Africa and the furtherance of world peace. In contrast, the USSR was alleged to use newly independent countries as "feeders" for its economy and pawns in the Cold War rivalry.[39]

Upon the announcement of US technical assistance for Indonesia's malaria eradication program, Soekarno critiqued the piecemeal nature of technical assistance by stating that "man does not live on bread alone."[40] Instead, Indonesia expected greater moral support from the US in the resolution of the West Irian dispute with the Netherlands.

In 1956, the US continued to focus on bread by providing surplus agricultural commodities worth US$97.6 million under the PL480 program.[41] The International Cooperation Administration (ICA)—predecessor to the United States Agency for International Development, that operated between 1955 and 1961—was instrumental in affiliating the Agricultural College at Bogor with the University of Kentucky.[42]

At the time, the US began to use universities as major resources for technical assistance due to their long association in the hurly-burly of American development.[43] Kentucky researchers had gained considerable experience working in the Appalachian areas of the state underlined by high poverty. The challenge of meeting the developmental needs of Kentucky led the state to select the faculty with motivation for and skill in development. Although the Kentucky faculty was unfamiliar with local agricultural conditions in Indonesia, conditioned by a tropical climate, it was skilled in the application of research findings to further agricultural production and enhance rural welfare. Many well-considered plans and policies to stimulate economic development and ameliorate facilities for rural health, education and welfare originated from

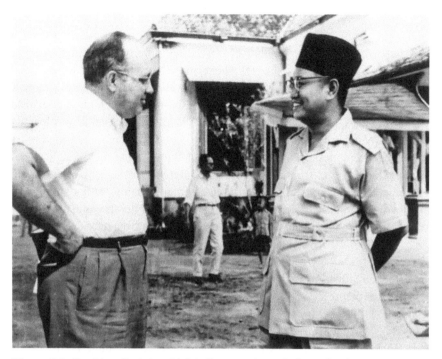

Figure 6.1. President Soekarno (right) discusses the malaria eradication program with United States Public Health Services (USPHS) officer Roy Fritz, c. 1959. NLM Unique ID: 101446992. Courtesy of the National Library of Medicine.

the University of Kentucky. During the 1950s, it was in the US's political interest that Indonesia would not fall behind the curtain of communism, either iron or bamboo. Technical assistance became a major plank of US foreign policy, particularly during the Eisenhower era (1953–61).

During the Eisenhower era, the malaria program remained of utmost importance to further US strategic interests in Indonesia. Technical aid to Indonesia consisted of high-impact demonstration programs such as the widespread use of the insecticide DDT against the anopheline species. Unfortunately, by the mid-1950s, the anopheline species turned resistant to DDT.[44] The US Assistant Secretary for Far Eastern Affairs, Walter S. Robertson (1953–59), issued a warning to the effect that if the US were to cease assisting the antimalarial program in Indonesia, resurgence of the disease would follow and provide a ready target for elements unfriendly to US interests (such as the PKI).[45] Due to Soekarno's reversion to the 1945 Constitution, which suspended parliamentary institutions, and the strengthening of Indonesia's bilateral ties with the USSR, the funding for malaria was reduced by 50 percent in 1959.[46]

In the aftermath of the Bandung Conference, the USSR became increasingly interested in providing technical assistance to Indonesia, although a decade earlier Soviet officials had offered no more than verbal support to Indonesian independence at the UN. The relations between the two were shaped by Soekarno's Marhaenist ideology, an uneasy coalescence between nationalist, Islamic and Marxist socialist elements.[47] Whereas the PKI and Soekarno (between 1955 and 1965) actively sought Soviet developmental assistance, the Masjumi, Nahdatul Ulama and the military were fearful of increasing Soviet influence in Indonesia. The Soviet premier, Nikita Khrushchev, sought to derive political capital from the Bandung Conference by signing bilateral aid agreements with countries not yet in the communist camp. Although Indonesia did not fit into the strict definition of a socialist state, its condemnation of colonialism at the Bandung Conference drew attention from the Soviet Union.[48]

By 1956, the USSR had appropriated the spirit of the Bandung Conference in terms of collaborating with Indonesia for the furtherance of the movement against colonialism and slavery, and raising people's living standards. In September 1956, the USSR signed an agreement with Indonesia to assist the latter country in implementing its Five-Year Plan.[49] To this effect, the USSR lent an advance of US$250 million without any strings attached to the loan. In its bid to check growing American influence in Indonesia, the USSR sketched a paradox that, although Indonesia was a rich country, it suffered from widespread hunger as its natural resources were exploited by foreigners (alluding to the Dutch colonial legacy and growing US intervention).[50] Soviet leader Nikita Khrushchev contrasted the Soviet health system from that of the US. He noted that public health received negligible attention in the US budget in contrast to centralized planning extant in the USSR that was directed at raising people's living standards and tackling poverty.[51]

By 1960, the Soviets were using public health as a tool of political propaganda. Soviet Deputy Health Minister D.D. Venediktov's vision of international health was translated into Bahasa Indonesia.[52] He contended that the question of health in the newly independent nations of Asia and Africa was essentially a socio-economic one. These countries lacked an adequate health infrastructure to deal with the burden of infectious diseases such as smallpox, cholera and plague. The Soviet Union was keen to share its technical expertise in public health with newly independent nations. To this effect, it launched preventive health initiatives, such as educating public health personnel, and provided aid for mass campaigns against smallpox across Asia and Africa. In the case of Indonesia, the Soviets sponsored the then Minister of Health Satrio's visit to Moscow to study the Soviet health system in 1961.[53] In Asia, Indonesia was by far the largest recipient of Soviet aid between 1959 and 1965, amounting to

789 million roubles.[54] The Soviets offered loans to Indonesia at low rates of interest with the hope of stimulating economic growth. Indonesia prioritized USSR technical assistance in the fields of large-scale development projects, particularly hydroelectric projects, coal mines and the exploration of non-ferrous mineral ore deposits. The Indonesians were given considerable leeway in how to utilize the Soviet aid.

Despite considerable Soviet investment in Indonesia, the Indonesians managed to complete only one project, the Soviet-Indonesian Hospital of Friendship (Rumah Sakit Persahabatan).[55] Between 1959 and 1965, Soekarno diverted 90 percent of Soviet aid towards the development of the Indonesian military on two fronts: (a) campaign against Malaysia, and (b) the campaign to press Indonesia's claims to West Irian.[56] Indonesian economic development during the 1950s was severely handicapped by a shortage of capital. In the case of US economic assistance to Indonesia, major drawbacks included Indonesian suspicion of technical assistance, hypersensitive nationalism and bureaucratic inefficiency.

Physicians as Architects of Post-colonial Indonesian Science

There are evident dangers in focusing entirely on Soekarno, of exaggerating the contribution of one individual to post-colonial Indonesian science. As the architect of modern Indonesia, he introduced *pembangunan*, a shared nation-building endeavor transcending political ideologies. It could be argued that Soekarno appropriated the scientific agenda of Indonesian physicians and gave them a definite form through *pembangunan*. During the Soekarno era, nationalist physicians, particularly M. Sardjito, Sarwono Prawirohardjo, and Soedjono Djoened Poesponegoro became influential players in Indonesian science. Since the turn of the 20th century, physicians in the East Indies, given their ability to appropriate biological metaphors derived from medical training, were able to diagnose independent Indonesia's *shortcomings* in science, and prescribe suitable policy interventions.[57]

M. Sardjito's Utopian Vision for Science

M. Sardjito, a 1915 School tot Opleiding van Inlandsche Artsen or the School for the Training of Native Doctors (STOVIA) alumnus, undertook his first research project on the outbreak of influenza in the Dutch East Indies. STOVIA—founded in 1902—was the only place in the Dutch East Indies where indigenous people could receive advanced training in scientific and experimental methods. In 1922, the Rockefeller Foundation offered him a fellowship to undertake further studies in epidemiology at Johns Hopkins University.[58] In the mid-1920s, he returned to Indonesia to work in the Central Laboratory of Medicine at Weltevreden and subsequently served in the Dutch East Indies Medical Service (Dienst der Volksgezondheid). In 1943, at the height of the Japanese occupation, he was active in Izi Hoko Kai (the Association of Indonesian Physicians, which was active during the Japanese occupation of Indonesia, 1942–45), which promoted research on effective indigenous herbal remedies (*djamu*). Shortly after the defeat of Japan and the Proclamation of Indonesian Independence (1945), he headed the Pasteur Institute in Bandung before it was relocated to Klaten in central Java during the Dutch occupation. In 1946 he founded Balai Perguruan Tinggi, the precursor to Universitas Gadjah Mada (UGM, established in 1949) and the first Indonesian academy of higher education of its kind in Jakarta, which was subsequently relocated to central Java during the revolutionary period. Subsequently he officiated as the president of UGM from 1949 to 1961. Sardjito's vision was that Indonesia would transform itself from an underdeveloped nation to a developed one by raising the levels of literacy and the technical skills of the population.[59]

In April 1946, during his inaugural lecture to medical students at Surakarta, Sardjito contrasted research in the Dutch East Indies to research that would be undertaken in post-colonial Indonesia.[60] In 1931, the Geneeskunde Hoogeschool (the Medical Faculty in Jakarta, established in 1927), under the leadership of professor C.D. de Langen, had undertaken a nutritional survey in the central Javanese village of Kutawinangun, which became famous as the Gobang Report (1935).[61] The investigations revealed that every individual in the village existed on less than 2.5 cents per day.[62] Sardjito lamented that little had changed since 1935. He critiqued the Gobang Report, and indirectly colonial medical research, for ostensibly focusing on a research investigation that did not lead to a practical solution to the problem of malnutrition. Sardjito had envisioned a unique niche for Indonesian physicians in resuscitating a strong and healthy population and addressing the problem of malnutrition. He exhorted Indonesian medical students to follow in the footsteps of bacteriologists, particularly Robert Koch (who discovered the cholera bacillus), and Louis Pasteur (whose discovery of the chicken cholera vaccine revolutionized the field of bacteriology). Sardjito's lecture pointed out the urgency and necessity for Indonesia to undertake research in endemic diseases ("penjakit rakjat") such as yaws, leprosy and tuberculosis that vitiated the overall productive capacity of the population.[63]

Towards the end of his inaugural lecture, Sardjito lamented that Indonesia did not produce scientists of the calibre of Pasteur and Koch.[64] He diagnosed the chief drawback of Indonesian [medical] science as the relatively low research output in international journals and the shortage of physicians in relation to the total population. Sardjito's speech ended on an optimistic note that, despite hurdles imposed by the Dutch military blockades such as the translocation of the Pasteur Institute to Klaten, or the shortage of bacterial cultures, Indonesian bacteriologists continued with their research uninterrupted.[65]

Sardjito identified natural resources, a skilled and literate population, a strong work ethic, and a glorious past as key ingredients that would lead Indonesia to national glory.[66] As Indonesia was a young nation, he prescribed raising the population's literacy levels and technical skills, minimizing political differences through the promotion of *Pantjasila* (the philosophical underpinnings of the Indonesian state), and utilizing centralized Five-Year Plans. As president of UGM, Sardjito sought to nurture both research and teaching that demanded coordination between different faculties,[67] and envisioned that each city in Indonesia would establish a university.

Sardjito identified a strong and healthy population as a critical ingredient in *pembangunan*. He had a holistic understanding of public health and attributed the prevalence of disease to a host of socio-economic factors. The construction of Indonesian science as the antithesis of Western (colonial) science, the appropriation of biological metaphors, and the extensive use of Javanese symbolism were three strategies used by Sardjito in articulating his utopian vision for science, which was aimed at transforming Indonesia into a developed country.

Sarwono Prawirohardjo and the Institutionalization of Science

Sarwono Prawirohardjo (b. 1906) was a 1929 STOVIA alumnus. Between 1929 and 1937 he served as a government health officer in the Riau archipelago. Between 1937 and 1939 he specialized in gynecology under the supervision of Professor Remmelts at the Geneeskunde Hoogeschool (GH, the Faculty of Medicine at Jakarta).[68] In 1942, at the height of the Japanese occupation, he became assistant professor in the Medical Academy at Jakarta (Ika Dai Gaku). In 1945, along with Sardjito, he was the co-founder of Balai Perguruan Tinggi. After the Proclamation of Indonesian Independence on 17 August 1945, Prawirohardjo was co-opted into the National Committee for Indonesian Independence. He was faced with the challenge of nurturing Indonesian science, given the exodus of Dutch scientists to the Netherlands between 1945 and 1949.

In 1948, Lt. Governor General van Mook established the Organisatie voor Natuurwetenschappelijk Onderzoek (OSR, or the Organization for Scientific

Research), which was the umbrella organization that coordinated research in all branches of natural sciences in Indonesia. With the transfer of sovereignty to the Indonesian republic, the *OSR News* ceased publication.[69] The exodus of several Dutch scientists to the Netherlands created vacancies in research positions. The revolutionary government's Nationalization Decree (1946)—which mandated that all lectures in higher education be delivered in Bahasa Indonesia—was probably a reaction to the domination of Dutch professors in higher education. In 1950, Prawirohardjo founded the Ikatan Dokter Indonesia (IDI, or the Indonesian Medical Association). The establishment of IDI immediately terminated the activities of the 99-year-old Society for the Furthering of Medical Sciences in Indonesia (Vereenigiging tot Bevordering der Geneeskundige Wetenschappen in Indonesie). The reasons for the abrogation of this society could be attributed to the exclusion of several Indonesian doctors from its membership.[70] Prawirohardjo was undoubtedly the most influential member of the IDI, given his standing as Professor of Obstetrics and Gynaecology at Universitas Indonesia (UI). By 1954 he was instrumental in the transformation of the medical curricula at UI from the Dutch to the American model—a corrective measure that was intended to maximize the graduation of physicians from Indonesia's medical schools and address the adverse doctor-to-patient ratio, which was estimated at one doctor per 60,000 people during the early 1950s.[71]

In 1951, Prawirohardjo was chosen as the head of a nine-member committee appointed by Indonesia's Ministry of Education to establish the Indonesian Council of Sciences (Madjelis Ilmu Pengetahuan Indonesia, or MIPI). In April 1956, MIPI was formally established in accordance with Presidential Decree No. 118. The objectives of the MIPI included coordinating all scientific endeavors within Indonesia, establishing the country's imprint in science at the international level, and promoting science in Indonesia without undue interference from the government.[72] Although the organization's aims and objectives were lofty, the MIPI's objectives failed to fructify during the 1950s, given the low salaries drawn by academics and stringent foreign exchange regulations that hampered the purchase of textbooks from overseas.

Prawirohardjo observed that Indonesia suffered from three interrelated problems during the 1950s: internal security, international security and socio-economic development.[73] Indonesia, having tackled the first two issues, needed to mobilize its resources to achieve socio-economic development. Applied research, with an emphasis on the utilization of Indonesia's natural resources, was the means to achieve socio-economic development.[74] But Prawirohardjo contended that basic science was the lynchpin of applied research. To this end, he exhorted that Indonesia build up a critical mass in

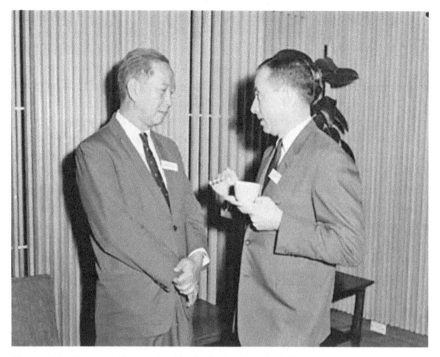

Figure 6.2. Sarwono Prawirohardjo (left), head of the MIPI, led the Indonesian delegation at the third regional meeting of National Scientific Research Organizations held
in Canberra from 17–21 February 1964. Professor Sarwono chats with Mr R.B.
Sheeks, who represented the Pacific Science Association at the meeting. Photographer,
Michael Brown. NAA: A1501, A4893/1. Courtesy: The National Archives of Australia.

the fields of life sciences, climatology and geology, in line with the United
Nations Educational, Scientific and Cultural Organization's (UNESCO)
prescriptions for the country.[75]

Prawirohardjo noted that the chief impediment to the furtherance of applied research was the shortage of trained personnel. At the time, Indonesian
universities were preoccupied with teaching and basic research and were not
robust enough to take on additional professional training and research. Indonesian research, prior to the establishment of MIPI, was uncoordinated and was
under the jurisdiction of various ministries. The only research institute affiliated with MIPI at the time was the National Biological Institute at Bogor.[76]

Prawirohardjo warned Indonesians that the country's centralized Five-
Year Plans contained elements detrimental towards creativity and facilitating
the spirit of inquiry.[77] He framed the country's bureaucracy as an "Indonesian
disease" that inhibited the growth of science.[78] For minimizing the deleterious

effects of the bureaucracy on Indonesian science, Prawirohardjo created a niche for intellectuals and university students, and established better coordination between MIPI and Bureau Perguruan Tinggi (the National Bureau for Higher Education). Furthermore, Prawirohardjo advocated socially relevant research, so that science and technology could percolate into the veins of Indonesians.[79]

Two major impediments to the realization of Prawirohardjo's vision of imbuing a scientific temper among the people were the Indonesian obsession with titles, particularly among the Javanese, and the dysfunction of higher education in the country. During the era of Dutch colonialism, the aristocratic Javanese (*prijaji*) learned to appreciate Western education in terms of its external status value while maintaining a deep reservation concerning its intellectual content.[80] The expansion of colonial rule across the East Indies archipelago at the turn of the 20th century created a demand for professionals, including physicians and engineers. The *prijaji* deprecation of manual labor greatly impeded the growth of technical and vocational education in the Dutch East Indies.[81] Indonesian nationalism provided the *prijaji* (who had varying degrees of schooling) with an avenue to satisfy their thirst for leadership, while Indonesian academicians from the medical school spent more time applying their professional skills to active politics than attending to patients. President Soekarno, one of the earliest graduates from the technical school at Bandung, only spent six years of his career as an engineer.[82] The white-collar fixation of Indonesian students during the 1950s did not translate into maximizing the number of technicians, who were badly needed for economic development.[83]

The non-utilitarian role of professionals, particularly physicians, had been accelerated by the expansion of the state apparatus during the 1950s that tended to withdraw specialists from continued practice in order to have them officiate in a supervisory capacity. Indonesia's increased participation in international organizations such as the WHO, UNESCO and UNICEF had turned its few specialists into traveling diplomats.[84]

Prawirohardjo maintained that, unlike Europe, newly independent nations in Asia, particularly Indonesia, had missed out on the scientific and industrial revolutions. As a catalyst to achieve economic growth, Indonesia resorted to technology developed in the West. This led to a state of scientific and technological neo-colonialism in which Indonesia was reduced to a state of dependency on Western technical knowhow.[85] Prawirohardjo exhorted Indonesia to realize its potential in science and technology through innovation.

Apart from his involvement in MIPI, Prawirohardjo was active in Indonesia's family planning program. In 1952, he established Yayasan Kesedjahteraan Keluarga (the Family Welfare Foundation) in Yogyakarta with an emphasis on maternal and child welfare. In 1957, aided by the Brush Foundation, Prawirohardjo founded Perkumpulan Keluarga Berentjana Indonesia (the Indonesian Family Planning Association, or PKBI). He tried to persuade Soekarno that birth control as a means of family planning was a preventive measure that could save mothers' lives.[86] But Soekarno seemed dismissive of Prawirohardjo's ideas in public. As president of Indonesia, he did not want to antagonize religious groups or uncritically accept the prescriptions of international agencies.[87] But, privately, Soekarno was sympathetic to the idea of birth control as a means to save mothers' lives.[88] Although Prawirohardjo's disagreements with Soekarno did not impede the functioning of MIPI, it cost the former his political career. He was excluded from the newly established ministerial portfolio for research.

Soedjono Djoened Poesponegoro: Pediatrics and Afro-Asian Solidarity

Soedjono Djoened Poesponegoro's notions of science converged with those of President Soekarno. Poesponegoro was able to relate pediatrics to Soekarno's conceptualization of the Indonesian Revolution as a period of investment in the human skills of the population. After graduating from the GH in 1934, he undertook a four-year specialization in pediatrics at Leiden University. Between 1938 and 1945, he practiced as a private pediatrician in Semarang. Soon after the transfer of sovereignty to the Indonesian republic (1949), Poesponegoro realized that with the deteriorating Indonesian–Dutch relationship and the exodus of Dutch academics and scientists to the Netherlands, Indonesia would suffer from a leadership vacuum that would inhibit the training of scientists and other skilled professionals. As a part of his commitment to develop Indonesia's research capabilities in medicine, in 1950 he joined the newly established Universiteit van Indonesie (UI, subsequently renamed Universitas Indonesia in 1954 to reflect the Indonesian character of the university) as a lecturer of pediatric diseases.[89] He was instrumental in introducing pediatrics as an academic specialty in UI. Due to his leadership, he was appointed as Dean of the Faculty of Medicine at UI between 1952 and 1960; UI Rector, 1958–62; and the Minister of Research between 1962 and 1966.

Poesponegoro's notion of undergraduate medical education was influenced by *pembangunan*. Based on the assumption that *pembangunan* was a dynamic process and involved socio-economic change, Poesponegoro maintained that such changes would have repercussions for public health. To this end, he emphasized the training of undergraduate students in the social, psychological and cultural problems that impacted public health,[90] and sought to nurture scientific curiosity among his medical students. Poesponegoro subscribed to the dictum "science for stakeholders."[91] He suggested that faculties

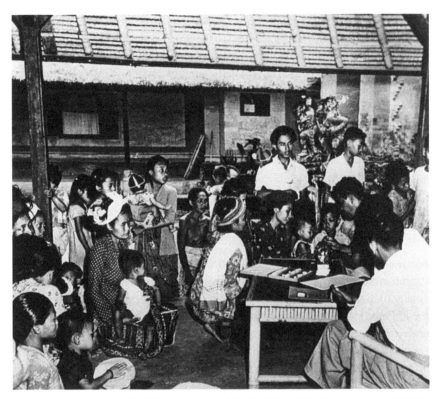

Figure 6.3. Women and children gather at a field office of the Department of Public Health and Preventive Medicine, Universitas Indonesia, c. 1961. Courtesy: USAID National Archive.

of medicine at Indonesian universities liaise with the Ministry of Health for the identification of dominant health issues affecting the community.

Poesponegoro sought to link pediatrics to *pembangunan* in his inaugural lecture delivered at UI on 7 February 1953. In his lecture, Poesponegoro appealed to Indonesian pride by stating that a nation could not be considered strong and healthy if it had a high prevalence of infant mortality.[92] In his speech, he expressed hope no less than four times (*mudah mudahan*) that with the advancement of pediatrics as an academic specialty in Indonesian schools, members of the Indonesian Dewan Perwakilan Rakjat (Indonesian House of Representatives) would become sensitized towards the problem of children's health. With women's organizations mobilizing society on the question of child health, the Ministry of Health would no longer have to deal with neonatal and infant mortality.[93] Poesponegoro's speech was indicative of the mobilization mindset underlying Soekarnoist science in the 1950s.

The Department of Paediatrics at the UI, under the leadership of Poesponegoro, initiated interdisciplinary research into nutrition in conjunction with the Nutrition Institute (*Lembaga Makanan Rakjat*, an autonomous research institute established in 1950) in Jakarta, which was directed by Poorwo Soedarmo. The aim was to discover cost-effective substitutes for milk that would help to combat kwashiorkor (protein energy malnutrition) and xerophthalmia (vitamin A deficiency) in Indonesian infants. This collaboration, in effect, initiated and demonstrated a model of collaboration between Indonesian universities and research institutes.[94] At the Nutrition Institute, Poorwo Soedarmo developed fish flour as a protein substitute for milk. Subsequently, the Department of Paediatrics at UI unsuccessfully conducted clinical trials using fish flour to treat kwashiorkor patients. Pediatricians at the UI, who attributed the prevalence of kwashiorkor and vitamin A deficiency to the colonial period, appealed to the medical profession, saying that if Indonesians sought to create a strong and healthy citizenry free of nutritional deficiencies, they needed to intensify their efforts to increase the production of animal protein and foods rich in vitamin A.[95]

Pediatrics provided cultural capital to Indonesia in terms of realizing Soekarno's political aspirations articulated at the Asian African Conference in Bandung (1955) that sought to project Indonesia as the leader of the Third World. The Second Afro-Asian Congress of Paediatrics, convened in Jakarta in 1964, built upon the social solidarity forged by delegates at the Bandung Conference convened a decade earlier. In his opening address, Poesponegoro observed that pediatrics was a powerful force in emancipating the people of the newly independent nations of Asia and Africa from the scourge of poverty. To quote Poesponegoro:

> Our successful struggles in advancing political independence have the effect that the Afro-Asian countries are now capable of striking off the bonds of ill health and misery, of freeing their people from the scourges of poverty, and of fully developing the creative potentialities of the forces imbedded in the children, the youth and the nation as a whole.
>
> For it is through our determined and continued efforts alone that we are destined to lift our nations out of the miserable stage of poverty, ill health and sufferings. Thus it is our task to examine microscopically the scientific and moral significance of medical science and its most important branch of pediatrics within a total setting of political independence and increasing Afro-Asian solidarity.[96]

The Congress approached the question of pediatric health from an interdisciplinary perspective that emphasized the social, physical and psychological factors affecting the prevalence of the disease. The Congress noted that malnutrition was not only a medical problem but also a social, agricultural and educational problem that could be ameliorated with self-help initiatives by the people themselves while minimizing international assistance.[97]

Poesponegoro was appointed as Minister for Research in 1962, a position that he held until 1966. As Minister for Research, he was head of the Departemen Urusan Nasional (DURENAS or Department of National Research) that sought to coordinate research undertaken in Indonesian universities with the activities of research institutes, particularly the Nutrition Institute, the National Institute of Biology and the Department of Agriculture, all three of which were under the jurisdiction of MIPI.[98]

Since the heads of both MIPI and DURENAS were physicians, Poesponegoro was able to achieve good working relations with Prawirohardjo by establishing a liaison between Indonesian universities and research institutes affiliated with MIPI. During Poesponegoro's tenure as Minister for Research, science policy decisions were suspended except for the holding of technology exhibitions. His ministerial position in the three Working Cabinets between 1962 and 1966 was of a short duration.[99] In 1962, given Indonesia's confrontation with Malaya and the mobilization of the military on the West Irian question, Soekarno promised that, following the normalization of the political situation, the government would allocate a greater proportion of the budget to research. Despite an assurance from Soekarno, the Ministry of Research remained severely underfunded due to the seventeen-fold depreciation in the value of the Indonesian rupiah.[100]

Conclusion: Was Soekarnoist Science a Variant of Post-colonial Science?

In his article entitled "Asia as a Method in STS Studies," Warwick Anderson observes that, since the 1970s, active debate about the meaning of science, technology and medicine has taken place within an Indian context, much of it occurring within the Gandhian, Marxist, subaltern and post-colonial frameworks.[101] A major research question raised by this study is whether Soekarnoist science was a variant of post-colonial science (in the Indian sense), or whether it embodied a distinctive national flavour? It implies locating the "post-colonial" moment in Indonesian history. The post-colonial moment, however, does not mean commemorating important dates in Indonesian history, such as the foundation of the Indonesian Medical Association in 1950 or the Indonesian

Council of Sciences in 1956. Instead, it involves asking the right kinds of questions, such as what the passing of colonialism signified and when, in relation to science, it effectively ended.[102]

This chapter has outlined a notion of Soekarnoist science that can be summed up in a few points. First, Soekarnoist science attempted to wrest science from a Western monopoly and situated it in the country's past. Second, science was packaged as a comprehensive program of socio-economic delivery. Third, Soekarno understood science functionally in terms of Indonesia's national needs—with particular reference to increasing the country's self-sufficiency in the production of rice—and strategically while establishing the country's niche in the Cold War as the leader of the Non-Aligned Movement. The country sought to maintain an equilibrium between increased receptiveness to technical assistance from the US and the USSR while maintaining its political sovereignty. In contrast, Philippine presidents, particularly Ramon Magsaysay (1953–57), understood science functionally in terms of furthering the country's aspirations to be leader of the free world in Southeast Asia.[103] Seen from the features outlined above, it can be inferred that Soekarnoist science was a variant of post-colonial science and shared several parallels with Nehruvian science in India (1947–64).[104]

What imbued Soekarnoist science with a distinctive Indonesian flavour was the niche occupied by physicians in the institutional growth of science. Another distinguishing feature of Soekarnoist science was the urgency of revolution that was directed towards the achievement of a just and prosperous society, where Soekarno stressed the need for reordering, reshaping and retooling. The speeches of Soekarno—enriched with Javanese aphorisms and underlying symbolism—were unique to Indonesia. The act of name-giving, such as naming universities after heroes (for example, Airlangga and Gadjah Mada), signified the production of scientific knowledge within the context of Indonesian history. New beginnings in a variety of prosaic activities were ceremonially made with urgent-sounding names such as *Operasi Makmur* (Prosperity Operation, 1959–60)—intended to increase rice production—and *Operasi Pemberantasan Buta Gizi* (Operation to Eradicate Ignorance in Nutrition, 1964).[105] A mobilization mindset suffused the practice of Soekarnoist science, in that the pursuit of knowledge would not only address national concerns, such as attaining self-sufficiency in food, but also broader socio-economic and political ones associated with the Cold War, such as Afro-Asian solidarity in health.

But the 1960s signalled an end to the non-aligned vision of Soekarnoist science. The exigencies of the Cold War had made such a form of post-colonial science a chimera.[106]

Notes

1. Soekarno, *Applied Sciences and Nation-Building: Speech Delivered by H.E. Soekarno at the Closing Reception of the Indonesian National Science Conference in Malang, 8 August 1958* (Jakarta: Ministry of Information Republic of Indonesia, 1958).
2. Unlike physics or chemistry, medicine is not a pure science. When we call it an applied science, it implies only principles of pure science are applied to address a medical problem. See S.C. Panda, "Medicine: Science or Art?" *Mens Sana Monographs* 4, 1 (2006): 127–38.
3. Soekarno, "Mobilizazi Dokter," *Berita Ketabiban* 1, 2, 3 and 4 (2604 [1944 of the Gregorian calendar]): 28.
4. Pramoedya Ananta Toer, *Footsteps* [Jejak Langkah] Buru Quartet, vol. 3, trans. Max Lane (New York: Penguin, 1990), p. 128.
5. Warwick Anderson and Hans Pols, "Scientific Patriotism: Medical Science and National Self-Fashioning in Southeast Asia," *Comparative Studies in Society and History* 54, 1 (2012): 93–113.
6. Vivek Neelakantan, "The Campaign against the Big Four Endemic Diseases and Indonesia's Engagement with the WHO, 1950s," in *Public Health and National Reconstruction in Post-War Asia: International Influences, Local Transformations*, ed. Liping Bu and Ka-Che Yip (Abingdon: Routledge, 2014), pp. 154–74.
7. Warwick Anderson, "Introduction: Postcolonial Technoscience," *Social Studies of Science* 32, 5 and 6 (2002): 643–58.
8. Anderson, "Introduction," p. 651. See also Sujit Sivasundaram, "Sciences and the Global: On Methods, Questions, and Theory," *ISIS* 101 (2010): 146–58. Sujit Sivasundaram contends that making a nation implied the need for the history of science of that particular nation. The transnational origins of science have been lost in the literature because of the stamp of anti-colonialism on contemporary writings. A historiographic question raised by Sivasundaram is whether nationalists appropriated the imperial powers' obsession with science, aiming to mimic it with a view to establishing their own political capabilities. Modernity is at the heart of post-colonial science. To be modern in the 20th century meant using science and technology to intervene in the problems of hunger, disease and development.
9. Itty Abraham, "The Contradictory Spaces of Postcolonial Technoscience," *Economic and Political Weekly* 41, 3 (2006): 210–17.
10. Abraham, "The Contradictory Spaces," p. 213.
11. See also Jennifer Lindsay, "Introduction," in *Heirs to World Culture: Being Indonesian, 1950–1965*, ed. Jennifer Lindsay and Maya H.T. Liem (Leiden: KITLV Press, 2012), pp. 1–30.
12. Vivek Neelakantan, "The Medical Spur to Postcolonial Indonesian Science during the Soekarno Era," *IIAS Newsletter* 70 (2015): 14–15.
13. Soekarno, *Soal Hidup atau Mati* (Djakarta: Kementerian Penerangan, 1952), p. 3.

14. Soekarno, *Soal Hidup atau Mati*, p. 6.

15. Soekarno, *Soal Hidup atau Mati*, p. 8.

16. Soekarno, *Soal Hidup atau Mati*, p. 7.

17. See also Nick Cullather, *The Hungry World: America's Cold War Battle against Poverty in Asia* (Cambridge, MA: Harvard University Press, 2010), p. 2. Challenges to the American vision of world order came from the Asian heartland: communist expansionism, nationalist expansionism and what social scientists termed as the revolution of "rising expectations," a collective aspiration for land, food and change. For the United States, the "revolution of rising expectations" represented an existential danger.

18. Soekarno, *Soal Hidup atau Mati*, p. 21.

19. Soekarno, *Persambahan Hidupmu Kepada Tanah dan Bangsa: Tjeramah Presiden Soekarno didepan pada Para Mahasiswa Universitas Gadjah Mada di Sitinghinggil Jogjakarta, 22 Oktober 1962* (Jakarta: Departemen Penerangan, 1962). For reversal of familiar racial hierarchies, especially around the trope of civilization, Gandhi's *Hind Swaraj* equated European civilization with the excesses of technological modernity that had resulted in the erosion of Europe's collective soul. Gandhi prescribed Asian knowledge as the sole panacea to global political disorder that European domination had led to. See Itty Abraham, "From Bandung to NAM: Non-Alignment and Indian Foreign Policy, 1947–1965," *Commonwealth and Comparative Politics* 46, 2 (2008): 195–219.

20. Soekarno, *Persambahan Hidupmu Kepada Tanah dan Bangsa*.

21. "Amanat PJM Presiden Soekarno pada Resepsi Pembukaan Kongres Ilmu Pengetahuan Nasional Kedua di Jogjakarta pada Tanggal 22 Oktober 1962," *Pidato Presiden Republik Indonesia*, Inventaris 429, Arsip Nasional Republik Indonesia (The National Archives of Indonesia or ANRI).

22. "Amanat PJM Presiden Soekarno pada Resepsi Pembukaan Kongres."

23. Soekarno, "Lecture by President Soekarno to Students of the Padjadjaran University in Bandung on 17 November 1958," *Presidential Lecture Series* (Jakarta: Ministry of Information Republic of Indonesia, 1959).

24. Soekarno, "Lecture by President Soekarno to Students of the Padjadjaran University."

25. Soekarno, "Lecture by President Soekarno to Students of the Padjadjaran University." For a comparison with India, see Gyan Prakash, *Another Reason: Science and the Imagination of Modern India* (Princeton, NJ: Princeton University Press, 1999), p. 106.

26. Soekarno, "Lecture by President Soekarno to Students of the Padjadjaran University."

27. Christopher Lee, "At the Rendezvous of Decolonization," *Interventions: International Journal of Postcolonial Studies* 11, 1 (2009): 81–93.

28. Joshua Barker, "Beyond Bandung: Development Nationalism and (Multi)Cultural Nationalism in Indonesia," *Third World Quarterly* 29, 3 (2008): 521–40.

29.   Vivek Neelakantan, *Science, Public Health and Nation-Building in Soekarno-Era Indonesia* (Newcastle upon Tyne: Cambridge Scholars, 2017), p. 9.
30.   Benjamin Higgins, "Indonesia's Development Plans and Problems," *Pacific Affairs* 29, 2 (1956): 107–25.
31.   David Webster, *Fire and the Full Moon: Canada and Indonesia in a Decolonizing World* (Vancouver: University of British Columbia Press, 2010).
32.   Neelakantan, *Science, Public Health, and Nation-Building*, p. 8.
33.   Arjun Appadorai, "The Bandung Conference," *India Quarterly: A Quarterly Journal of International Affairs* 11, 3 (1955): 207–35.
34.   Appadorai, "The Bandung Conference," p. 217.
35.   "Opening Address Given by Soekarno: 18 April 1955, Bandung," *Asia Africa Speak from Bandung* (Djakarta: The Ministry of Foreign Affairs, Republic of Indonesia, 1955).
36.   "Opening Address Given by Soekarno: 18 April 1955, Bandung."
37.   "Item 7: Progress Report on Indonesia," Meeting dated 7 May 1957, NSC 5518, *White House Security Council Staff Papers: NSC Papers, 1953–61*, Special Staff File Series Box 3, A 82-18 Series, Dwight Eisenhower Presidential Library.
38.   Draft of Eisenhower's Speech, "Security and Peace," White House Correspondence: General 1955 (2), *John Foster Dulles Papers: White House Memoranda Series* Box 5, Dwight Eisenhower Presidential Library.
39.   Draft of Eisenhower's Speech, "Security and Peace."
40.   "Telegram from the Embassy in Indonesia to the Department of State dated February 25, 1955," Document 87, *Foreign Relations of the United States (1955–1957): Southeast Asia*, vol. 22, ed. Robert McMahon, Harriet Schwar and Louis Smith (Washington, DC: United States Government Printing Office, 1989), *Office of the Historian*. Available at: https://history.state.gov/historicaldocuments /frus1955-57v22/d87 [accessed 27 August 2019].
41.   "Outline of Plan of Operations with Respect to Indonesia dated 21 September 1956," *White House Office National Security Council Staff Papers (1948–1961): OCB Central File Series* 91 Indonesia, Box 42, A 82-18 Series, Dwight Eisenhower Presidential Library.
42.   "Outline of Plan of Operations with Respect to Indonesia dated 21 September 1956."
43.   See, for example, Howard Beers, *An American Experience in Indonesia: The University of Kentucky Affiliation with the Agricultural University at Bogor* (Lexington: University of Kentucky Press, 1971).
44.   Neelakantan, "The Campaign against the Big Four Endemic Diseases," p. 161.
45.   "Memorandum from Assistant Secretary of State for Far Eastern Affairs (Robertson) to the Undersecretary of State (Hoover) dated January 25, 1955," Document 84, *Foreign Relations of the United States (1955–1957): Southeast Asia*, vol. 22, ed. Robert McMahon, Harriet Schwar and Louis Smith (Washington, DC: United States Government Printing Office, 1989), *Office of the Historian*.

Available at: http://history.state.gov/historicaldocuments/frus1955-57v22/d84 [accessed 27 August 2019].
46. Neelakantan, "The Campaign against the Big Four Endemic Diseases," p. 162.
47. Ragna Boden, "Cold War Economics: Soviet Aid to Indonesia," *Journal of Cold War Studies* 10, 3 (2008): 110–28.
48. Boden, "Cold War Economics."
49. Nikita Chrusjtjov, *Uni Sovjet Sahabat Setia Bagi Rakjat 2 jang Sedang Berdjoeang Untuk Kemerdekaanja* (Djakarta: Kedutaan Besar URSS, 1960).
50. Chrusjtjov, *Uni Sovjet Sahabat Setia Bagi Rakjat.*
51. *Untuk Perdamaian dan Kesedjahteraan Rakjat* (Djakarta: Bagian Penerangan Besar URSS, 1960).
52. D.D. Venediktov and V.I. Petrov, *Untuk Taraf Kesehatan jang Tertinggi* (Djakarta: The Soviet Embassy, 1960).
53. Satrio and Mona Lohanda, "Perjuangan dan Pengabdian: Mosaik Kenangan Professor Dr Satrio, 1916–1986," *Penerbitan Sejarah Lisan* 3 (Jakarta: Arsip Nasional Republik Indonesia, 1986).
54. Boden, "Cold War Economics," p. 116.
55. Boden, "Cold War Economics." See also Satrio and Lohanda, "Perjuangan dan Pengabdian."
56. Boden, "Cold War Economics," pp. 120–1.
57. For a nuanced understanding of the niche physicians occupied in decolonization in the Dutch East Indies, see Hans Pols, *Nurturing Indonesia: Medicine and Decolonisation in the Dutch East Indies* (Cambridge: Cambridge University Press, 2018), p. 12.
58. "M Sardjito: Netherlands East Indies Country Card," Rockefeller Foundation Fellowship Records: Medical and Fellowship Recorder Cards, 1917–1970s, Record Group 10.2, Rockefeller Archive Center (RAC).
59. M. Sardjito, *Bangsa Indonesia Seharusnja Dikemudian Hari Mendjadi Bangsa Jang Besar: Tjeramah Diutjapkan Dimuka Para Mahasiswa Baru pada Bulan September 1956* (Jogjakarta: Universitas Gadjah Mada, 1956).
60. M. Sardjito, *Kewadjiban Para Ilmoe Ahli Bakteri dan Ahli Ilmoe Hajat Didalam Djaman Pembangoenan Indonesia Merdeka* (Soerakarta: Pergoeroen Tinggi Kedokteran, 1946).
61. "De Oekonomische Toestand van den Desamen," *Het Vaderland*, 1 February 1935.
62. Sardjito, *Kewadjiban.*
63. Sardjito, *Kewadjiban.*
64. Sardjito, *Kewadjiban.*
65. Sardjito, *Kewadjiban.*
66. Sardjito, *Bangsa Indonesia.*
67. *Menyingkap Pemikiran Professor Dr Sardjito* (Yogyakarta: UGM Press, 2006).

68. Aswi Warman Adam, *Sarwono Prawirohardjo: Pembangunan Institusi Ilmu Pengetahuan di Indonesia* (Jakarta: LIPI, 2009).
69. Adam Messers, "Effects of the Indonesian National Revolution and Transfer of Power on the Scientific Establishment," *Indonesia* 58 (1994): 41–68.
70. Messers, "Effects of the Indonesian Revolution," p. 48.
71. Neelakantan, *Science, Public Health and Nation-Building*, p. 189.
72. Neelakantan, *Science, Public Health and Nation-Building*, p. 183.
73. "Indonesian Council of the Sciences: Sarwono Prawirohardjo," Indonesian Council of the Sciences, File 652, Lucien Gregg Diary, 4 September 1963, RAC.
74. "Indonesian Council of the Sciences: Sarwono Prawirohardjo."
75. Sarwono Prawirohardjo, "Beberapa Pikiran Tentang Perkembangan Ilmu Pengetahuan dan Penjelidikan di Indonesia," in *Laporan Ilmu Pengetahuan Nasional Pertama*, ed. Madjelis Ilmu Pengetahuan Indonesia (Jakarta: MIPI, 1958) n. p.
76. "Indonesian Council of Sciences."
77. Prawirohardjo, "Beberapa Pikiran."
78. Prawirohardjo, "Beberapa Pikiran."
79. Prawirohardjo, "Beberapa Pikiran."
80. Justus van der Kroef, "The Cult of the Doctor and Its Indonesian Variant," *The Journal of Educational Sociology* 32, 8 (1959): 381–91.
81. Kroef, "The Cult of the Doctor." After World War I, the colonial authorities established engineering, law and medical colleges. Towards the end of Dutch colonialism (1940), of the 637 Indonesian students enrolled in various colleges, only 60 attended engineering colleges in contrast to 308 in medicine and 241 in law.
82. Kroef, "The Cult of the Doctor."
83. Between 1945 and 1955, Indonesia graduated only seven engineers per annum, in contrast to 35 physicians and 50 lawyers.
84. See also Andrew Goss, *Floracrats: State-Sponsored Science and the Failure of the Enlightenment in Indonesia* (Madison: University of Wisconsin Press, 2011), pp. 164–9. Under Soekarno, it was expected that Indonesian science would not blindly follow the scientific practice of foreign science but would be oriented to problems specific to Indonesia. Scientists retooled their disciplines in order to make them appear to be productive tools for Indonesian national development while also trying to preserve the ideals of science, a practice that Goss terms as "Desk Science."
85. Neelakantan, *Science, Public Health and Nation-Building*, p. 184.
86. Adam, *Sarwono Prawirohardjo.*
87. Terence Hull and Valerie Hull, "From Family Planning to Reproductive Healthcare," in *People, Population and Policy in Indonesia*, ed. Terence Hull and Valerie Hull (Jakarta: Equinox Publishing, 2005), pp. 1–69.
88. See also Adam, *Sarwono Prawirohardjo.*
89. Dhurudin Mashad, *Tahun Penuh Tantangan; Soedjono Djoened Poesponegoro, Menteri Riset Pertama di Indonesia* (Jakarta: LIPI, 2008), p. 43.

90. Mashad, *Tahun Penuh Tantangan*, p. 48.

91. Mashad, *Tahun Penuh Tantangan*, p. 51.

92. Soedjono Djoened Poesponegoro, *Masalah Kesehatan Anak di Indonesia* (Jakarta: Jajasan Pembangunan, 1953).

93. Soedjono Djoened Poesponegoro, *Masalah Kesehatan Anak.*

94. Neelakantan, *Science, Public Health and Nation-Building*, p. 186.

95. Poey Seng Hin, "Defisiensi Protein Kalori (Kwashiorkor) dan Penjakit Defisiensi Vitamin A," in *Research di Indonesia*, ed. M. Makagiansar and Poorwo Soedarmo (Djakarta: Departemen Urusan Research Nasional Republik Indonesia, 1965), p. 276.

96. Soedjono Djoened Poesponegoro, "Address at the Opening Ceremony of the Second Afro-Asian Congress of Paediatrics, August 19, 1964," *Paediatrica Indonesiana* 4 (1964): vii–xii.

97. "Resolutions Adopted at the General Session of the Second Afro-Asian Congress of Paediatrics, Jakarta," 26 August 1964, *Paediatrica Indonesiana* 4 (1964): xxxvi–xxxix.

98. Mashad, *Tahun Penuh Tantangan*, p. 160.

99. Mashad, *Tahun Penuh Tantangan*, p. 167.

100. Neelakantan, *Science, Public Health and Nation-Building*, p. 188.

101. Warwick Anderson, "Asia as a Method in STS," *EASTS* 6, 4 (2012): 445–51.

102. See, for example, David Arnold, "Nehruvian Science and Postcolonial India," *ISIS* 104 (2013): 360–70, 360.

103. For a contrast with the Philippines, see Vivek Neelakantan, "No Nation Can Go Forward When It Is Crippled by Disease: Philippine Science and the Cold War, 1950s," *Southeast Asian Studies* 10, 1 (2021): 53–89.

104. Arnold, "Nehruvian Science," p. 365.

105. Herbert Feith, "Indonesia's Political Symbols and Their Wielders," *World Politics* 16 (1963): 79–97.

106. See, for examples, Guy Pauker, "Indonesia in 1964: Toward a People's Democracy," *Asian Survey* 5, 2 (1965): 88–97. By 1960, the Soviets had hoped that assisting Indonesia in liberating West Irian from the Dutch would result in bringing the PKI closer to the center. At the same time as Indonesia was suffering an economic crisis, precipitated by the military confrontation with Malaysia and the West Irian question, First Minister Djuanda attempted an economic stabilization program recommended by the International Monetary Fund. But the program was withdrawn due to opposition from the PKI. On 25 March 1964, President Soekarno's statement before US Ambassador Howard Jones, "go to hell with your aid," indicated that foreign aid was a luxury that Indonesia could ill afford to have. At the time, Soekarno's quest for economic autarky was to shield the country against the kind of economic pressure experienced in China. Following the 1 October 1965 attempted coup, Indonesia gravitated into the US orbit.

CHAPTER 7

The Cholera Pandemic, the Chinese Diaspora and Cold War Politics in Southeast Asia and China during the 1960s

Xiaoping Fang

Introduction

Since the early 19th century, imperialist penetrations, trade expansion, political violence, military conflict and religious pilgrimages have facilitated the intensification of population movements and the spread of diseases and epidemics in Southeast Asia and China.[1] These diseases were given different sociopolitical, cultural, and even racial meanings and interpretations, which further led to various control and prevention measures. Since the late 1940s, Cold War politics in the decolonization and nation-building contexts significantly impacted transnational population movement and the transmission of epidemics, while highly politicizing connotations of disease and control practice.

This chapter aims to explore the dynamics between population mobility, disease prevalence and Cold War politics based on the study of the Chinese diaspora in Southeast Asia and China. It first examines the Chinese diaspora, disease transmission and its interpretation and control from the early 19th century to the mid-20th century. It then explores under what circumstance Indonesian Chinese returned to China and how the movement of the Indonesian Chinese coincided with the outbreak and transmission of the cholera pandemic in 1960 and 1961. It further investigates why and how the Chinese government privileged returning Chinese members of the diaspora in the large-scale but clandestine anti-cholera campaign in terms of epidemiological interpretation, quarantine and stool tests. In the end, the chapter discusses how China isolated itself from the international health community and events and how medical humanitarian donations and the media were deliberately used as political tools to justify its sociopolitical and ideological legitimacy in the military and geopolitical tensions of the Cold War.

The Chinese Diaspora and Disease before the Cold War

From the early 19th century onwards, millions of Chinese left southeast coastal China for destinations around the world. Prompted by the hunger, famine, war and chaos that plagued China, they sought to make their living elsewhere and departed as coolies and indentured laborers.[2] Southeast Asia was the key destination as a result of the huge demand for labor generated by the rapid development of its cities and plantations,[3] and around 20 million people from China arrived there in the century after 1840. Some were self-funded, others were recruited by labor-hire foremen, others traveled on debt-servitude credit tickets (in which a broker paid the cost of passage but retained control of the traveler's labor until the debt had been repaid in full), and a further group were indentured to European employers.[4]

However, the history of the Chinese diaspora in Southeast Asia and elsewhere is accompanied by a parallel history of disease. These migrant workers, regardless of whether they traveled on sailing ships or steamships, were affected by disease from the outset of their miserable sea journeys. During the voyage, each passenger was usually restricted to carrying only a single water bottle, two pairs of clothes, one bamboo hat and a straw mat.[5] The cabins were airless and stuffy and offered only limited sunshine. The drinking water provided was insufficient and often contaminated, and the food was poor quality and lacking in nutrition. The terrible living conditions in the cabins resulted in rampant diseases. The combined death rates from illness, whippings, hangings and beatings on some of these sea voyages were extremely high. For example, maritime statistical data from 1847 to 1859 reveals that, on average, each year there were 14.5 boat departures to Cuba across the Pacific Ocean, carrying a total 6,265 coolies going to work in the plantations, 15.21 percent of whom died en route.[6]

As the movement of the Chinese diaspora correlated to the transmission of epidemic diseases, the members of the Chinese diaspora soon became identified or suspect as being disease carriers in their host countries regardless of whether or not this was true. For example, it was argued that a cholera epidemic spread from Guangdong Province, China, to Manila in the Philippines via Chinese passengers in 1882. From August to October, cholera claimed about

20,000 victims in Manila, among a total population of around only 400,000. In 1902, the disease was reintroduced into the Philippine archipelago from Guangdong, through a shipment of fresh vegetables that were thrown into the harbor from a boat that was refused landing in Manila.[7] It was also argued that an influenza epidemic broke out in China and was spread to the British and French troops in Europe by Chinese coolies who were working on World War I's Western Front during the winter of 1917. From the trenches in France, it ultimately spread to a US army base in Kansas.[8]

The movements of the Chinese diaspora and the complicated patterns of epidemic transmission were further entangled with social and racial prejudice in host countries that produced a narrative in which the Chinese were seen as a diseased race. For instance, the Chinese Exclusion Act in the USA and the White Australia policy basically used the fear of Chinese people as disease carriers as an argument to keep them out.[9] Some diseases were even labeled with Chinese names: the 1917 influenza outbreak earned the name "Chungking fever," for example.[10]

In many cases, Chinese residents were quarantined when there was an epidemic not because of their disease status but because of their race.[11] Chinese migrants' quarantine experience on St John Island, Singapore, was a typical case. The island is about two miles away from Singapore and all passengers arriving in Singapore by boat had to undergo a medical examination. The first- and second-class passengers, who were usually rich people, would be released to go to Singapore after a brief examination. However, all third-class passengers, who were generally poor laborers, would be disembarked and held on St John Island for up to two weeks' quarantine whenever there was a sick passenger among them.[12]

Worse still, the racial identification of the Chinese as being disease carriers jeopardized the stability of the fragile relationships with local communities in the host countries. In Manila, the Chinese monopolized enterprise and industry and filled "the commercial space between ruler and ruled" in their work as merchants and artisans, but when the cholera epidemic broke out in 1820, both Chinese immigrants and mestizos of mixed Chinese and Filipino ancestry bore the brunt of local Filipino hostility, becoming the chief victims of the Manila massacre.[13]

At the same time, the movement of Chinese diaspora and the transmission of diseases were not unidirectional.[14] Instead, the returning Chinese laborers also brought diseases back to China. For example, there was close, regular contact between the many sea ports of southeastern Fujian Province, such as Xiamen, and Southeast Asia. Around 2.55 million people migrated overseas from Quanzhou, Zhangzhou, Xinghua, Fuzhou and Yongchun in the late

19th and early 20th centuries. This large-scale population movement exacerbated the speed and frequency of the spread of plague. The returning overseas Chinese triggered outbreaks of epidemics in their places of origin, while merchants doing business in Xiamen and other ports returned to their hinterland hometowns and prompted outbreaks of plague among residents who had never left.[15] In all, the mobility of the Chinese diaspora in Southeast Asia and elsewhere has been the history of disease.

Transnational Politics, the Indonesian Chinese and the Cholera Pandemic[16]

At the same time as the Chinese migrant workers headed to Southeast Asia and other parts of the world via the South China Sea and the Pacific, another group of mobile people were making their own voyages between the Hejaz (the Red Sea and the Arabian and Yemeni coasts) and the Indian Ocean. These were Southeast Asian Muslim pilgrims who were traveling to Mecca via the Red Sea port city of Jeddah to perform the Hajj, a journey their communities had been making annually since the 14th century as a gesture of religious devotion. Voyages of Chinese migrant workers and Southeast Asian pilgrims are examples of population mobility and disease transmission in the South China Sea and the Indian Ocean, respectively, before the mid-20th century. However, the Indonesian Chinese unexpectedly connected these two seemingly unrelated social and medical events in the early 1960s when the transnational politics of the Cold War highly politicized population mobility, transmission of disease, and its interpretation and control. The seventh global cholera pandemic (*Vibrio cholerae* El Tor) broke out and spread in Indonesia, Southeast Asia and China against this background in 1960–61.

Like the classical biotype strains of cholera, the El Tor biotype strains also first occurred in South Asia. It was then spread to Mecca by pilgrims and then transmitted to El Tor on the Sinai Peninsula, 120 miles south of Suez on the eastern shore of the Gulf of Suez and other areas in the Middle East by pilgrims prior to 1900. From there, returning pilgrims took the strain to the Indonesian port of Makassar, Sulawesi, by 1925. Makassar was a major center for international shipping during this period and it was there that El Tor cholera gained its foothold and developed its various potent mutations.[17] Soon after 1937, cholera broke out around Makassar, with patients showing clinical signs of the hemolytic (El Tor) biotype of *V. cholerae*.[18] By 1958, there were four major outbreaks of cholera in Indonesia, but all were basically confined to Makassar.[19] Makassar became the starting point for the El Tor strain after undergoing 12 additional mutations.[20] From here, El Tor cholera evolved into a pandemic by 1961, one that would spread to other areas of Indonesia, Southeast Asia and the world.[21] More significantly, the outbreak and transmission of the El Tor cholera strain coincided with the return of Indonesian Chinese to China around the same time.

After the Dutch East India Company was established in the 17th century, the Chinese moved to Indonesia on a large scale. Because of the economic changes brought by the expansion of plantation crops, their numbers increased steadily from the late 19th century onwards and reached around 2 million by 1951.[22] However, the Chinese communities in Indonesia remained distinct and preserved their cultural heritage. Furthermore, the history of Chinese collaboration with the colonial regime in the Dutch East India era, their distinct racial and cultural practices, and the wealth of some community members meant that feelings of distrust and animosity toward the Chinese prevailed through much of the 20th century.[23]

The specific and distinct features of the Chinese community in Indonesia were soon complicated by the changes in the geopolitics between Indonesia and China during the Cold War. After the Republic of Indonesia and the People's Republic of China established diplomatic relations in April 1950, one of the disputes was about determining the nationality of Indonesian citizens who were also Chinese nationals. After intensive negotiations, the Chinese premier and foreign minister, Zhou Enlai, and the Indonesian foreign minister, Sunario, signed the Agreement on the Issue of Dual Nationality between the Republic of Indonesia and the People's Republic of China on 22 April 1955 during the Bandung conference. The agreement stipulated that "anybody with both the citizenship of the Republic of Indonesia and of the People's Republic of China shall choose between the two citizenships on the basis of his or her own will."[24] It further regulated that the agreement came into force when the documents were ratified and exchanged by the two governments.[25]

Nonetheless, the ongoing and deep suspicions towards the Chinese in Indonesian communities remained. Soon, a series of factors combined to place the Indonesian Chinese in mortal danger, including the rise of communist China's political influence in Indonesia, the Chinese premier's visit to Indonesia, the vast funds held by communist supporters, and the expanding activities of the Embassy of the People's Republic of China in the world of education. These factors were further complicated by changes in US–Indonesia relations during the Cold War. All these factors facilitated the anti-left-wing sympathies and fueled anti-Chinese feeling.[26]

On 3 November 1959, Presidential Regulation No. 10 banned alien retailers, the vast majority of whom were Chinese, from operating in rural areas, although this did not apply to the capitals of first- and second-tier autonomous districts. Soon, the regulations about the residential rights of the Chinese in rural areas came into effect. This decree and other related policies affected at least 300,000 Indonesian Chinese and caused 100,000 of them to lose their liveli-hoods.[27] Meanwhile, beginning in December 1959, the Chinese government initiated a series of broadcasts inviting overseas Chinese who either no longer wished to stay in Indonesia or who had suffered persecution from the Indone-sian government to return to China. On 20 January 1960, the Chinese and Indonesian governments exchanged the ratified Agreement on the Issue of Dual Nationality in Beijing, which finally brought this fully into effect.[28] The Chi-nese government then initiated a repatriation scheme for those ethnic Chinese who opted for People's Republic of China (PRC) citizenship. By the end of 1960, around 94,000 Indonesian Chinese had returned to mainland China.[29] Among these Indonesian Chinese who returned to China, some were from Makassar on the island of Sulawesi.

However, cholera, whose spread had largely been confined to that locality between 1937 and 1958, would reach epidemic proportions in Makassar by Jan-uary 1961, in an outbreak that was different from earlier episodes because the cholera spread beyond Makassar and quickly escalated into a global pandemic.

Around 1960, Makassar was experiencing huge population movements, including troop movements to and from the area to suppress local military re-bellions, unprecedented high-scale Chinese emigration from Indonesia, and considerable unsupervised smuggling by small boats.[30] Of these movements, the movement of Indonesian Chinese is believed to have been particularly important. During the anti-Chinese campaigns, the Indonesian Chinese started leaving Makassar for Java from December 1959 to join the ocean liners going to mainland China.[31] The outward emigration reached its peak in the summer of 1960 and continued into 1961, which coincided with the outbreak of cholera in Makassar. During this process, asymptomatic and convalescent carriers of El Tor cholera played an important role in transmission.[32] In all, the disease had spread far and wide from Makassar to Java and then on to other outer is-lands of Indonesia. Cholera was first reported in Java in May 1961, in a seaside community that had been visited by residents from Makassar, and then spread to Semarang in Central Java and then infected Jakarta in June.[33] Spreading to Java, the cholera bacteria found ideal conditions in which to establish a foot-hold and flourish.[34] The cholera also spread northbound to Kuching in Sarawak and British North Borneo.

Simultaneously, the Indonesian Chinese were still leaving for China in 1961, mainly to Guangdong and Fujian Provinces, which had been designated as disembarking points. Around 18–23 June, the "vomiting and diarrhea ill-ness" emerged in a few coastal communes of Yangjiang County. From 22 June to 20 August, there were a total of 2,226 cases and the death toll reached 150. While the government launched the anti-cholera campaign quickly, the disease had already spread beyond Yangjiang County by early July. The cholera quickly spread from Guangdong Province to Macau and Hong Kong on 11 and 15 August 1961 respectively.[35] Hong Kong soon came to play a similar role to Guangzhou in spreading this cholera epidemic. The same patterns marked the spread of cholera from Hong Kong to Manila in 1961. From Sulu Island, a second wave of cholera spread to British Northern Borneo.[36]

The cholera spread back into Southeast Asia in this way. Eight months later, in February 1962, cholera re-emerged in Guangdong and from July 1962 onward affected southeastern coastal China, spreading rapidly through Zhejiang, Fujian, Shanghai and Jiangsu. Following a large-scale but clandestine medical campaign, the pandemic was contained by 1965. By this time, the WHO had announced that cholera had spread to almost all Asian countries and was on the verge of reaching the Middle East and Eastern Europe.[37]

The Returned Diaspora in the Pandemic: Epidemiological Interpretations, Quarantine and the Stool Test in China

During the cholera pandemic and after 1961, the Indonesian Chinese had triple identities: they were fleeing aliens in Indonesia, a returning diaspora in China, and suspected cholera carriers in a pandemic that spread across Southeast Asia, China and the world. Among them, the identity of the returning diaspora was of ideological and economic significance for the Chinese government. In the late 1950s and early 1960s, the returned overseas Chinese served important sociopolitical goals for the Communist government. The returned overseas Chinese represented the patriotism of the Chinese diaspora, but the Communist Party, in displaying benevolence to them in their hour of need, was able to promote its own political and ideological legitimacy, and demonstrate its political superiority over the Nationalist Party as the defender of Chinese people's interests. Thus, overseas Chinese affairs became a major focus of ideological propaganda and of the United Front work on the part of the Chinese Communist government, which competed with the Nationalist government based in Taiwan during the Cold War of the 1950s and 1960s. The Nationalist government ordered its consular officials to withdraw from Indonesia as a result of the country's recognition of the Chinese Communist government in 1950.[38] However, pro-Nationalist sympathizers and organizations were still important forces in the Indonesian Chinese community, from which the Nationalist government aimed to win support.

Overseas Chinese affairs also involved practical economic needs because remittances from overseas Chinese were a key source of foreign currency for national industrialization projects in the early 1960s. However, after 1958, during the People's Commune campaign, some local governments confiscated houses and furniture and opened locked houses owned by the returned overseas Chinese. Some cadres confiscated other means of subsistence held by families of the overseas Chinese and returned overseas Chinese, such as sewing machines, and asked them to donate money, jewelry and gold to local governments.

In Zhejiang Province, the Provincial Department of Overseas Chinese Affairs pointed out in an internal report, "these local policies have seriously affected the activeness of the families of overseas Chinese in procuring foreign currency remittances. Some relatives of overseas Chinese and returned overseas Chinese have written letters to their families abroad asking them to stop sending money."[39] For example, remittances began dropping in late 1958 in key counties in Wenzhou Prefecture, which is the main hometown of the overseas Chinese in Zhejiang Province, decreasing by 30 percent compared with 1957. Instead of currency, the overseas Chinese began to send staple foods to support their hungry families in Wenzhou.[40] There was a corresponding drop in overseas Chinese visitors around this time, including those from Hong Kong and Macau. It therefore became imperative for the government to enhance its image among the overseas Chinese to boost remittances.

Meanwhile, the foreign currency brought by overseas visitors was an important factor, so their mobility was not restrained, but was instead guaranteed and facilitated. For example, the Zhejiang Provincial Government regulated that if overseas Chinese and Hong Kong and Macau residents paid for transport (taxis, buses and chartered buses) and accommodation in foreign currency, they would only pay 80 percent of the standard prices provided they showed a letter of proof issued by the Overseas Chinese Travel Agency in each locale. The differences between these two prices would be covered by the work unit in each locale. Likewise, they were given priority access to tickets, grain, non-staple foodstuffs and daily commodities.[41]

Ideological and economic factors also further facilitated the Chinese government to privilege returned overseas Chinese during the anti-cholera campaign. While the central government, the Guangdong Provincial Government, and the Zhanjiang Prefectural Committee dispatched a large number of epidemic prevention staff to Yangjiang County to prevent the further spread of cholera after 6 July 1961, the Guangdong Provincial Epidemic Prevention Headquarters' Work Team started to investigate the etiology of this pandemic.

In view of the fact that cholera had not occurred in Yangjiang County over the preceding 18 years, the investigations mainly focused on external factors, targeting the returned Indonesian Chinese.

However, the government was extremely careful with the etiological investigation and interpretation during this process. In the epidemiology report about the cholera outbreak in Yangjiang County submitted to the Guangdong Provincial Party committee on 24 August 1961, the investigation team pointed out: "Because there had been outbreaks of this cholera in Indonesia, we conducted vibrio examinations among returned Indonesian Chinese who had settled on national farms. To prevent suspicion, we conducted a total of 462 vibrio tests on both Indonesian Chinese and local residents throughout the farms." This preliminary investigation concluded that "No cholera vibrio was identified among returned Indonesian Chinese."[42]

But the subsequent etiological investigations concluded that the returned Indonesian Chinese were the suspected cholera carriers during the pandemic, and this was disclosed by the Chinese government at internal meetings of senior medical and health officials. In December 1962, Qian Xinzhong, the deputy minister of the Ministry of Health from the mid-1950s to 1966, gave a speech at a cholera prevention and treatment meeting attended by many representatives from southeast coastal provinces: "This cholera pandemic must have been transmitted from overseas. However, the transmission paths are still not clear. There is a great possibility that returned Indonesian Chinese brought cholera to China. Of course, we must not rule out the possibility that our enemies [used cholera] to sabotage us."[43] By 1964, he explicitly confirmed that:

> The cholera pandemic in Guangdong Province in 1961 was brought by cholera carriers from foreign countries. We first identified that suspected cholera patients were in areas where returning Indonesian Chinese congregated . . . Epidemiological surveys indicate that mild patient cases and cholera carriers were the main spreaders of epidemic diseases from one province and one area to another province and another district.[44]

Nonetheless, this definitive statement about the etiology of the cholera pandemic was only announced by the Deputy Minister of Health. This statement only appeared in the secret, internal official files of the central government, which could be accessed by senior party and government officials. Those at lower levels could not read this etiological interpretation, not to mention the public. Keeping the etiological interpretation as secret disentangled returning diaspora from the suspected cholera carriers and maintained their patriotic images.[45]

Returned Chinese diaspora members also experienced unique quarantine and isolation practices in the anti-cholera campaign. As the two basic interventionist methods used to respond to the cholera pandemic, quarantine and isolation were strictly implemented among the mass residents in the cholera-stricken southeast coastal areas of China. Integrated with the concurrent social restructuring campaign, these schemes greatly strengthened the highly immobile and sedentary nature of Chinese society at the time.

In contrast, quarantine involving overseas Chinese visitor groups was more unusual, because local governments made specific quarantine regulations for the returned overseas Chinese, visitors, Hong Kong and Macau residents, and foreign guests and visitors, extending quarantine waiver privileges and other specific treatment. For example, there were many foreign guests visiting Xin'anjiang Hydraulic Station, Shaoxing, and other areas of Zhejiang Province, while quarantine checks were imposed on passengers and vehicles on major roads and highways during the pandemic. In a report submitted to the Zhejiang Provincial Health Department in October 1963, the Foreign Affairs Office of Hangzhou City pointed out that quarantine staff requested that foreign visitors stop for these checks and proposed that such procedures should be done away with:

> In order to avoid such occurrences in the future, it is proposed that, if foreign guests and overseas Chinese vehicles pass the quarantine station, staff should not require them to undertake examinations. Vehicles should make the following signals: during the daytime, its parking lights should be switched on and the drivers should wave a newspaper. At night, vehicles should flash their headlights three times.[46]

Such privileges were also extended to the stool sample examination. After the arrival of overseas Chinese visitors, the Zhejiang Provincial Government regulated that:

> Overseas Chinese Affairs Departments, police substations, and travel agencies were to register and report the arrivals to local health departments, which in turn informed each relevant medical and healthcare unit. After receiving this notice, each unit would quickly dispatch staff to conduct three consecutive stool examinations and five days of medical observations. Anything suspicious would be reported to the health bureau.[47]

In the stool examinations, "if any cholera patients or suspected carriers were identified, they would be persuaded to accept isolation at hospitals in order to prevent the transmission of infection." In particular, for those with social, political and economic influence, the Provincial Health Department stipulated that "medical staff may conduct brief feces examinations in toilets by persuading ordinary people to leave stool samples for further thorough examination following the standard approach. During this process, the medical staff should be patient and persuasive."[48]

The privileges of quarantine waiver and the specific stool examination procedure offered to overseas Chinese visitors during the 1962–65 cholera pandemic contrasted with the treatment of their ancestors who migrated to Southeast Asia in the 19th and early 20th centuries. Chinese migrants were usually targeted as suspected disease vectors and suffered racial prejudice in quarantine at that time.[49] Their historical memories and personal experience of these returned overseas Chinese in the previous quarantine were usually highlighted and compared with their current experience in China, by which the Communist Party intended to demonstrate fraternity and benevolence to the overseas Chinese and further justify its ruling legitimacy over their motherland.

However, this attitudinal change was not concurrent with medical and scientific knowledge of cholera bacteriology. In fact, El Tor cholera often appeared in a mild clinical form and resulted in many symptomless carriers moving around while unaware that they were spreading the disease. The majority of individuals infected with cholera either had no symptoms or just showed mild diarrhea. For classical cholera, the ratio of severe cases that require hospitalization to either mild or asymptomatic infection is 1:5 to 1:10. For El Tor cholera, this figure reached 1:25 to 1:100. Thus, quarantine was not advocated by international medical and health communities, such as the World Health Organization (WHO).[50] As discussed earlier, however, the Chinese government strictly implemented quarantine for cholera in 1961–65. The similar cases in Mao's era were plague and tuberculosis control, for which quarantines were strictly applied too.[51] Thus the privileges of quarantine waiver and specific stool examination procedures were significant for the Chinese government and those returned overseas Chinese.

Pandemic Politics between China and Southeast Asia during the Cold War

While the returned overseas Chinese received specific treatment in China during the pandemic, China's role in the pandemic politics between China and Southeast Asia was unique. When the cholera pandemic broke out in Southeast Asia and China in 1961, the global epidemic reporting network had actually already been operating in Northeast and Southeast Asia for nearly four decades. As early as 1925, the Eastern Bureau of the League of Nations Health Section was established in Singapore to collect and disseminate epidemiological information in the East or the Far East. After World War II, the bureau was renamed the Epidemiological Intelligence Station of the WHO.[52] According to the WHO program, "each state recognizes the right of the Organization to communicate directly with the health administration of its territory or territories."[53]

However, the WHO is an intergovernmental organization with no supra-governmental authority. Furthermore, it cannot execute policies which override the will of its members' governments.[54] From 1948 to 1972, the PRC was not a member country of the WHO and remained isolated from the international epidemic reporting network. The Chinese government was therefore absent from the increasingly strengthened cooperation of the international epidemic surveillance network. This specific relationship between the international organization and a non-member country shaped the features of the politics of the cholera pandemic during the Cold War, particularly when China defined this as being a national secret. During this pandemic, the Chinese government did not share epidemic information with the international community at the government level. The WHO therefore could not obtain direct information from China after the cholera pandemic broke out in Guangdong Province in June–July 1961.

In view of the serious pandemic situation in Asia, the WHO Western Pacific Regional Office convened an interregional meeting on cholera control in Manila, the Philippines, on 16–19 April 1962. At this meeting, the participants came from the countries in the Western Pacific Region, including Hong Kong, Japan, Korea, Macao, Malaya, Netherlands, North Borneo, Philippines, Ryukyu Islands, Sarawak, Singapore and Vietnam. Indonesia and Thailand as the member states of the Southeast Asia Region and Pakistan as the member state of the East Mediterranean Region also attended the meeting. In addition, representatives from the US Agency for International Development/the United States Operations Mission, the United States Air Force, the Clark Air Force Base in the Philippines, and Silliman University Mission Hospital attended the meeting as observers. The government of the Republic of China based in Taiwan similarly attended the meeting—the representative was Dr C.H. Yen from the Department of Health of the Taiwan Provincial Government. The government of the People's Republic of China based in mainland China did not attend the meeting.

Dr I.C. Fang, Director of the WHO Regional Office for the Western Pacific, delivered the opening speech. As the meeting report pointed out:

> This unprecedented occurrence in the region of epidemics caused by the El Tor cholera vibrios has pointed to the urgent need for a better understanding of the epidemiology, prevention and control of the disease.

It was accordingly arranged that an ad hoc meeting should be held in Manila under sponsorship of the Western Pacific Regional Office of the World Health Organization for an exchange of information between senior officers of the health administrations of the countries either affected by epidemic or at risk of the introduction of the infection. The purpose of the meeting was to pool knowledge and experience of the clinical management of patients suffering from El Tor infections, of the prevention of the spread of the disease and of its control, once established. It was also thought desirable to invite advisers in the various fields of cholera treatment, research and control so that the health administrators concerned would have available to them a wide range of experience and information of the present state of knowledge of cholera.[55]

In 1964, a follow-up meeting was also held in Manila, with delegates from all over the world.[56] The government of the People's Republic of China did not attend these global health community meetings. Its absence impacted cholera prevention. By the late 1960s, the adoption of the cordon sanitaire and the requirement of inoculation certificates at frontiers were no longer encouraged, as they did not significantly prevent the spread of cholera. Instead, close cooperation and exchange of epidemiological information between infected countries and non-infected neighboring countries came to play crucial roles in preventing the global spread of cholera.[57] As Dr Marcolino Gomes Candau, then the WHO's second director-general, claimed in 1962, the WHO faced difficulties in combating disease in Asia due to lack of first-hand knowledge of the health situation in mainland China.

Though the government of the PRC did not attend the international health meetings, it participated in the politics of the pandemic against the specific background of the Cold War in different ways. Following the debacle of the Great Leap Forward and the ensuing Great Famine, the government also encountered serious external challenges in 1962, including border clashes with India in the southwest, the radically worsening relationship with its ally the Soviet Union in the north, and Chiang Kai-shek's "Reclaim Mainland" plan to attack in the southeast. In particular, both the cholera pandemic and military confrontation across the Taiwan Strait broke out in June 1962.[58]

According to China Xinhua News Agency's report:

On January 27, 1962, China's Red Cross sent a telegraph message to the Philippines Red Cross and expressed its concern with the prevalence of cholera in the Philippines and informed them: China Red Cross had decided to donate 500,000 ml cholera vaccine (for 333,000 person), to assist the Philippines to eradicate this infectious disease. Cholera started to spread in the Philippines since last September. In the demand of the Philippines Red Cross, the League of Red Cross Societies called for help from Red Cross Societies of many countries to donate cholera vaccines.[59]

It was reported that the China Red Cross had received a telegraph message from the Chairman of the Philippine Red Cross on 14 February, in which he expressed his gratitude to the China Red Cross.[60] Through this medical humanitarian donation, the Chinese government showed its commitment to the international anti-cholera campaign to the Chinese society.

The Chinese official media also reported the outbreak and spread of cholera in Taiwan under the Nationalist government. On 21 July 1962, *The People's Daily*, which is the mouth-piece of the Central Committee of the Communist Party of China, first reported: "Jiayi, Yunlin, and Tainan in southern Taiwan broke out cholera. The Department of Health, puppet Taiwan Provincial Government (伪台湾省政府卫生处) announced on July 17 to classify 26 townships in southern Taiwan as the urgent area of cholera."[61] In the report, *The People's Daily* referred to the government of the Republic of China in Taiwan as the "puppet Taiwan provincial Government." This terminology not only refuted the political legitimacy of the Nationalist government but also claimed it was a provincial-level government.

In the second report, released three weeks later, *The People's Daily* noted that:

> According to the Taiwanese newspapers, due to the indifferent attitude of the Chiang Kai-shek bandit gang to the prevention and treatment of the paracholera epidemic (i.e., El Tor cholera) in Taiwan, the epidemic area has rapidly expanded and the number of patients has continued to increase. Paracholera spreads so quickly in Taiwan, but the director of the "Taiwan Provincial Health Department" of the Chiang bandit gang is still living a life of feasting. Taiwan's "Gong Lun Pao" published a report on July 20 under the title of "Cholera Spreading Day, the Chief Is Whirling." When asked whether the "Provincial Department of Health" had adopted "fighting" measures, "Director" Yan Chunhui "danced and drunk in a nightclub in Taichung for two consecutive days." *The Taipei Evening News* also reported that Lin Yanhui, the first index case in Tainan City, became ill due to repeated delays by the "health authorities." Three days after the incident, his condition was still not diagnosed and he was not given medical treatment. He died quickly. Then, Lin Yanhui's grandmother and four siblings were also knocked down and the cholera quickly spread to other people. The Taiwanese newspapers revealed that the "health authorities" of the Chiang Bandit Gang in Taiwan paid little or no

attention to the disinfection of water and fertilizers, the removal of garbage, the dredging of sewers, and the injection of vaccines. They only "advised residents to eat carefully." The disinfection of the epidemic area is nothing but lime. Some vaccination stations even inject several people without disinfecting one needle.

Taiwan newspapers also revealed that the Chiang Kai-shek Bandit Gang does not care about the health of the people at ordinary times, and the residents' environmental hygiene is extremely poor, which is one of the important reasons for the occurrence of paracholera. *The Gong Lun Bao* published a letter from a group of "poor citizens" on Dongyuan Street in Taipei City on the 3rd of this month, saying: They live there with a population of more than 1,000, and there is only one garbage bin. Since the garbage bin installed two years ago, the "city sanitation brigade" has never collected it once. The water ditch on the roadside is stinky, mosquitoes flies, the smell is suffocating, and the sewage overflows after the rain, rushing into their houses and draft wells. The Chiang Kai-shek bandits "shut their eyes to" this.[62]

These two reports were issued in July and August 1962 when the cholera was ravaging the southeast coastal areas of mainland China, including Guangdong Province, Fujian Province, Zhejiang Province, Shanghai Municipality and Jiangsu Province. The government strictly controlled the information concerning the cholera pandemic in national and local media, which kept the people across the country in the dark about the pandemic, particularly those in non-cholera-affected areas. In the cholera-infected area, on the one hand, the government conducted hygiene and prevention education to provide local residents with basic knowledge concerning the cholera; on the other hand, the government gathered information to compare the handling of epidemics, medicine, and doctors before and after 1949, following the principle of praising the new communist society and criticizing the old nationalist society.

Under this dichotomic discourse, epidemics and pandemics in the old society were described as miserable and devastating. The portrayal of the frustrated and hopeless sufferings of Taiwanese society under Nationalist rule in *The People's Daily* further sharply contrasted the official media coverage of the benevolence the people received under Communist rule. Therefore, the historical and contemporary comparison served to enhance the national image of the Communist government and demonstrate its legitimacy. Together with the medical humanitarian donation, the media reports concerning the cholera pandemic were highly politicized in the geopolitics of the Cold War during the early 1960s.

Conclusion

Beginning in the early 19th century, war, turmoil, hunger and famine caused by incompetent and chaotic politics in China prompted Chinese laborers from southeast coastal areas to emigrate overseas in search of a living. The history of Chinese migrants is a parallel history of disease to some extent, one that is usually entangled with racial and political issues in host countries. In the early 1960s, changing national and transnational politics impacted the origin, outbreak and spread of the El Tor cholera pandemic in Southeast Asia and China. The return of the Indonesian Chinese to the People's Republic of China was a major factor in escalating endemic cholera into a global pandemic. The movement of the Indonesian Chinese across the South China Sea occurred in the context of nation-building and international relations in Indonesia and China following the end of World War II. In the geopolitics of the Cold War, ideological and economic factors facilitated the Chinese government's extension of privileges to the returning Chinese diaspora in the large-scale but clandestine anti-cholera campaign. While isolated from the international health community and events, the Chinese government participated in cholera pandemic politics through the medical humanitarian donation to the Philippines and media coverage of the pandemic in Taiwan, which was intended to enhance the national image of the Communist government and demonstrate its legitimacy. In all, the cholera pandemic was highly politicized in the context of the Cold War politics.

Notes

1. Mark Harrison, *Contagion: How Commerce Has Spread Disease* (New Haven, CT: Yale University Press, 2012); Sunil S. Amrith, *Migration and Diaspora in Modern Asia* (Cambridge: Cambridge University Press, 2011), pp. 5–7.
2. Adam McKeown, "Conceptualizing Chinese Diasporas, 1842 to 1949," *Journal of Asian Studies* 58, 2 (1999): 313–15; Xiaoping Fang, "Teji xuyan: Jindai xinma huaren yiliao weisheng yu jibingshi yanjiu" [Introduction to Special Issue: Historical Research on Chinese Diaspora, Medicine, Health, and Disease in Modern Singapore and Malaysia], *Huaren yanjiu guoji xuebao* [International Journal of Diasporic Chinese Studies] 13, 1 (2021): 1–4.
3. Sunil S. Amrith, "Migration and Health in Southeast Asian History," *The Lancet*, 384, 9954 (2014): 1569.
4. Amrith, *Migration and Diaspora in Modern Asia*, p. 38.
5. Chen Da, *Nanyang huaqiao yu minyue shehui* [Nanyang Overseas Chinese and Guangdong Fujian Society] (Shanghai: Shangwu yinshuguan, 1937), p. 45.

6. Peng Jiali, "Shijiu shiji xifang qinlüezhe dui zhongguo laogong de lulüe" [Plundering and Looting of Western Invaders in China during the Nineteenth Century], in *Huagong chuguo shiliao huibian* [A Compilation of Historical Documents Concerning Chinese Laborers Overseas], ed. Chen Hansheng (Beijing: Zhonghua shuju, 1981), vol. 4, p. 209.

7. Reynaldo C. Ileto, "Cholera and the Origins of the American Sanitary Order in the Philippines," in *Discrepant Histories: Translocal Essays on Filipino Cultures*, ed. Vincente L. Rafael (Manchester and New York: Manchester University Press, 1988), pp. 125–8.

8. Robert Peckham, *Epidemics in Modern Asia* (Cambridge: Cambridge University Press, 2016), p. 258.

9. Angela Ki-Che Leung, *Leprosy in China: A History* (New York: Columbia University Press, 2009), p. 142.

10. Peckham, *Epidemics in Modern Asia*, p. 258.

11. Alison Bashford and Peter Hobbins, "Rewriting Quarantine: Pacific History at Australia's Edge," *Australian Historical Studies* 46, 3 (2015): 399.

12. Feng Banba, "Qizhangshan jianyizhan" [Quarantine Station of St John Island], *Xifeng* [Western Wind] 13, 115 (1949): 18–20.

13. Peckham, *Epidemics in Modern Asia*, pp. 61–2.

14. Regarding disease of Chinese migrants after their arrival in their destinations, see Amrith, "Migration and Health in Southeast Asian History," p. 1569; Amrith, *Migration and Diaspora in Modern Asia*, p. 41; James Francis Warren, *Ah Ku and Karayuki-San: Prostitution in Singapore, 1870–1940* (Singapore: Oxford University Press, 1993), p. 306; and Peckham, *Epidemics in Modern Asia*, pp. 44–94.

15. Li Yushang, "Heping shiqi de shuyi liuxing yu renkou siwang—yi jindai Guangdong, Fujian weili" [Plague and Death Tolls in Peacetime: An Example from Modern Guangdong and Fujian], *Shixue yuekan* [Journal of Historical Science] 9 (2003): 91–4. As to how returning overseas Chinese spread diseases among their home communities, such as venereal disease, see Chen, *Nanyang huaqiao yu minyue shehui*, pp. 257–8.

16. The following three sections reuse and revise some texts of chapters 1, 2, 4 and 7 of the monograph Xiaoping Fang, *China and the Cholera Pandemic: Restructuring Society under Mao* (Pittsburgh, PA: University of Pittsburgh Press, 2021).

17. Dalong Hu and Bin Liu, et al., "Origins of the Current Seventh Cholera Pandemic," *Proceedings of the National Academy of Sciences of the United States of America* 113, 48 (2016): E7730–2.

18. W.H. Mosley, "Epidemiology of Cholera," in *Principles and Practice of Cholera Control*, ed. World Health Organization (Geneva, 1970), pp. 23–4.

19. A.M. Kamal, "The Seventh Pandemic of Cholera," in *Cholera*, ed. Dhiman Barua and William Burrows (Philadelphia: Saunders, 1974), pp. 1–14.

20. Weishengbu gongzuozu [Work Team of the Ministry of Health], "Jin 25nianlai shijie fuhuoluan de liuxing he fangzhi gaikuang (1937.9–1962.9)" [Survey of El

Tor Cholera Transmission, Prevention and Treatment in the Last 25 Years], November 1962, Zhejiang Provincial Archives (ZJA), J166-2-160.

21. Dalong Hu and Bin Liu, et al., "Origins of the Current Seventh Cholera Pandemic," E7730.

22. Australian Embassy in Jakarta, "The Chinese in Indonesia," 15 December 1952, National Archives of Australia (NAA), A1838/280, 3034/2/5/1.

23. Jemma Purdey, *Anti-Chinese Violence in Indonesia 1996–1999* (Singapore: NUS Press, 2005), pp. 4–11.

24. Fang, *China and the Cholera Pandemic*, p. 32.

25. Walter H. Mallory, "Chinese Minorities in South East Asia," *Foreign Affairs* (New York), January 1956, NAA, A1838/280, 3034/2/5/1.

26. Bradley R. Simpson, *Economists with Guns: Authoritarian Development and U.S.-Indonesian Relations, 1960–1968* (Stanford, CA: Stanford University Press, 2010).

27. Liang Yingming, *Jinxiandai dongnanya 1511–1992* [Modern Southeast Asia, 1511–1992] (Beijing: Beijing daxue chubanshe, 1994), pp. 394–5.

28. Australian Embassy in Jakarta, "The Sino/Indonesian Dual Nationality Treaty, 1957–1962," NAA, A1838/280, 3034/2/5/1 Part 2.

29. At the same time, roughly 17,000 Indonesian Chinese went to Taiwan. Mozingo, *Chinese Policy toward Indonesia, 1949–1967* (Ithaca, NY: Cornell University Press, 1976), p. 175.

30. Herbert Feith and Daniel S. Lev, "The End of the Indonesian Rebellion," *Pacific Affairs* 36 (Spring 1963): 32–46.

31. Oscar Felsenfeld, "Some Observations on the Cholera (El Tor) Epidemic in 1961–1962," *Bulletin of World Health Organization* 28, 3 (1963): 290.

32. Tagliacozzo, "Pilgrim Ships and the Frontiers of Contagion: Quarantine Regimes from Southeast Asia to the Red Sea," in *Histories of Health in Southeast Asia: Perspectives on the Long Twentieth Century*, ed. Tim Harper and Sunil S. Amrith (Bloomington, IN: Indiana University Press, 2014), p. 48.

33. Felsenfeld, "Some Observations," p. 290.

34. Felsenfeld, "Some Observations," pp. 289–96.

35. Felsenfeld, "Some Observations," p. 290.

36. Zhonghua renmin gongheguo shanghai weisheng jianyisuo, "Shijie huoluan yiqing de zhangwo, fenxi yu yingyong," October 1963, ZJA, Vol. J166-2-199.

37. S.L. Kotar and J.E. Gessler, *Cholera: A Worldwide History* (Jefferson, NC: McFarland, 2014), p. 276.

38. Australian Embassy in Jakarta, "Chinese Nationalist Government Closed Down Consulate in Indonesia," August 1950, NAA, A1838, 406/9/2/12.

39. Fang, *China and the Cholera Pandemic*, p. 62.

40. Yongjiaxian qiaowuke [Department of Overseas Chinese Affairs of Yongjia County], "1961niandu diyi jidu qiaowu gongzuo xiaojie" [Summary of Overseas Chinese Affairs Work in the First Quarter of 1961], 2 May 1961, Yongjia County Archives, Zhejiang Province, Vol. 7-11-31.

41. Zhejiangsheng renmin weiyuanhui bangongting [The General Office of Zhejiang Provincial People's Commission], "Guanyu huaqiao he gang'ao tongbao yi waihui zhifu lüefei, qi jiaotong zhusu feiyong shixing bazhe youdai de tongzhi" [Circular on Offering 20% Discount to Overseas Chinese and Visitors from Hong Kong and Macau Paying Transport and Accommodation Fees in Foreign Currency], 27 January 1964, Pingyang County Archives, Zhejiang Province, Vol. 10-16-40.

42. Guangdongsheng fangyi zhihuibu Yangjiang gongzuozu [Work Team of Guangdong Provincial Epidemic Prevention Headquarters], "Liuxingbing diaocha baogao" [Investigation Report of the Epidemic in Yangjiang County, Guangdong Province], 24 August 1961, Yangjiang County Archives, Guangdong Province, Vol. X38.A12.1.36.

43. Qian Xinzhong, "Fuhuoluan fangzhi gongzuo de qingkuang ji jinhou renwu: Qian Xinzhong tongzhi zai fuhuoluan fangzhi gongzuo huiyishang de baogao," 12 December 1962, WZA, Vol. 38-14-7.

44. Qian Xinzhong, "Fuhuoluan fangzhi gongzuo huiyi zongjie" [Summary of the El Tor Cholera Prevention and Treatment Meeting], December 1964, ZJA, Vol. J166-1-80.

45. The government confirmed the role of returned Indonesian Chinese in the transmission of the cholera vibrio in its official publication in 1984. See *Dangdai zhongguo de weisheng shiye* [Health Development in Contemporary China], ed. Huang Shuze and Lin Shixiao (Beijing: Dangdai zhongguo chubanshe, Xianggang zuguo chubanshe, 2009), vol. 1, p. 268.

46. Hangzhoushi renmin weiyuanhui waishi bangongshi [Foreign Affair Office of Hangzhou City People's Commission], "Dui waibin he huaqiao cheliang tongguo ke mianjian fangxin de yijian" [Instructions on Exempting Quarantine Examination and Clearing Vehicles Carrying Foreign Guests or Overseas Chinese], 14 October 1963, ZJA, Vol. J166-2-175.

47. Shaoxingxian weishengju [Shaoxing County Health Bureau], "Guanyu jiaqiang dui fuhuoluan fabing diqu de wailai ji waichu renkou de jianyi he guanli gongzuo de tongzhi" [Circular on Strengthening Quarantine Management Work over Populations Coming into and Going Out of Cholera-affected Areas], 7 April 1965, Keqiao District Archives, Shaoxing City, Zhejiang Province, Vol. 105-8-13.

48. Zhejiangsheng weishengting [Zhejiang Provincial Health Department], "Guanyu dui huaji chuanyuan, guiguo huaqiao, gang'ao tongbao he shuqi fanxiao shisheng kaizhan yiyuan jiansuo de tongzhi" [Circular on Launching the Search for Epidemic Sources among Overseas Chinese Boatmen, Returned Overseas Chinese, Hong Kong and Macau Residents, and Students on Summer Vacation], 24 July 1964, ZJA, Vol. J166-2-206.

49. Valeska Huber, "The Unification of the Globe by Disease? The International Sanitary Conferences on Cholera, 1851–1894," *The Historical Journal* 49, 2 (June 2006): 474.

50. By the early 1970s, the WHO had further explicitly pointed out that inoculation was usually of no help for cholera control. Fang, *China and the Cholera Pandemic*, pp. 37–8, 113.
51. Liu Shaohua, *Mafeng yisheng yu jubian zhongguo: Hou diguo shiyanxia de jibing yinyu yu fangyi lishi* [Leprosy Doctors in China's Post-Imperial Experimentation: Metaphors of a Disease and Its Control] (Xinbei: Weicheng chuban, 2018); Guo Ruiqi (Rachel Core), "Laizi feijiehebing de jingyan: faxian he geli bingli yi kongzhi chuanranbing chuanbo" [Lesson from Tuberculosis: Identifying and Isolating Cases to Control Infectious Disease], *Zhonggong dangshi yanjiu* [CPC History Studies] 1 (February 2022): 92–5.
52. World Health Organization, *Guidelines for Cholera Control* (Geneva, 1993).
53. Charles L. Briggs and Clara Mantini-Briggs, *Stories in the Time of Cholera: Racial Profiling during a Medical Nightmare* (Berkeley, CA: University of California Press, 2003), p. 256.
54. Sung Lee, "WHO and the Developing World: The Contest for Ideology," in *Western Medicine as Contested Knowledge*, ed. Andrew Cunningham and Bridie Andrews (New York: Manchester University Press, 1997), pp. 25–8.
55. World Health Organization Regional Office for the Western Pacific, Report on Meeting for the Exchange of Information on El Tor Vibrio Paracholera, Manila, Philippines, 16–19 April 1962, WHO WPRO Archives, 1.
56. Willie T. Ong, "Public Health and the Clash of Cultures: The Philippine Cholera Epidemics," in *Public Health in Asia and the Pacific: Historical and Contemporary Perspectives*, ed. Milton J. Lewis and Kerrie L. MacPherson (Abingdon and New York: Routledge, 2008), p. 217.
57. Karel Raška, "Surveillance and Control of Cholera," in *Principles and Practice of Cholera Control*, ed. The World Health Organization (Geneva, 1970), p. 116.
58. Fang, *China and the Cholera Pandemic*, p. 56.
59. Xinhuashe [Xinhua News Agency], "Xiezhu feilübin pumie fuhuoluan, Wo hongshizihui jueding zengsong yipi huoluan yimiao" [To Assist the Philippines in Eradicating Cholera, Our China Red Cross Society Decided to Donate a Batch of Cholera Vaccines], *Renmin ribao* [The People's Daily, *RMRB*], 30 January 1962.
60. Xinhuashe [Xinhua News Agency], "Wo juanzeng de huoluan yimiao yundi feilübin" [Cholera Vaccines Donated by Our Country Have Reached the Philippines], *RMRB*, 16 February 1962.
61. Xinhuashe [Xinhua News Agency], "Taiwan nanbu fasheng fuhuoluan" [Cholera Broke Out in Taiwan], *RMRB*, 21 July 1962.
62. Xinhuashe [Xinhua News Agency], "Jiangfeibang mobuguanxin fangzhi gongzuo, Taiwan fuhuoluan yiqu xunshu kuoda" [Chiang Kai Shek Bandit Clique Did not Care about Epidemic Prevention and Treatment Work. Cholera Is Spreading Rampantly], *RMRB*, 14 August 1962.

CHAPTER 8

Managing Wartime Conditions: South Korean Developmental Ambitions, Public Health and Emerging Forms of Overseas Medical Outreach, 1964–73

John P. DiMoia

South Korean Military Medicine as Civic Outreach

The idea of cutting a soldier's hair to provide a standard appearance has long been a practice within military forces. By removing a significant portion of an individual's hair, the authority in charge reduces individuality, and begins the process of creating a new or replacement identity, one more in keeping with the ideals of the state. Moreover, the haircut fits nicely with public health concerns, as the removal of excess hair on the head, along with close grooming of the body, minimizes the risk of pests, reducing available territory in which parasites live and breed. For all of these reasons, the practice of the haircut suits the needs of the military, and scenes of fresh recruits undergoing such a ritual frequently dominate the literature and film imagery associated with the intake process for military life, with the accumulated hair clippings representing what has been left behind, the lingering traces of civilian identity.[1] Certainly the closely cropped skull of a fresh recruit is a familiar image, and allows outsiders to guess that the individual bearing such a look is undergoing boot camp or a similar form of rigorous training.[2]

Prior to these more recent (military) associations, there is a much longer history within East Asia of hair as a marker of cultural identity. The cutting of the queue in the Chinese context, a sign of the transition from the Qing to Republican China, has received a great deal of attention, and there are similar examples for the greater region. For the Korean peninsula, more specifically, there has been less written about hair and modernity per se, the transition to the late Joseon, and the arrival of Japanese colonialism. However, Shin Dong Won's "Hygiene, Medicine, and Modernity in Korea, 1876–1910" nicely locates the "top-knot controversy" of the 19th century in the context of emerging debates about hygiene.[3] Similarly, and in keeping with the seminal work of Ruth Rogaski, Jeong-ran Kim explains the Korean circumstances surrounding this conversation about hygiene, with port cities such as Incheon and Busan falling under Japanese quarantine practice as early as the 1870s (1876), even prior to the start of formal colonialism in 1910.[4]

South Korea Re-emerges after 1954

If these brief accounts of hair/the haircut fall within the domain of the familiar, the comparable use of the haircut for civilians holds less clarity as a form of practice. For nearly a decade, South Korean troops based in Vietnam (1964–73) offered "free haircuts" to children in Vietnamese villages, carefully documenting these encounters through a series of photographs, cartoon images and carefully compiled statistics.[5] Officially, the haircut was offered under the broad rubric of "civic actions," a series of public outreach campaigns mobilized specifically to provide a message of goodwill to complement the Korean military presence (Figure 8.1).[6] Such actions typically took two forms: either as military medicine, or as work activities related to construction and labor contexts. In the first case, well-known examples included vaccination campaigns for newborns, along with free health exams for village elders, that is, targeting the two most vulnerable populations, the youngest and the most senior cohorts. The Republic of Korea (ROK) military was acutely aware of the disruption it might cause in Vietnam, and offered a good deal of advice to its members regarding how to behave in the country, especially in terms of eliciting a positive reception precisely through these neighborly types of gestures.[7] In this setting, the haircuts marked such a form of outreach, embodying Korean developmentalist impulses, along with the desire for neighborly relations and the possibility of undertaking future projects together.

For its part, the South Korean army had existed for less than two decades as an institution, evolving from a constabulary force in the late 1940s as part of anti-communist nation-building.[8] Initially designed to handle the difficult transition from the US occupation to independence (September 1945–August 1948), the ROK military faced its first significant test dealing with civil disturbances in

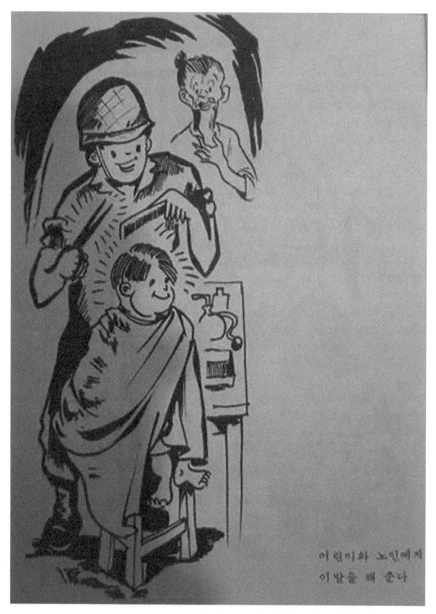

Figure 8.1. The caption reads "a child (and senior) receives a barber's favor," *Civic Actions*, p. 42.

the southwest portion of the peninsula in Yeosu (October 1948), before address-ing the outbreak of the Korean War, a conflict in which the very nature of society was put to the test. Facing a takeover by combined North Korean (June 1950) and Chinese forces (October–November 1950), South Korean troops received significant anti-communist training in keeping with the nationalist ideology under President Syngman Rhee (1948–60), justifying the state upon an affirma-tion of what the nation was not, and could never possibly be.[9]

In this context, medicine and public health formed a core part of the mis-sion of rebuilding, both during wartime and its aftermath. In fact, the transition to a greater reliance on biomedicine began, arguably, as early as the occupation, with the initial focus placed on public health as an outbreak of disease across the region was feared.[10] The use of models of biomedicine, whether inter-national or American, came to characterize South Korean military medicine over a period of more than a decade (1948–early 1960s), a process especially useful to those with prior (Japanese) training in the colonial education sys-tem. The desire to employ this form of practice in the Vietnamese context makes sense, in that Korean personnel were eager to display the products of their accumulated experience, and were highly familiar with the experience as recipients.[11] In Korean-language research materials, the mission is thus de-picted as one of benevolent outreach, with the ROK repaying its allies for their Korean War assistance.[12] In this version of events, South Vietnam found itself under threat from communist aggression, with the Koreans, drawing upon their own recent experience, willing to respond in turn.

This repayment of a debt figures prominently in Korean-language research materials, but this description does not necessarily reflect the Vietnamese perspective. At the same time, anxiety about the encounter runs palpably through the Korean materials, as the Koreans were highly concerned with, and eager to manage, the process of reception. In particular, this encoun-ter was not just about the haircut as an act or individual performance, but also about a diverse cluster of perceptions regarding the treatment of children, fo-cusing on their care and handling. A growing literature for the Korean War concerns the presence of children in the war zone, and how they became a means for changing the wartime scenario into a post-war, humanitarian mis-sion from the American standpoint. In brief, waifs or orphans in the field first became unofficial "mascots," linked to US GIs, before becoming formal adop-tees, patients and recipients of various forms of aid.[13] If South Korea was not yet equipped at this level to handle Vietnamese children, it nonetheless pos-sessed the motivation to understand how civil affairs combined with public health might transform an uncomfortable wartime scenario. In its own case, South Korea used transnational adoption to handle its post-war social problems (single mothers, mixed-race children), while crafting a new image abroad, with healthy children strategically placed with specific demographics, generally white, Christian families.

To support this claim, it bears mentioning that a number of the parties previously involved in the Korean War also came to play prominent roles in the Vietnamese context. Dr Howard Rusk, renowned for his work with prosthetics and rehabilitative medicine at New York University (NYU), came to prominence in the Korean War and its aftermath, working especially with young children and injured soldiers.[14] Rusk later used his NYU position as a platform, writing a weekly column in *The New York Times*. In Vietnam, he would advise on burn injuries and the loss of limbs, just as he had in Korea. Similarly, a number of the Korean doctors working with parasites and pests in the domestic context took charge of the same range of issues on behalf of Korean soldiers in Vietnam.[15] The combination of American and Korean approaches to public health should not be taken as a strict determinant of health policy in Vietnam, but it highlights the reality that Koreans drew upon existing models when working with children in the field, models already familiar from a decade previously, and still being used domestically in Korean villages. In other words, haircuts represented much more than an isolated act, and embodied a range of core values undergoing transition during and following the Korean War.

Managing the Encounter with Developmental Attitudes

This chapter considers the "free haircuts" encounter in Vietnam as a combination of public health, civic outreach and formative developmentalism, while seeking to place this set of questions within the larger context of renewed diplomatic relations between the south and its close neighbors in East and Southeast Asia. With the renewal of diplomatic relations to its regional partners, such as Taiwan (1948), the Philippines (1949), South Vietnam (1956), Thailand (1958) and others in proximity, South Korea began to construct a context for itself, a network of trade partners and allies, beginning in the late 1950s.[16] At the same time, the ROK had to work through the novelty of conducting this business as an emerging, post-colonial partner, whereas previously, it had interacted with many of these same sites in its capacity as either Chosŏn Korea (1392–1910), or more recently as a colony, part of the Japanese Empire (1910–45). It should not be surprising that the "new" network, provisional and labeled as the "Free World," closely resembled the previous Japanese imperial network, and a number of scholars have begun to comment upon this historical correspondence.[17] At the same time, the previous East Asian order had changed dramatically, and as many of the chapters in this volume illustrate, emerging post-colonial nations also had to address questions of legitimacy, with claims about health serving as a useful metric.

Along with this temporal transition comes the imagined relationship of kinship or proximity between South Korea and South Vietnam, two post-colonial nations holding provisional status, with sovereignty still very much in question.[18] A significant amount of energy went into providing legitimation for the sovereignty of each of these two nations. In fact, the Korean experience of more than a decade served as a potential model for South Vietnam, an analogy present in (Korean) propaganda materials across linguistic and cultural lines.[19] For its part, specifically, South Korea frequently used the trope of a symbolic relationship between the 38th parallel (North/South Korea) and the 17th (North/South Vietnam), suggesting that here was an opportunity to return the debt incurred during the Korean War. On the ground, this meant that the Korean military presence was complemented by a diverse set of outreach activities, including infrastructure, medical aid and even Taekwondo demonstrations, with the last of these offering a condensed version of Korean culture expressed in a concentrated, masculinist form.[20]

If this vision of Korean dynamism was constructed to convince the Vietnamese of their partner's power within a wartime context, much of this activity was also designed with the domestic context as its primary audience. Newsreels and the beginnings of Korean broadcasting offered an opportunity to display the mission abroad, albeit in a carefully filtered form.[21] For medicine in particular, the campaigns for public health not only offered a symbolic link between the Korean village and its Vietnamese counterpart but, in fact, a material connection. In the case of anti-parasite activity, as previously mentioned, many of the same personnel (doctors, parasitologists) ran the campaigns in both locations, overseeing national campaigns at home, while also running outreach initiatives overseas.[22] This approach allowed for comparative data to be gathered and, in fact, Korean medical teams, along with their Filipino and Taiwanese allies, were asked to subsidize South Vietnamese public health during the later stages of the war, as Americans did not trust the Vietnamese health infrastructure.[23]

If the Korean role in the war ended with the departure of armed forces in 1973, to be followed by the fall of Saigon in 1975, these dates do not mark a terminal point for the effects of outreach. In 1974, Korean medical representatives, along with their colleagues from Japan, joined to form the Asian Parasite Control Organization (APCO), a group which brought together East and Southeast Asian partners to share information about a wide variety of pests.[24] For the Korean side, many of the leading figures had served in Vietnam and participated in the Korea Preventive Medicine (KOPREM) initiative and comparable outreach efforts, meaning that the overseas experience was very much one of cumulative learning carried forward. Again, while the focus here begins modestly with the haircut scenario, the meeting site between Korean soldiers and Vietnamese children, the larger point remains one of recognizing the long-term implications, especially for Korea and Southeast Asia, with diplomatic normalization between South Korea and Vietnam resuming in 1992. Framed as an act of civic outreach, and embedded within notions of psychological warfare, acquired in part from the Americans during the 1950s, the haircut rested within a larger set of concerns about how to mobilize Korean developmental ambitions.

Constructing a "Free World" Network (1952–Early 1960s)

The gradual erosion of 1945 as a dividing line has taken place within a cluster of related fields, including Japan Studies, Korean Studies and Development Studies. This remark does not deny the political and symbolic significance of the year, but recognizes that imperial structures continued to play a critical role throughout the region, and continued doing so for at least the next several decades (1945–early 1970s), especially during post-war Japan's period of rapid economic growth. For South Korea, this claim means that the transformation of its institutions coinciding with the Korean War represented outreach in at least two directions: towards an international model, and towards a Japanese/imperial model, with the second case often restoring prior relationships dating back to colonial rule. For public health specifically, the construction of basic infrastructure possessed, at least nominally, the appearance of a completely "new" set of structures, especially those facilities and practices associated with new sources of funding deriving from international partners.

The initial gesture towards building a public health network dates back to the Korean War, with combat confined largely to the center of the peninsula from the middle of 1951. The United Nations Korea Reconstruction Agency (UNKRA) and other UN affiliates began to address subsistence issues, seeking to limit the spread of disease, and to house and care for displaced populations, especially the large numbers of refugees living in or close to Pusan.[25] The American-Korean Foundation (AKF), an organization linking Korean mission interests with American East Coast foundations and universities, became one of the major actors bridging this kind of work, constructing housing for orphans, and focusing in particular on disability.[26] In this last case, Dr Howard Rusk, already well-known for his work with wounded veterans during World War II, saw an opportunity through providing prosthetic limbs to Koreans, those suffering from war-related injuries, polio and a variety of congenital ailments.[27]

To offer a generalization, building upon the work of Rusk, the multilateral forms of aid coming to South Korea during wartime, and continuing after 1953, effectively subsidized the construction of a health network during the second half of the decade (1954–60), with new work appearing under the auspices of the World Health Organization (WHO) and other partners.[28] Whereas Korea had previously worked within a Japanese network, it now replaced these ties with a set of international actors. From wartime contingencies (cholera, typhus, hemorrhagic fever), the post-war focus shifted to treating problems of chronic disease, an issue that might be handled while building a network, starting with the major cities, and reaching out into rural areas. Such problems included tuberculosis and leprosy, and, in these cases, the issues had already been addressed previously by missionaries and by Japanese physicians.[29] In terms of potential models, the international partners drew upon knowledge from the previous context, often sending specialists familiar with other imperial situations. At the same time, those Koreans with prior Japanese training were able to assert their "ownership" of the network and its resources, a critical development for nation-building.

In the process of connecting beyond the domestic to the East and Southeast Asian regions, South Korea normalized its diplomatic relations with many of its neighbors. In the case of South Vietnam, dating to the late 1950s, there was a prior context: first as a country with a similar history in the Sino-centric world and, equally, as a space (very briefly) under Japanese rule. The new partnership in the Cold War setting explains in part the "Free World" network, where regional partners—Thailand, Taiwan, South Korea, Hong Kong and South Vietnam—nominally shared a certain language borrowed from the American and European imperial contexts. In fact, what many of these countries shared was a history as former colonies, especially under the influence of either China or Japan. The process of reconnecting, therefore, was accelerated when existing networks could be mobilized to enhance the process. Certainly this was the case for public health and biology, where many former Korean students (imperial or colonized subjects) now held positions as leading national figures in South Korea.

In particular, Korean entomologists and biologists were able to further their career ambitions in the post-war and Syngman Rhee periods by leveraging these types of relationships, sometimes with previous Japanese partners, and, at other times, with new partners. In 1962, a national campaign against malaria began with considerable assistance from the WHO, and this initiative continued throughout the decade (1959, 1962–70).[30] Two years later, in 1964, a diverse group formed the Korea Anti-Parasite Eradication (KAPE) program, and this started a national school-based campaign late in the decade distributing anthelminthics to young children suffering from roundworm infestation (1969–late 1980s). In both cases, the perceived "success" of these campaigns provided Korean doctors, scientists and political figures with the confidence to begin mobilizing a message blending post-colonial ambitions and public health to their partners, no longer exclusively to a domestic constituency.

More importantly, this perception of success was not held by Koreans alone, but was often shared by their partners. Whereas previously, American medicine had worked in the region primarily through Filipino partners, given a lengthy historical relationship, this pattern would begin to change by the early 1960s. In Laos, American doctors had created a loose network to assist rural communities, and this program was augmented by Operation Brotherhood (OB), an initiative run by Filipino Jesuits.[31] By 1964, the ROK sent its first actors to Vietnam—a medical unit designed to aid Vietnamese civilian patients, based southeast of Saigon in Vung Tau.[32] The desire to avoid contact with the North Vietnamese (and Vietcong) forces shaped the reality of this civic mission. It also indicated the presence of surrounding violence, as fighting had continued, despite the end of the French War in 1954.

To link the end of the Korean War and the intervention in Vietnam (1953–64), the attention devoted to building a domestic health infrastructure would carry implications as the Koreans began to move beyond the peninsula. As mentioned previously, the National Malaria Eradication System (NMES) had its origins in a 1962 WHO-sponsored initiative, with a preliminary study dating to 1959.[33] Throughout this program, attention was specifically devoted to rural public health, ensuring the availability of basic infrastructure at the provincial and village levels. This initiative held great possibilities, as it served multiple functions: many of the new and refurbished clinics attended to not only the issue of malaria, but to an overlapping series of campaigns, including tuberculosis and family planning. In brief, nearly a decade of experience yielded a good deal of confidence for the Korean medical personnel, and this carried over into the Vietnam context, with Koreans eager to demonstrate their skills.

This connection, the imagined relationship between the Korean rural village and its Vietnamese counterpart, helped to shape the medical relationship that carried over for nearly a decade. If Korean communities experienced tension with respect to biomedicine, perhaps deriving from the previous colonial relationship, it helps to remember that the Vietnam context also held a heightened degree of ambivalence. In general, Korean medical personnel arrived only after a village had been "pacified," that is, rendered sufficiently safe to be occupied by troops interested in establishing a long-term presence. Korean troops such as the Tiger Division were known for their harsh responses to any suspected Vietcong presence. This factor meant that villagers were unsure whether to expect more violence, while, in turn, the Korean medics hoped to provide a message of reassurance, combined with some pragmatic measures. It was in this context that haircuts likely became a means of establishing contact and ensuring goodwill, by attempting to return to a basic gesture of human interaction, a simple strategy of seeking solidarity.

Although these perceptions relate to the Korean side, and not necessarily to the reactions of the Vietnamese, the common trope of the village runs deeply through American and Korean documents from the period, especially in relation to the deployment of public health. South Korean personnel were already penetrating the rural (domestic) countryside as late as the second half of the 1950s, working with leprosy and, later, malaria. In effect, the problem of chronic disease, along with baseline health maintenance for the military recruits, formed the core of Korean public health, providing a level of uniformity to a population still largely based in rural communities. This powerful mechanism of cultural change is what the Koreans brought to Vietnam through their participation in "Free World" medical assistance. In fact, the Americans believed that there might be common elements to village life, despite the obvious differences in context. This logic formed part of the motivation for placing Asians partners (Filipinos, Koreans and, to a degree, Thai, though less so in the case of medical doctors) in these settings.

Moreover, the barbershop, or *ibalso*, was one of the first provisions associated with the arrival of the Koreans, even before our consideration of the "free haircut." The Dove (or Pigeon) Brigade of the Korean military, specifically its civil affairs component, undertook a good deal of building upon arrival at a location, seeking to mobilize the benefits of living in proximity to such a community.[34] Common features included housing structures, some sort of facility for work training (typing, sewing and so on), schools and orphanages. A quick survey of these facilities, typically featured in newsreels promoted under the heading of "Vietnam News," notes the similarities with the Korean context a decade earlier, especially the period immediately following the war.[35] In other words, without suggesting any conscious effort to copy, it should not be surprising that the civil affairs forces worked with familiar tools and methods, using comparable experiences drawn from the Korean context. This remark refers to wartime, but especially to the period of post-war rebuilding.

Mobilizing (Korean) Civil Affairs in Vietnam (1964–73)

Prior to its military role, South Korea was already reaching out to Southeast Asia. Following the normalization of relations with Thailand and South Vietnam, the ROK began to transition from an import substitution economy to establishing a modest set of export ambitions. With this gesture, South Korea opened the first Korea Overseas Trade Agency (KOTRA) offices in 1962, a government agency tasked specifically with paving the way for Korean business and trade overseas. The first four offices included two in the surrounding region (Bangkok and Hong Kong) along with two in the United States (New York and Los Angeles).[36] In 1964, a Saigon office would follow, further indicating interest in Southeast Asia, along with several Japanese offices (Tokyo and Osaka), with these last two tied to the normalization of relations in 1965. This frenzy of activity runs counter to the realities of war, or so it would appear, pairing war with commerce.

This last observation emphasizes a central feature of the Korean role in Vietnam, one often overlooked in historical accounts: logistics and infrastructure. Along with other allies recruited under the rhetoric of "Many Flags," South Korean forces undertook the diverse tasks related to the conduct of the war, especially the work of transporting, building and housing, whether in reference to material goods, services or human beings.[37] Given its prior relationship with the US military, and especially in port cities such as Incheon and Busan during and following the Korean War, the Korean military, along with private firms, became a trusted partner, one whose primary function was not strictly military, at least in the limited sense of conducting battles in the field.[38] If the first Korean contingent to arrive in Vietnam was medical (September 1964), the second group (February 1965) was devoted almost exclusively to civil affairs, combining the Dove/Pigeon Brigade (비둘기) with a group of Taekwondo instructors. This second group frequently conducted demonstration lessons for Vietnamese villagers, showcasing the best of Korean athletic ability, culture and masculinity.

The Korean role in Vietnam was complicated by the proximity of American troops—although Korean forces generally conducted their affairs on an independent basis—and by their interactions with Vietnamese villagers, often following a conflict. Given these tense relations, the medical role was carefully restricted from the start, and specifically tied to the treatment of civilian injuries, thus avoiding the appearance of any direct involvement in the war. These rigid restrictions changed after 1965 but, nonetheless, the notion of treating only the South Vietnamese, whether civilians or soldiers, remained part of the rhetoric. Moreover, the medical presence was tied to the care of a diverse range of groups: first, to individual military units; next, to the care of the increasing number of private contract workers arriving for construction; and finally to the Dove/Pigeon Brigade, the official branch of the Korean military representing the civil affairs presence.

With this array of at least three different groups in the country, we will restrict discussion to the last of these, while recognizing that interactions took place in a variety of circumstances. Arriving in early 1965, the Dove/Pigeon Brigade combined the tasks of construction and civil affairs, with the second category perhaps generating the greatest attention in terms of shaping the unit's reputation. In a booklet distributed to the Korean troops, titled "Civic Actions," the rationale for reaching out to the Vietnamese civilians is carefully justified as a form of psychological warfare, a means by which locals might be persuaded to understand the Korean point of view.[39] In the image shown in Figure 8.2, three circles represent the vertices of a triangle: one in which Koreans fight for the Vietnamese (morale), one in which Koreans provide support and assistance (to the Vietnamese citizens), and a third in which the Koreans contest the enemy directly.[40] The last image is not necessarily set in opposition to the first two, but rather depicted as part of a cycle, a relationship in which the Vietnamese, regardless of ideological persuasion, come to know and respect the Koreans based upon their actions.

Although this series of relationships is framed specifically in terms of "psychological warfare," it does not appear to preclude the notion of human contact, nor the possibility of engaging with others even during a contentious war. Along with its focus upon children, the volume provides a wide range of vignettes concerning Vietnamese elders and women, as soldiers encounter them in different social situations. In this context, the volume seeks to provide a comprehensive guide to Vietnamese social mores, consistently emphasizing the need to adapt to local conditions. If the geography is not specified beyond the locale of Vietnam, the city of Saigon and its surroundings appear to form the default backdrop, as many of these imagined encounters depict urban scenes rather than rural. On the whole, the images dedicated to medicine and haircuts represent a small fraction of the content, as the volume's major premise links to minimizing social friction and getting along on Vietnamese terms. The assumptions within which these civil affairs activities appear, moreover, derive from the lessons learned previously in Korean villages.

If these relations come across as idealized, they do so not only within the Vietnam context, but also likely draw upon the experiences of the Korean War, whether positive or negative. In this context, the focus upon children makes perfect sense, as the presence of refugees and camp followers was a common phenomenon in Korea, especially within the Pusan perimeter and its surroundings. Here, a large number of orphans, displaced families, war widows and others fled during the outbreak of war in the summer of 1950 (June 1950–spring 1951), and many would not return to Seoul (or other locations)

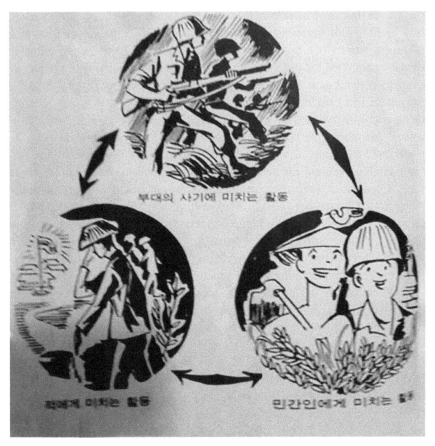

부대의 사기에 미치는 활동

적에게 미치는 활동   민간인에게 미치는 활동

Figure 8.2. *Civic Actions*, p. 4. The relationships among morale, support and combat.

until 1954. A second wave of refugees appeared with the second fall of Seoul in early 1951. With a growing body of literature concerning the practice of international adoption, specifically during and following the Korean War, scholars have commented on how certain American units informally "adopted" young Korean boys, those left without means and with no sign of family support.[41] In some cases, these arrangements became more formalized as some of these children were eligible for adoption, with American patrons willing to assume responsibility.

Without beginning a discussion on the complicated politics of adoption on the American side, for which there is a rich and growing literature, it is easy to see how these children complicated the conduct of war.[42] At the very least, security around American bases was subject to numerous "camp followers," who depended economically on leftovers, whether in the form of food, shelter or other provisions.[43] In the Vietnamese context, these types of concerns carried over, even more so for those fighting positions situated in or near jungle sites, where there was no clear "front line," a set of circumstances much murkier than in previous conflicts. For large storage sites, such as Cam Ranh Bay on the east coast, the American military favored other Asians over Vietnamese to staff the warehouses, acknowledging that it might be "difficult" to distinguish Vietnamese civilians from any Vietcong seeking to gain entry. In other words, if identity and tropes of race had previously caused confusion in Korea, these issues again played a major role in Vietnam, with the presence of additional actors heightening tensions.

Structuring/Ordering Civilian Life

With civic actions, Korean forces made some attempt to bring order to this situation, at least in terms of establishing a stable form of community. The building campaigns associated with the Dove/Pigeon Brigade typically included an orphanage and housing as part of the package, and these measures presumably sought to deal with the issue of those with unclear status. Next, the public health campaigns brought a necessary check to the problem of disease outbreak, keeping such incidents to a minimum, and ensuring a safe environment for Korean troops living nearby. Finally, other forms of outreach—whether expressed as culture, Taekwondo, and similar demonstrations and performances—built better relations with the community, indicating good intentions on the part of these visitors. As for haircuts, this activity accomplished several goals simultaneously, with public health enforcement only representing the most obvious.

The Pigeon/Dove Brigade arrived as the second part of the Korean presence, following the dispatch of medical forces in September 1964. Devoted specifically to civil affairs, the brigade brought a diverse program to the Vietnam context, featuring in particular an ambitious building program, along with related medical and public health activities (Figure 8.3). It is the building program which received a great deal of attention in the official publications

Figure 8.3. The unit patch for the Dove Brigade, featuring an olive branch and Korean script in *hangul*, indicating the mission: "Construction."

emerging from the war, along with newsreels intended for domestic distribution. As stated previously, there are numerous points of comparison between the building/relief activities associated with the Korean War and its aftermath and the Vietnam context, whether in terms of materials, personnel or thematic approaches. Certainly both wars introduced a great deal of civil disorder, with refugees forced to relocate due to the circumstances. In the Korean context, emerging international and United Nations institutional structures created during and following World War II found a test environment in which models and practices could be tried out and improved accordingly, especially in terms of providing relief and basic forms of sustenance.

In this scenario, the period of post-Korean War reconstruction (1954–60) links neatly to the construction ambitions in Vietnam, as Korean firms sought to continue their rapid growth, whether in terms of contracts or skill acquisition. Vietnam, and Southeast Asia more broadly, provided an experimental setting, a context in which technical learning would be ongoing, with lucrative results available as a fringe benefit. As in the case of KOTRA (1962), these ambitions preceded the war, with Korean firms such as Hyundai opening a Bangkok office as early as 1964. Though unsuccessful, Korean firms had begun to bid for contracts in the region at least two years previously, recognizing the opportunity. Geographers Jim Glassman and Young-Jin Choi, for example, cite a case where Korean firms were informed about the building of airfields in northern Thailand, sites later to be used as the bases for B-52 bombers carrying out strikes over Vietnam.[44] Positioned as an intermediary, or sub-imperial role, Korean firms sought to surpass the niche assigned to them, overtaking the Filipino and Cambodian workers in similar situations, and competing directly with the Japanese.

The first successful contract bids went through in 1965 (Hyundai and Daerim), with construction commencing later that year through early 1966. If this activity was directed through private firms, the Korean military also participated very actively in the war zone, especially Vietnam, taking charge over a significant number of infrastructure projects. During much of this activity, Korean workers earned the trust of their partners, while also directing work teams from Southeast Asia, including many Vietnamese. Here, as with the civil affairs teams in the villages, the critical importance of relationships with colleagues became part of the process—that is, working in an international environment, with a multi-national workforce.

The larger point motivating this discussion is twofold: whatever form it took, Korean civil affairs in its institutional version emerged out of the context of the Korean War and its aftermath, therefore likely drawing upon a wealth of resources, including domestic, Japanese and international models. Along with this observation, the growth of the practice, while officially framed in terms of Korean–Vietnamese relations, actually took place within a much larger set of relationships. Korean building and construction for this period occurred in several different locations throughout Southeast and East Asia—Thailand (1965–68), Vietnam (1964–73) and Guam (1969)—and, at these sites, encountered an extremely diverse population. So while Vietnam remains the primary object of this inquiry, it is clear that the Koreans were seeking to establish a notion of order not only in the village context, but also in respect of themselves, aware of how they might be perceived by onlookers.[45]

In other words, even as there remain important factors to consider (public health, demography) as constituent parts of the encounter, the most conspicuous thread of the narrative rests with the establishing of South Korean–Southeast Asian neighborly relations, a set of ideals with critical importance to the growing Korean economy. Moreover, if economy remained a major part of the story, this process of outreach also connected to issues of sovereignty and legitimacy, as indeed it did for other "Free World" partners. For "divided nations" in competition over a contested national category—East and West Germany, South and North Korea, South and North Vietnam, and Taiwan (Republic of China) and China (People's Republic of China), the Cold War competition for allies and legitimacy often determined survival over the long-term, certainly shaping how the nation was perceived, and with whom it might interact.[46] In the South Korean case, the investment in South Vietnam was not merely symbolic, therefore, but possessed a sense of genuine interest in the viability and longevity of the project, having undergone a similar set of experiences in the late 1940s and early 1950s.

Public Health, Demography and Model-Building

To this point, the discussion has been framed in terms of civic outreach, and the set of humanitarian values implicit to the encounter. While this approach holds value, it is unlikely to cover the entirety of the official rationale underlying the campaigns. In terms of their public roll-out, the haircuts appeared in two forms: in numerous photographic images and in statistical charts, with the latter compiled and appearing in annual reports issued by the Korean military.[47] In these two forms, the campaigns assumed a more official stance, especially in statistical form, with the ease of display and the possibility of drawing inferences, although this second possibility does not seem to have been a goal. Given these forms, what was the intent behind the haircuts, here framed in public health and biomedical terms? The reports generally do not offer a detailed rationale, and merely present the cumulative work on its own terms, suggesting that the message was sufficiently clear, at least to its target demographic, presumably civil servants who might come across such a report.

In the absence of an official rationale, our answer has to be necessarily framed as partial and speculative, but there are a number of avenues which suggest a response. At the very least, the desire to cut the hair of Vietnamese children formed a core part of outreach, suggesting friendly relations following a period of combat. Moreover, as already suggested, Korean soldiers likely retained a historical memory of American soldiers undertaking similar forms of outreach a decade previously, via housing, food and other goods distributed to neighboring camp towns.[48] Given these circumstances, the most likely explanation of the haircuts lies with public health and the desire to minimize the spread of disease, especially among populations living in close proximity. In 1945, much of northeast Asia witnessed mass sprayings of DDT—especially in Korean and Japanese port cities—as repatriation brought thousands of soldiers "home" in the aftermath of the Japanese empire.[49] For many Koreans, this uncomfortable and invasive process formed their first impressions of Americans, and, indeed, there is a rich photographic record of the period, with this activity continuing throughout the Korean War.[50]

Along with familiarity, the desire of Korean officials to generate and exert control over their own statistical information should not go without mention. Imperial Japan ran its first empire-wide census in 1925, with Korean participation only at the ground level. This activity continued throughout 1940, with the war then interrupting the process, followed by the major disruption of the Korean War. It was not until 1955 that South Korea, a new post-colonial nation, was able to conduct its own census, an exercise holding much greater significance.[51] Besides the need for reliable data internally, these figures provided a comparison with North Korea in the contest for legitimacy. Korean statistics also had to be shared with partner nations, and the combination of American aid and Japanese funds (starting as of 1965) meant an opportunity, assuming the numbers and data looked appropriate, to demonstrate the "right" forms of progress to its patrons. In this sense, these statistics were integral to ROK nation-building, and, again, Vietnam offered an opportunity to gather comparative data.

Public Health and Hair Length

As noted at the outset, the issue of hair—aesthetically, culturally—figures in military regulations, although here again the problem of capturing distinct Korean and Vietnamese voices presents itself. Certainly Korean masculinity was often tied to shorter, closely maintained hairstyles by the mid-1960s, even outside of military life. Famously, following the suspension of the constitution

(1972–79), the government would send police to monitor hair length—and the length of women's skirts—during the Yusin period of the early 1970s.[52] In these cases, it was also well-known for the police to tug the hair of offenders, and sometimes to pull them off the street for an impromptu hair trim. Although these encounters took place shortly after the period under focus here, the point remains that masculinity and short hair were closely linked, in contrast to the much more diverse styles of the present.

In the case of Vietnam, the images do not suggest any one standard haircut, but rather a generic style suited to young children, approximating the well-known "bowl cut." In other words, the haircut was not the military induction style familiar to recruits, nor was it the "high and tight" style typical of many troops following basic training. A suitable description might be "short and neat," a haircut ensuring that Vietnamese children retained their identity while encountering Korean troops in a controlled situation. From a public health standpoint, the haircut permitted a quick check for head lice/parasites, and the short hairstyle likely provided a visual marker of those who had already been checked or cleared. In particular, the presence of head lice seems to have been a major factor of interest, given the possibility of typhus or other epidemic diseases.

If the factor of controlling disease in the Vietnamese population was not stated explicitly, the goal certainly informed a great deal of the Korean approach, as indeed this kind of approach typifies public health in many combat situations. Living in close proximity to another group or population entails an overlap of diet, sanitation and living spaces. Logically, a possible exchange of microbes and the microbial environment (biome) follows from these factors. In preparation for Vietnam, and during the Korean mission overseas, the majority of domestic campaigns for disease—especially for parasites and malaria—saw the medical personnel in charge extend their research to Southeast Asia, enabling comparative work with Vietnamese soldiers and villagers. In this respect, the Vietnamese children offered another possible demographic, and although this aim was not necessarily advertised as such, it is still worth pointing out, namely, that medical outreach and disease prevention represented complementary goals, with typhus probably representing the target.

Although "counting" does not receive any explicit mention in the form of a proper demographic survey, it does appear to be utilized in the statistical figures associated with haircuts issued annually by the ROK military. In the ROK domestic context, the use of demography shaped population concerns, family planning and urban planning up until the early 1960s. In particular, Korean rural areas were targeted for family planning, as these areas constituted high growth areas, and there was the added difficulty of reaching the population through newspaper adverts or print and with radio and TV promotions not always penetrating these sites.

Moreover, internal migration became a major concern for much of the 1960s and 1970s, with major cities serving to drive rural to urban patterns of movement, especially for those seeking jobs and hoping to leave the agricultural sector. While South Korea never strictly policed individual provinces, nor forbade such types of movement, the internal migration represented a concern which the government hoped to track. With the Vietnam effort happening almost simultaneously, it is reasonable that military officials wanted some idea of the surrounding populations to which Korean troops were living in proximity, especially in terms of their health conditions and the potential for the outbreak of disease.

The recent work of Mark Harrison hints at the possibility of greater ambitions, as programs like Korean Preventive Medicine (KOPREM)—with Korean public health officials subcontracting their work to United States Agency for International Development (USAID), and thereby subsidizing the work of Vietnamese officials—reached out to the countryside, supplementing existing efforts achieved via American aid. When Korean forces withdrew from Vietnam in 1973, the plans for KOPREM indicated a desire to continue beyond the period and, in fact, indicated a scope comparable to that for South Korea. In other words, Korean health officials, given their experience in rural villages, felt that their experience could be beneficial to the Vietnamese, and saw the potential to achieve similar results in peacetime, assuming the war could be brought to a conclusion. If these ambitions never reached fruition, they nonetheless underscore an alternative vision for Vietnam, one in which the post-1975 communist nation held a distinct trajectory, perhaps more closely resembling the path taken by South Korea and Taiwan in the late 1980s.

To hint beyond the scope of this chapter, similar ambitions extended to other parts of the developing world, including the recently decolonizing nations of Africa. As early as 1968, South Korea sent small medical teams to select new nations, asking for diplomatic recognition in return for medical assistance.[53] If this activity was explicitly political in its motives, there was nonetheless a set of related economic motives, aiming at promoting trade and exchange once relations had been established. In the case of South Vietnam, specifically, Korean identification with a close partner, one for which it held ambitions similar to its own, was not merely about forming symbolic ties. The Republic of Vietnam figured in Korean trade figures almost immediately following the Korean War, and offered a ready market for Korean exports throughout the 1960s. Again, the ties between the two nations can be seen at multiple levels—the village, public health, trade—as South Korea continued to expand its developmental ambitions.

To be clear, these ambitions never happened, and much of what South Korea anticipated has to be considered as counterfactual, a fantasy of democratic allies working together throughout the 1970s with expanding economies. At the same time, the Korean desire to reach out to Vietnam and normalize relations, a drive beginning at some point in the mid-1980s, loses some of this ideological edge, while retaining much of the ambition. South Korea normalized relations with the Vietnamese (in 1992) prior to the United States, and did the same with other communist nations. This later increasingly meant the movement of Korean factories, construction and infrastructure ambitions to Vietnam at the close of the century, and into the next, where Vietnam and Southeast Asia now stand at the center of Korean ambitions to negotiate a space for itself between the United States and China. If the majority of the chapters here reflect Cold War circumstances, with a subset of post-colonial nations finding their way, the region now wrestles with the US–China divide in political and material terms. If Korean ambitions have to change, moreover, at least part of the early 1960s optimism and impulse remains.

The haircuts reflect concerns both about Vietnam and about emerging patterns for Korean developmentalism, as the Vietnam experience proved to be the origins for what soon became a road map to the Middle East and beyond. The institutions, practices and beliefs tested in Southeast Asia provided a tentative way out of the domestic context and back into the region, and a way of negotiating the spaces between the Japanese and American empires. Specifically, haircuts rhetorically and materially connected Korean health officials with an approach to Vietnamese public health, one bridging the Korean experience and the new context. If the assumptions underpinning the haircuts were not always made explicit, it is possible that the actors themselves did not always hold fully formed notions concerning their ambitions, choosing instead to translate some version of what they had experienced in their own relationship to the American presence in post-war "rehabilitation" Korea (1954–60). These "civic actions" formed the basis for what would become, by the early 1990s, a set of institutions and practices (including the Korea International Cooperative Agency, 1991) to sell the Korean developmental vision to the larger world.

Notes

1.   Shin Dong Won, "Hygiene, Medicine, and Modernity in Korea, 1876–1910," *East Asian Science, Technology and Society* 3, 1 (2009): 5–26.
2.   John P. DiMoia, "Providing Reassurance and Affirmation: Masculinity, Militarization and Refashioning a Male Role in South Korean Family Planning: 1962

to the Late 1980s," in *Gender, Health, and History in Modern East Asia*, ed. Angela Leung and Izumi Nakayama (Hong Kong: Hong Kong University Press, 2018), pp. 244–70. See also Won Kim, "The Race to Appropriate 'Korean-ness': National Restoration, Internal Development, and Traces of Popular Culture," in *Cultures of Yusin: South Korea in the 1970s*, ed. Youngju Ryu (Ann Arbor: University of Michigan Press, 2018), p. 30.

3. Shin Dong Won, "Hygiene, Medicine, and Modernity in Korea, 1876–1910."

4. Jeong-ran Kim, "The Borderline of 'Empire': Japanese Maritime Quarantine in Busan c.1876–1910," *Medical History* 57, 2 (April 2013): 226–48; Ruth Rogaski, *Hygienic Modernity Meanings of Health and Disease in Treaty-Port China* (Berkeley: University of California Press, 2014).

5. Chuwŏl Han'gukkun Saryŏngbu (Republic of Korea, Military Headquarters), *Civic Actions* (Saigon: 1966), p. 42.

6. Chuwŏl Han'gukkun Saryŏngbu, *Civic Actions.*

7. Chuwŏl Han'gukkun Saryŏngbu, *Civic Actions.* The volume contains numerous points of advice on how to behave towards a wide variety of Vietnamese civilians, especially women and the elderly.

8. Allen Millett, *The War for Korea: A House on Fire, 1945–1950* (Lawrence, KA: University of Kansas Press, 2015).

9. Anti-communist education became compulsory with the transition to Yusin under Park Chung Hee (1972–79), and probably peaked in the 1980s under Chun Du Hwan.

10. John P. DiMoia, *Reconstructing Bodies: Biomedicine, Health, and Nation-building in Korea since 1945* (Stanford, CA: Stanford University Press, 2013). See chapters 1 and 2 for the 1945–48 period. For the context of the socialist world and medicine, see Dora Vargha's *Polio across the Iron Curtain: Hungary's Cold War with an Epidemic* (Cambridge: Cambridge University Press, 2018), and the project "Connecting Three Worlds," overseen by Dora Vargha (Exeter), Sarah Marks (Birkbeck) and Edna Suarez-Diaz (UNAM). Available at: https://connecting3worlds .org [accessed 17 February 2022].

11. Chuwŏl Han'gukkun Saryŏngbu주월한국군사령부 (HQ. POKF. V), *Peace and Construction*, 평화와건설P'yŏnghwa wa kŏnsŏl, Saigon: HQ. POKF. V [196–]. The phrase "Peace and Construction" is one associated with the ROK government's series of annual volumes covering activities in Vietnam.

12. Chuwŏl Han'gukkun Saryŏngbu주월한국군사령부 (HQ. POKF. V), *Peace and Construction*, pp. 50–2. A series of cartoons depicts Koreans crossing the 17th parallel, a clear reference to the 38th parallel and the Korean War.

13. Susie Woo, *Framed by War: Korean Children and Women at the Crossroads of US Empire* (New York: New York University Press, 2019). Na Sil Heo, "Rearing Autonomous Children in Cold War Korea: Transnational Formations of a Liberal Order, 1950s–1960s" (PhD dissertation, University of Toronto, 2020).

14. Howard Rusk, *A World to Care For: The Autobiography of Howard A. Rusk, M.D.* (New York: Random House, 1972).

15. Mark Harrison and Sung Vin Yim, "War on Two Fronts: The Fight against Parasites in Korea and Vietnam," *Medical History* 61, 3 (July 2017): 401–23. Thanks to Professor Sung Vin Yim for generously sharing materials from the collection of Kyunghee University. When Korean doctors served in Vietnam, they also traveled to Laos to observe conditions in field hospitals.

16. Hiromi Mizuno, Aaron S Moore and John P. DiMoia, *Engineering Asia: Technology, Colonial Development, and the Cold War Order* (London: Bloomsbury, 2018).

17. Barak Kushner and Sherzod Muminov, *The Dismantling of Japan's Empire in East Asia: Deimperialization, Postwar Legitimation and Imperial Afterlife* (New York: Routledge, 2016).

18. Jessica Elkind, *Aid under Fire: Nation-Building and the Vietnam War* (Lexington: University of Kentucky Press, 2016). See also James Carter, *Inventing Vietnam: The United States and State Building, 1954–1968* (Cambridge: Cambridge University Press, 2008); Jessica Chapman, *Cauldron of Resistance: Ngo Dinh Diem, the United States, and 1950s Southern Vietnam* (Ithaca, NY: Cornell University Press, 2013); Edward Miller, *Misalliance: Ngo Dinh Diem, the United States, and the Fate of South Vietnam* (Cambridge, MA: Harvard University Press, 2013); and Heonik Kwon, *Ghosts of War in Vietnam* (Cambridge: Cambridge University Press, 2008).

19. *Peace and Construction* contains a series of cartoons illustrating the imagined relationship, with Koreans bringing "freedom" to the Vietnamese.

20. *Peace and Construction.*

21. Available at: http://www.ehistory.go.kr/page/view/movie.jsp?srcgbn=KV&mediaid=10683&mediadtl=22814&gbn=MH [accessed 13 June 2020].

22. Aya Homei and John DiMoia, "Integrating Parasite Eradication with Family Planning: The Colonial Legacy in Post-war Medical Cooperation in East Asia," *Social History of Medicine* 34, 4 (November 2021): 1094–115.

23. Mark Harrison and Sung Vin Yim, "War on Two Fronts." The Korean part of this program was called Korea Preventive Medicine (KOPREM).

24. Jun-ho Jung and Ock-Joo Kim, "'It All Started from Worms': Korea–Japan Parasite Control Cooperation and Asian Network, 1960s–1980s," *Korean Journal of Medical History* 27, 1 (2018): 49–88. See also Aya Homei and John DiMoia, "Integrating Parasite Education with Family Planning."

25. United Nations Korea Reconstruction Agency (UNKRA), *UNKRA in Action* (New York: United Nations, 1956).

26. "Tongnae Rehabilitation Center," Box 344, File 16. United Nations ARMS, New York; John P. DiMoia, "From Ruin to Revival: Mobilizing the Body, Child Welfare, and the Hybrid Origins of Rehabilitative Medicine in South Korea, 1954–1961," in *Future Yet to Come: Sociotechnical Imaginaries in Modern Korea*, ed. Sonja Kim and Robert Ji-Song Ku (Honolulu: University of Hawai'i Press, 2021), pp. 132–54.

27. DiMoia, "From Ruin to Revival." Howard Rusk's materials are at NYU Bobst Library, and his main collection of papers is held at the University of Missouri, Columbia, Western Historical Collection (WHC).

28. Kyuri Kim and Buhm Soon Park, "Infrastructure-building for Public Health: The World Health Organization and Tuberculosis Control in South Korea, 1945–1963," *Korean Journal of Medical History* 28, 1 (2019): 89–138.

29. Sonja M. Kim, *Imperatives of Care: Women and Medicine in Colonial Korea* (Honolulu: University of Hawai'i Press, 2019).

30. WHO materials for both South and North Korea cover the expected range of diseases (cholera, leprosy, malaria). Where the WHO encountered trouble was with AIDS (in the early 1980s), which both Koreas wanted to deny.

31. Miguel Bernad, *Adventure in Viet-Nam: The Story of Operation Brotherhood, 1954–1957* (Manila: Operation Brotherhood International, 1974). See also Simeon Man, "Colonial Intimacies and Counterinsurgency: the Philippines, South Vietnam, and the United States," chapter 2 of *Soldiering through Empire: Race and the Making of the Decolonizing Pacific* (Berkeley: University of California Press, 2018); see also Kathryn Dawn Sweet, "Limited Doses: Health and Development in Laos, 1893–2000" (PhD dissertation, National University of Singapore, 2015).

32. Chuwŏl Han'gukkun Saryŏngbu. 월남전선 2 년간의발자취 [Korean Forces in Vietnam: Two Years in Vietnam] (Saigon, 1967).

33. John P. DiMoia, "Parasites and the Postcolonial: Renewed Japan–Korea Medical Collaboration and South Korean Developmentalism, 1964–Early 1970s," Paper Presented to the History of Science Society Annual Meeting, Utrecht, July 2019.

34. Available at: https://www.youtube.com/watch?v=4bga2dIm3hY [accessed 13 June 2020].

35. Available at: https://www.youtube.com/watch?v=4bga2dIm3hY [accessed 13 June 2020].

36. 세계를 향한 KOTRA 50: 1962~2012 / KOTRA [편] 서울: KOTRA, 2012 [50 Year History of KOTRA].

37. Simeon Man, *Soldiering through Empire*. See also Jin-kyung Lee, *Service Economies: Militarism, Sex Work, and Migrant Labor in South Korea* (Minneapolis: University of Minnesota Press, 2018).

38. Patrick Chung, "From Korea to Vietnam: Local Labor, Multinational Capital, and the Evolution of US Military Logistics, 1950–97," *Radical History Review* 133 (2019): 31–55. John P. DiMoia, "Reconfiguring Transport Infrastructure in Postwar Asia: Mapping South Korean Container Ports, 1952–1978," *History and Technology* 36, 4 (2020): 382–99.

39. *Civic Actions*, p. 4.

40. *Civic Actions*, p. 4.

41. Susie Woo, *Framed by War: Korean Children and Women at the Crossroads of US Empire.* In addition to Woo, there is a growing body of literature regarding adoption

and Korean children, as in the work of Eleanna Kim, Arissa Oh, Sujin Pate and many others. See Kori Graves, *A War Born Family: African American Adoption in the Wake of the Korean War* (New York: New York University Press, 2020).

42. Woo, *Framed by War*; Graves, *A War Born Family.*

43. Woo, *Framed by War*; Graves, *A War Born Family.*

44. Jim Glassman and Young-Jin Choi, "The *Chaebol* and the US Military–Industrial Complex: Cold War Geopolitical Economy and South Korean Industrialization," *Environment and Planning A: Economy and Space* 46, 5 (2014): 1160–80.

45. Simeon Man, "Working the Sub-Empire," chapter 4 in *Soldiering through Empire.*

46. Young Sun Hong, *Cold War Germany, the Third World, and the Global Humanitarian Regime* (Cambridge: Cambridge University Press, 2017); Dora Vargha, *Polio across the Iron Curtain*; James Lin, "Sowing Seeds and Knowledge: Agrarian Development in the US, China, Taiwan, and the World, 1920–1980" (PhD dissertation, University of California Berkeley, 2017); Benjamin Young, *Guns, Guerillas, and the Great Leader: North Korea and the Third World* (Stanford, CA: Stanford University Press, 2021).

47. Available at: www.vietvet.co.kr [accessed 13 June 2020]. There are digitized versions of the entire series at this site.

48. Susie Woo, *Framed by War: Korean Children and Women at the Crossroads of US Empire.*

49. Kim, Jeong-ran, 김정란, "제국의 흔적 지우기: 패전 후 일본에서의 귀환자 검역", 최해별 편, 『질병 관리의 사회문화사: 일상생활에서 국가정책까지』, 서울, 이화여자대학교출판문화원 / "jegugui heunjeok jiugi': paejeon hu ilboneseoui gwihwanja geomyeok', choehaebyeol pyeon, 『jilbyeong gwalliui sahoemunhwasa: ilsangsaenghwareseo gukgajeongchaekkkaji』," [Erasing the Traces of Empire: Quarantine of Returnees in Japan after Defeat], in *Social and Cultural History of Disease Management: From Daily Life to National Policy*, ed. Hae-byeol Choi (Seoul: Ewha Womans University Press and Cultural Center, 2021), pp. 291–321.

50. Kim, Jeong-ran, 김정란, "제국의 흔적 지우기: 패전 후 일본에서의 귀환자 검역", 최해별 편, 『질병 관리의 사회문화사: 일상생활에서 국가정책까지』, 서울, 이화여자대학교출판문화원.

51. Major Korean universities did not yet have their own demographic centers in 1955, but they did by the 1960s and 1970s, corresponding to Family and Economic Planning.

52. Won Kim, "The Race to Appropriate 'Korean-ness.'"

53. Youngsu Park, "Tempoethics: Envisioning Asian Modernities and Enacting Global Health Projects in Ethiopia" (PhD dissertation, Stanford University, 2018); Benjamin Young, *Guns, Guerillas, and the Great Leader.*

Glossary

Animism: A variety of "indigenous" cosmologies that at one end of the spectrum posit an agentive, all-animate, or partly-animate, world, and at the other end, identify dead kin or totem figures (for example, plants and animals) as spirits or spirit ancestors; in both cases, ritual is required to communicate with and supplicate these supernatural beings.

Anopheles: A genus of mosquito, comprising more than 450 identified species. Less than 100 of these species can transmit plasmodia parasites to humans. Each of these Anopheles species has a specific habitat and requirements.

Asian–African Conference (also known as the Bandung Conference): Convened at Bandung, Indonesia, in April 1955 at the initiative of the then Indonesian Prime Minister Ali Sastroamidjojo. It was sponsored by five Asian nations: India, Pakistan, Burma, Indonesia and Ceylon. At the close of the conference, 29 participant nations jointly issued a communiqué that included a range of concrete objectives. These goals included promotion of economic and cultural cooperation among participating newly decolonized Asian and African nations, minimization of international aid from either the US or the Soviet Union and denunciation of colonialism. The conference and the communiqué contributed to the emergence of the Non-Aligned Movement.

Cochinchina: One of the five regions of Indochina, a political unit constructed by the French. It corresponds roughly to the south central and southern regions of modern Vietnam.

Colombo Plan: A regional intergovernmental organization headquartered in Sri Lanka, which focuses on human resources development in South and Southeast Asia. It is best known for its long-term scholarship program which began operations in 1951. Originally comprised of seven countries from the British Commonwealth plus the United States of America, Cambodia, Laos and South Vietnam, the Colombo Plan now has 28 member states.

Confucian: An intellectual tradition based on the writings of Kongzi and his followers. After its diffusion in Vietnam under Chinese rule before the tenth century, it was adapted to the Vietnamese context and used by the Nguyễn Dynasty as an ideological underpinning for its rule.

Coolies: A derogatory term used mainly to refer to Chinese who came from southern China and labored in plantations, mines and wharfs in Southeast Asia, Oceania and the Americas in the 19th century. They usually suffered from violence, coercion and high mortality rates.

Dove/Pigeon Brigade: The civic affairs branch of the South Korean military, famous for its "civic actions" conducted in Vietnam, and later replaced by the Construction Support Group as the war intensified.

Estado Novo: Specifically, the Portuguese Salazar dictatorship that ran from 1933 to 1972; the term may be used as a gloss referring to the entire period of dictatorship from 1926 to 1974.

Gandhian: Refers to the movement centered on Mahatma Gandhi, sometimes considered the central figure of the Indian independence movement. The Gandhian approach to science—centered on the community—was attentive to alternative non-Western forms of knowledge that could not be validated by the scientific method but as ways of living that had their own cognitive validity.

Joseon: The period of Korean history covering 1392–1910, generally associated with long-term stability, a turn to Confucianism (away from the Buddhism of the preceding Koryo period), and with the peninsula strongly influenced by Chinese (Ming) culture and models.

Kampong: A Malay term for village.

Kinta Valley Home Guard: An all-Chinese security force formed in 1953, with the sponsorship of Perak Chinese Tin Mining Association and the approval of British colonial administration, to protect the tin mines in Kinta Valley, Malaya.

KOICA: The Korean International Cooperation Agency is South Korea's overseas aid and Official Development Assistance (ODA) coordinating agency, and has been so since the early 1990s. It was preceded by KODCO (Korean Overseas Development Corporation), 1965–91, which represented the first overseas workers sent out in the mid-1960s.

Korean dynamism: A term mobilized to represent Korean spirit or strength ("him" in Korean), and adopted as a national slogan to publicize Korean commercial and political ambitions.

MCA: Malaysian Chinese Association (initially Malayan Chinese Association), a pro-British administration, race-based political party formed in 1949 to represent the interest of ethnic Chinese. Its founding members consisted of rich Chinese businessmen in Malaya.

Mestizos: A Spanish and Portuguese term originally referring to a person of mixed European and Indigenous American ancestry. In the Philippines, Mestizos could also refer to a person of mixed Chinese and Filipino ancestry.

Nguyễn Dynasty: Vietnamese dynasty that ruled from 1802 to 1945. After the French conquest in 1883, the Nguyễn emperors ruled as symbolic heads of state until 1945.

Orang Asli: A Malay term for "aboriginal people."

Oro-hydrographical: Refers to both the topographic relief and the surface-water distribution of a place or a region.

Pasteur Institute: A private, non-profit institution, based in Paris and founded in 1887 by the French scientist Louis Pasteur, dedicated to the study of infectious diseases, the production of vaccines and the development of other practical medical applications. Today it is a biomedical research organization, at the center of a global network, partially inherited from branches created in former French colonies as well as those existing in some other foreign countries.

***Pembangunan*:** An Indonesian word meaning development in the framework of nation-building. During the Soekarno era, *pembangunan* was holistic as it embraced advances in public health, improvements in communications, the construction of monuments, the growth of a strong military and a favorable balance of trade. These advancements were invested with symbolic meaning as they articulated Indonesia's aspirations for a brighter future after the country endured three-and-a-half centuries of Dutch colonialism and indicated to the world that the country was capable of standing on its two feet (Bahasa Indonesian: "berdiri di atas kaki sendiri").

***Plasmodia* species:** A genus of unicellular eukaryotes, obligate parasites of insects and vertebrates. Their life cycle includes two different stages, the first one evolving in a blood-feeding insect which then injects the parasites into a vertebrate. There are six species currently known to cause malaria in humans: *P. falciparum*, *P. vivax*, *P. malariae*, *P. ovale curtisi*, *P. ovale wallikeri* and *P. knowlesi*.

Quelicai: A small town (and a sub-district) in central Timor, set on the flanks of Mount Matebian in central East Timor.

Rural Industrial Development Authority (RIDA): A program established in 1951 by the British colonial administration to provide economic assistance and support to Malay farmers and rural inhabitants.

SAPT (Sociedade Agrícola Patria e Trabalho): A network of (predominantly) coffee plantations established in the Ermera district under the governorship of Celestino da Silva (1894–1908).

Semai: An indigenous tribe of Peninsular Malaysia.

Senoi Pra'aq: A Semai term, which refers to a military unit formed during the Malayan Emergency and made up of aboriginal people to deter communist guerrillas in the jungle.

Shaman: Witchdoctor or local, usually animist, medical practitioner incorporating both medicines and magic.

Splenomegaly: An enlargement of the spleen, which can be detected by palpation of the left hypochondria. In areas with endemic malaria, it often derives from a chronic antigenic spleen stimulation due to the disease parasite.

Straits Settlements: A group of British colonies consisting of Singapore, Penang, Malacca, Christmas Island and the Cocos Islands in Southeast Asia under the governance of the British Empire from 1826 to 1946.

Swidden agro-system: A "small-scale" agricultural system, characterized by the shifting or rotation of agricultural plots, diversity of crops and cultivars, and highly variable and localized practices and knowledge; often pejoratively framed as slash-and-burn agriculture, and juxtaposed with modern agriculture.

Tetum: One of many local languages of Timor, which in Portuguese Timor became the dominant and most widespread local language in the late colonial period, as it is today.

Traditional/Vietnamese medicine/Eastern medicine: A set of relational terms that describe healing practices in Vietnamese society. Traditional medicine is used in opposition to modern biomedicine. Vietnamese medicine, or Southern medicine, is used in opposition to Chinese, or Northern medicine. Moreover, Eastern medicine is used in opposition to Western medicine. Traditional Vietnamese medicine continues to be differentiated from traditional Chinese medicine in today's Vietnam.

Bibliography

Abraham, Itty. "From Bandung to NAM: Non-Alignment and India's Foreign Policy, 1947–65." *Commonwealth and Comparative Politics* 46, 2 (2008): 195–219.

———. "The Contradictory Space of Postcolonial Technoscience." *Economic and Political Weekly* 41, 3 (2006): 210–17.

Agência Geral do Ultramar. *Timor: Pequena Monografia* [Timor: Short Monograph]. Lisbon: Agência Geral do Ultramar, 1970 [1965].

Aldeia, Fernando Alves. "Timor na Esteira do Progresso. Discurso Proferido na Sessão de Abertura da Assembleia Legislativa e da Junta Provincial, em Dili, no dia 14 de Maio de 1973" [Timor on the Way to Progress. Speech Delivered at the Inaugural Session Legislative Assembly and the Provincial Council in Dili, 14 May]. Lisbon: Agência Lusitânia, 1973.

Amrith, Sunil S. "Migration and Health in Southeast Asian History." *The Lancet* 384, 9954 (2014): 1569–70.

———. *Migration and Diaspora in Modern Asia*. Cambridge: Cambridge University Press, 2011.

Anderson, Robert S., Edwin Levy and Barrie M. Morrison. *Rice Science and Development Politics: Research Strategies and IRRI's Technologies Confront Asian Diversity, 1950–1980*. New York: Oxford University Press, 1991.

Anderson, Warwick. "Asia as a Method in STS." *East Asian Science, Technology and Society (EASTS): An International Journal* 6, 4 (2012): 445–51.

———. "Introduction: Postcolonial Technoscience." *Social Studies of Science* 32, 5–6 (2006): 643–58.

Anderson, Warwick and Hans Pols. "Scientific Patriotism: Medical Science and National Self-Fashioning in Asia." *Comparative Studies in Society and History* 54, 1 (2012): 93–113.

Anonymous. *Laos Mil neuf cent cinquante. Le Royaume du Laos, ses institutions et son organisation générale* [Laos 1950. The Kingdom of Laos, Its Institutions and Its General Organization], no publication details, no date.

———. "Kham-hay-samphad khong thao Bounlap" [Interview with Mr Bounlap]. *Sai Kang* 97, 7 (March 1964): 10–11.

———. "Hang lay-ngane saphab viak-ngane sathalanasouk you kongpasoum-ngay khang thi I tae 1 ha 12 toula 1979" [Draft Report on the Health Situation for the

First Conference of Health from 1–12 October 1979]. Vientiane: Ministry of Health, 1979.

———. Former NLHX and retired Lao PDR doctor, in Vientiane, Lao PDR, November 2012 and August 2013.

———. *60 pi heng kane-teub-nyay khong lao-hob Senahak, 1.11.1954–1.11.2014* [60 Years of Development of the Military Health Service, 1.11.1954–1.11.2014]. Vientiane: Lao People's Army, 2014.

Appadorai, Arjun. "The Bandung Conference." *India Quarterly: A Quarterly Journal of International Affairs* 11, 3 (1955): 207–35.

Arnold, David. *Colonizing the Body: State Medicine and Epidemic Disease in 19th Century India.* Los Angeles: University of California Press, 1993.

———. "Nehruvian Science and Postcolonial India." *ISIS* 104 (2013): 360–70.

Aso, Michitake. "Patriotic Hygiene: Tracing New Places of Knowledge Production about Malaria in Vietnam, 1919–75." *Journal of Southeast Asian Studies* 44, 3 (2013): 423–43.

———. *Rubber and the Making of Vietnam: An Ecological History, 1897–1975.* Chapel Hill: University of North Carolina Press, 2018.

Aso, Michitake and Annick Guénel. "The Itinerary of a North Vietnamese Surgeon: Medical Science and Politics during the Cold War." *Science, Technology and Society* 18, 3 (2013): 291–306.

Australian Embassy in Jakarta. "The Chinese in Indonesia." National Archives of Australia (NAA), A1838/280, 3034/2/5/1, 1952.

———. "The Sino/Indonesian Dual Nationality Treaty, 1957–1962." National Archives of Australia (NAA), A1838/280, 3034/2/5/1 Part 2, 1962.

Azevedo, J. Fraga de, A. Franco Gândara and A. Pedroso Ferreira. "Missão de Estudo a Timor II—Contribuição para o Conhecimento da Endemia Malárica na Província de Timor" [Research Mission to Timor II—Contribution to the Knowledge of Endemic Malaria in the Province of Timor]. *Anais do Instituto de Medicina Tropical* 15, 1 (1958): 35–52.

Bain, Chester A. "The Persistence of Tradition in Modern Vietnamese Medicine." *Southeast Asia: An International Quarterly* 3, 1 (1974): 607–19.

Balashov, Yu.S. "Паразитология ШколаАкадемика Е. Н.Павловского в Зоологическом Институте РАН" [Academician E. N. Pavlovskiĭ's Parasitology School in the Zoological Institute RAS]. *Parazitologiia* 37, 4 (2003): 249–58.

Barata, Filipe Temudo. *Timor Contemporâneo: da Primeira Ameaça da Indonésia ao Nascer de Uma Nação* [Contemporary Timor: from Indonesia's First Threat to the Birth of a Nation]. Lisbon: Equilíbrio Editora, 1998.

Barker, Joshua. "Beyond Bandung: Development Nationalism and Multi(cultural) Nationalism in Indonesia." *Third World Quarterly* 29, 3 (2008): 521–40.

Bashford, Alison and Peter Hobbins. "Rewriting Quarantine: Pacific History at Australia's Edge." *Australian Historical Studies* 46, 3 (2015): 392–409.

Bayly, Christopher and Tim Harper. *Forgotten Wars: The End of Britain's Asian Empire.* London: Penguin, 2007.

Beers, Howard. *An American Experience in Indonesia: The University of Kentucky Affiliation with the Agricultural University at Bogor.* Lexington: University of Kentucky Press, 1971.

Bernad, Miguel A. *Adventure in Viet-Nam: The Story of Operation Brotherhood, 1954–1957.* Manila: Operation Brotherhood International, 1974.

———. *Filipinos in Laos, with 'Postscripts' by J 'Pete' Fuentecila.* New York: Mekong Circle International, 2004.

Birn, Anne-Emmanuelle and Nikolai Krementsov. "'Socialising' Primary Health Care? The Soviet Union, WHO and the 1978 Alma-Ata Conference." *BMJ Global Health* (2018). Available at: http://dx.doi.org/10.1136/bmjgh-2018-000992.

Boden, Ragna. "Cold War Economics: Soviet Aid to Indonesia." *Journal of Cold War Studies* 10, 3 (2008): 110–28.

Boletim Geral do Ultramar. "Apontamentos para a Monografia de Timor" [Notes for a Monograph on Timor]. *Boletim Geral do Ultramar* XLI, 480 (1965): 71–113.

———. "Relatório dos Peritos da Organizaçção Mundial de Saude que em 1962 se deslocaram às Provincias Ultramarinas de Guiné, Angola e Moçambique, a Convite do Governo Português" [Report of Experts from the World Health Organization, Who in 1962 Visited the Overseas Provinces of Guine, Angola, and Mozambique, by Invitation from the Portuguese Government]. *Boletim Geral do Ultramar* XXXIX, 456–57 (1963): 115–22.

Bounheng Banxalith. "Special Relationship between Laos and Vietnam in Military Medicine," in *History of Vietnam-Laos, Laos-Vietnam Special Relationship (1930–2007). Memoirs Volume II,* ed. Vietnamese and Lao Compilatory Steering Committees, Hanoi: National Political Publishing House, 2012, pp. 192–4.

Bounthan Bandavong. "Vietnam-Laos Special Solidarity in Military Medicine," in *History of Vietnam-Laos, Laos-Vietnam Special Relationship (1930–2007). Memoirs Volume II,* ed. Vietnamese and Lao Compilatory Steering Committees, Hanoi: National Political Publishing House, 2012, pp. 507–9.

Bounthanh Oudom. Retired Operation Brotherhood and Lao PDR nurse, interviewed in Vientiane, Lao PDR, 3 February 2012.

Bộ Y Tế. *Lịch sử Viện sốt sét ký sinh trùng và côn trùng (1957–1997)* [History of the Institute of Malariology, Parasitology and Entomology (1957–1997)]. Hà Nội: Nhà Xuất Bản Chính Trị Quốc Gia, 1998.

Bộ Y Tế. *Đặng Văn Ngữ. Một Trí Thức Lớn, Một Nhân Cách Lớn* [Dang Van Ngu. A Great Intellectual, a Great Man]. Hà Nội: Nhà Xuất Bản Y Học, 2010.

Branfman, Fred. *Voices from the Plain of Jars. Life under an Air War.* New York: Harper Colophon Books, 1972, pp. 46–56.

Brass, Alister. "The Importance of Foreign Medical Aid for South Vietnam." *The Australian Quarterly* 39, 2 (1967): 45–55.

Braun, Matthias. "From Landscapes to Labscapes: Malaria Research and Anti-Malaria Policy in Soviet Azerbaijan, 1920–41." *Jahrbücher für Geschichte Osteuropas* (2013): 513–30.

Briggs, Charles L. and Clara Mantini-Briggs. *Stories in the Time of Cholera: Racial Profiling during a Medical Nightmare*. Berkeley, CA: University of California Press, 2003.

Brown, Mervyn. *War in Shangri-La: A Memoir of Civil War in Laos*. London and New York: Radcliffe Press, 2001.

Bruce-Chwatt, Leonard J. "Malaria Research and Eradication in the USSR. A Review of Soviet Achievements in the Field of Malariology." *Bulletin of the World Health Organization* 21, 6 (1959): 737–72.

Bryant, John. "Communism, Poverty, and Demographic Change in North Vietnam." *Population and Development Review* 24, 2 (1998): 235–69.

Bui Van Y. "Public Health Support for Lao Friends during the Resistance against French Colonialists," in *History of Vietnam-Laos, Laos-Vietnam Special Relationship (1930–2007). Memoirs Volume II*, ed. Vietnamese and Lao Compilatory Steering Committees, Hanoi: National Political Publishing House, 2012, pp. 243–8.

Cardoso, João Jr. "Plantas medicinais da Ilha de Timor" [Medicinal Plants on the Island of Timor]. *Subsidios para a Materia Médica e Terapeutica das Possessões Ultramarinas Portuguezas* [Contribution to Medical and Therapeutic Information in the Overseas Portuguese Possessions]. Volume l, Lisbon, 1902, pp. 233–6.

Carpenter, Kathleen. *The Password Is Love.* London: The Highway Press, 1958.

Carter, Eric D. "State Visions, Landscape, and Disease: Discovering Malaria in Argentina, 1890–1920." *Geoforum* 39, 1 (2008): 278–93.

Carter, James. *Inventing Vietnam: The United States and State Building, 1954–1968*. Cambridge: Cambridge University Press, 2008.

Chamberlain, Ernest. "The 1959 Rebellion in East Timor: Unresolved Tensions and an Unwritten History." In *Proceedings of Understanding Timor-Leste*, ed. M. Leach, N.C. Mendes, A.B. da Silva, A. da C. Ximenes and B. Boughton. Melbourne: Swinburne Press/Timor-Leste Studies Association, 2010, pp. 174–9.

Chan, Kallista, Lucy S. Tusting, Christian Bottomley, Kazuki Saito, Rousseau Djouaka and Jo Lines. "Malaria Transmission and Prevalence in Rice-Growing versus Non-Rice-Growing Villages in Africa: A Systematic Review and Meta-Analysis." *The Lancet Planetary Health* 6, 3 (2022): 257–69.

Chanpheng Thongphimpha. *Botbanhtheuk: Xivit kanekheuanvay pakobsouan het kanepativat nay vongkanephet khong Pa Chanpheng Thongphimpha tae pi 1953 theung pi 2000* [The revolutionary Contribution of Aunt Chanpheng Thongphimpha to the Health Sector from 1953–2000]. Vientiane: self-published, 2013.

Chapman, Jessica. *Cauldron of Resistance: Ngo Dinh Diem, the United States, and 1950s Southern Vietnam.* Ithaca, NY: Cornell University Press, 2013.

Chen Da. *Nanyang huaqiao yu minyue shehui* [Nanyang Overseas Chinese and Guangdong Fujian Society]. Shanghai: Shangwu yinshuguan, 1937.

Chrusjitjov [Krushchev], Nikita. *Uni Sovjet Sahabat Setia Bagi Rakjat Rakjat Jang Sedang Berdjoeang Untuk Kemerdekannja* [Solidarity of the USSR with Nations Struggling for Independence]. Djakarta: Kedutaaan Besar URSS, 1960.

Chung, Patrick. "From Korea to Vietnam: Local Labor, Multinational Capital, and the Evolution of US Military Logistics, 1950–97." *Radical History Review* 133 (2019): 31–55.

Chuwol Hangukgun Saryŏngbu [Republic of Korea, Military Headquarters]. *Civic Actions.* Saigon, 1966, p. 42.

Chuwŏl Han'gukkun / 주월한국군. (HQ. POKF. V). *Peace and Construction*, 평화와건설 *P'yŏnghwa wa kŏnsŏl.* Saigon: HQ. POKF. V, 1966.

Chuwŏl Han'gukkun Saryŏngbu. 월남전선 2년간의발자취 [Korean Forces in Vietnam: 2 Years in Vietnam]. Saigon, 1967.

Ciucă, M. "Le paludisme en Roumanie de 1949 à 1955" [Malaria in Romania from 1949 to 1955]. *Bulletin of the World Health Organization* 15, 3–5 (1956): 725–51.

Clarence-Smith, William Gervase. *The Third Portuguese Empire, 1825–1975: A Study in Economic Imperialism.* Manchester, UK: Manchester University Press, 1985.

Comber, Leon. "The Malayan Emergency: General Templer and the Kinta Valley Home Guard, 1952–1954." *Journal of the Malaysian Branch of the Royal Asiatic Society* 85, 1 (302) (June 2012): 45–62.

Cousins, Judith and Alfred W. McCoy. "Living It Up in Laos. Congressional Testimony on US aid to Laos in the 1950s," in *Laos. War and Revolution*, ed. Nina S. Adams and Alfred W. McCoy. New York: Harper and Row, 1970, pp. 340–56.

Craig, David. *Familiar Medicine: Everyday Health Knowledge and Practice in Today's Vietnam.* Honolulu: University of Hawai'i Press, 2002.

Crush, Jonathan. *Power of Development.* London: Routledge, 1995.

Cueto, Marcos. "Appropriation and Resistance. Local Responses to Malaria Eradication in Mexico, 1955–1970." *Journal of Latin American Studies* 37, 3 (2005): 533–59.

Cullather, Nick. *The Hungry World: America's Cold War Battle Against Poverty in Asia.* Cambridge, MA: Harvard University Press, 2010.

Danaraj, Thamboo John. *Medical Education in Malaysia: Development and Problems.* Subang Jaya: Pelanduk, 1988.

de Bevoise, Ken. *Agents of Apocalypse: Epidemic Disease in the Colonial Philippines.* Princeton, NJ: Princeton University Press, 1995.

DiMoia, John P. *Reconstructing Bodies: Biomedicine, Health, and Nation-building in Korea since 1945.* Stanford, CA: Stanford University Press, 2013.

———. "Providing Reassurance and Affirmation: Masculinity, Militarization and Refashioning a Male Role in South Korean Family Planning: 1962 to the late 1980s," in *Gender, Health, and History in Modern East Asia*, ed. Angela Leung and Izumi Nakayama. Hong Kong: Hong Kong University Press, 2018, pp. 244–70.

———. "Parasites and the Postcolonial: Renewed Japan–Korea Medical Collaboration and South Korean Developmentalism, 1964–Early 1970s." Paper Presented to the History of Science Society Annual Meeting, Utrecht, July 2019.

———. "Reconfiguring Transport Infrastructure in Post-War Asia: Mapping South Korean Container Ports, 1952–1978." *History and Technology* 36, 4 (2020): 382–99.

———. "From Ruin to Revival: Mobilizing the Body, Child Welfare, and the Hybrid Origins of Rehabilitative Medicine in South Korea, 1954–1961," in *Future Yet to Come: Sociotechnical Imaginaries in Modern Korea*, ed. Sonja Kim and Robert Ji-Song Ku. Honolulu: University of Hawaii Press, 2021, pp. 132–54.

Đỗ, Tất Lợi. *Những Cây Thuốc và Vị Thuốc Việt Nam* [Vietnamese Medicinal Plants and Medicinal Flavors]. Hà Nội: NXB Nhà Xuất Bản Khoa Học và Kỹ Thuật, 2009.

Đoàn, Văn Quýnh. "Y Miếu Huế." [Hue Temple of Medicine]. *Nghiên Cứu Huế* 7 (2010): 443–6.

Dobby, E.H.G. "Resettlement Transforms Malaya: A Case History of Relocating the Population of an Asian Plural Society." *Economic Development and Cultural Change* 1, 3 (1952): 163–89.

Dooley, Thomas A. *Dr Tom Dooley's Three Great Books: Deliver Us from Evil, The Edge of Tomorrow [and] The Night They Burned the Mountain.* New York: Farrar, Straus and Cudahy, 1960.

Dubos, René J. and Fred L. Soper. "Their Contrasting Views on Vector and Disease Eradication." *Perspectives in Biology and Medicine* 41, 1 (1997): 138–49.

Ehnmark, Anders and Per Wästberg. *Angola and Mozambique: The Case against Portugal.* Trans. Paul Britten-Austin. London and Dunmow: Pall Mall Press, 1963.

Elkind, Jessica. *Aid under Fire: Nation-Building and the Vietnam War.* Lexington: University of Kentucky Press, 2016.

Engelbert, Thomas. "Vietnamese—Chinese Relations in Southern Vietnam during the First Indochina Conflict." *Journal of Vietnamese Studies* 3, 3 (2008): 191–230.

Escobar, Arturo. *Encountering Development: The Making and Unmaking of the Third World.* Princeton, NJ: Princeton University Press, 1995.

"E영상 역사관." e영상역사관 "영상보기 [E-Visual History Hall / e-Video History Museum/ View the video]. Available at: https://www.ehistory.go.kr/page/view/movie.jsp?srcgbn=KV&mediaid=10683&mediadtl=22814&gbn=MH [accessed 13 June 2020].

Fairbairn, Geoffrey. Review "Vietnam: The Roots of Conflict. By Chester A. Bain." *Journal of Southeast Asian History* 9, 2 (1968): 362.

Fang, Xiaoping. *China and the Cholera Pandemic: Restructuring Society under Mao.* Pittsburgh, PA: University of Pittsburgh Press, 2021.

———. "Teji xuyan: Jindai xinma huaren yiliao weisheng yu jibingshi yanjiu" [Introduction to Special Issue: Historical Research on Chinese Diaspora, Medicine, Health, and Disease in Modern Singapore and Malaysia]. *Huaren yanjiu guoji xuebao* [International Journal of Diasporic Chinese Studies] 13, 1 (2021): 1–4.

Farinaud, M.E. *Rapport sur le paludisme dans le Sud Viet-Nam et sur les activités de l'équipe antimalarienne de l'OMS* [Report on Malaria in South Vietnam and on the Activities of the WHO's Anti-malaria Team]. WHO, Project Files VNR/MRD/001, 1952.

Federation of Malaya Report of the Medical Department (FMRMD). 1949–58.

Feinsilver, Julie. "Fifty Years of Cuba's Medical Diplomacy: From Idealism to Pragmatism." *Cuban Studies* 41 (2010): 85–104.

Feith, Herbert. "Indonesian Political Symbols and Their Wielders." *World Politics* 16 (1963): 79–97.

Feith, Herbert and Daniel S. Lev. "The End of the Indonesian Rebellion." *Pacific Affairs* 26 (Spring 1963): 32–46.

Felgas, Hélio A. Esteves. *Timor Português* [Portuguese Timor]. Lisbon: Agência Geral do Ultramar, 1956.

Felsenfeld, Oscar. "Some Observations on the Cholera (El Tor) Epidemic in 1961–1962." *Bulletin of World Health Organization* 28, 3 (1963): 289–96.

Feng Banba. "Qizhangshan jianyizhan" [Quarantine Station of St. John Island]. *Xifeng* [Western Wind] 13, 115 (1949): 18–20.

Ferreira, A. Pedroso. "Relatório Anual da Missão Permanente de Estudo e Combate de Endemias de Timor: 1959" [Annual Report of the Permanent Research Mission for the Combat against Diseases in Timor]. *Separata dos Anais do Instituto de Medicina Tropical* 17, 3 (1960): 907–27.

————. "Estudos sobre a Endemia Malárica em Timor, com Vista a Estabelecer-se um Plano de Luta contra a Mesma: 1—Considerações Biogeográficas" [Research on Malaria in Timor, with the Aim to Establish an Action Plan against the Disease: 1. Biogeographical Considerations]. *Anais do Instituto de Medicina Tropical* 18, 1–2 (1961): 109–62.

Figueiredo, Antonio de. *Portugal and Its Empire: The Truth*. London: Victor Gollancz, 1961.

Forman, Shepard. "Spirits of the Makassae: The Vengeful Dead Hasten an Anthropologist's Departure." *Natural History* 85, 9 (1976): 12–18.

Foucault, Michel. *Power/Knowledge: Selected Interviews and Other Writings 1972–1977*. Hove, Sussex: The Harvester Press, 1980.

FRETILIN (Frente Revolucionária de Timor Leste-Independente). *Manual e Programa Políticos* [Policy Handbook and Program]. Dili, 1974.

Gabalon, Arnoldo. "Independent Path for Malaria Control and Public Health in the Tropics: A Lost 'Paradigm' for WHO." *Parassitologia* 40 (1998): 231–8.

Glassman, Jim and Young-Jin Choi. "The *Chaebol* and the US Military–Industrial Complex: Cold War Geopolitical Economy and South Korean Industrialization." *Environment and Planning: Economy and Space* 46, 5 (2014): 1160–80.

Gonçalves, M. Mayer, A.P. Silva Cardoso, N. Sui Siong and M. Si Min. "Melhoramento da Cultura do Arroz em Timor. Introdução e Selecção de Variedades e Primeiros Ensaios de Adubação" [Rice Improvement in Timor: Introduction and Selection of Varieties, and First Experiments with Fertilizers]. *Comunicações* 84, Lisbon: MEAU, 1974.

Goss, Andrew. *Floracrats: State-Sponsored Science and the Failure of the Enlightenment in Indonesia*. Madison, WI: Wisconsin University Press, 2011.

Graves, Kori. *A War Born Family: African American Adoption in the Wake of the Korean War*. New York: New York University Press, 2020.

Guangdongsheng fangyi zhihuibu Yangjiang gongzuozu [Work Team of Guangdong Provincial Epidemic Prevention Headquarters]. "Liuxingbing diaocha baogao" [Investigation Report of the Epidemic in Yangjiang County, Guangdong Province]. GYJA, X38.A12.1.36, 1961.

Guénel, Annick. "Malaria Control, Land Occupation and Scientific Developments in Vietnam in the XXth century." 1999. Available at: https://halshs.archives-ouvertes .fr/halshs-00137031 [accessed 09 October 2023].

Gurney, Henry. *Communist Banditry in Malaya: Extracts from Speeches by the High Commissioner Sir Henry Gurney.* Federation of Malaya: Department of Public Relations, 1949.

Guterres, Abel. "Life Was Good and Easy," in *Telling East Timor: Personal Testimonies, 1942–1992,* ed. Michele Turner. Kensington, NSW: The University of NSW Press, 1992, pp. 63–6.

Hägerdal, Hans. *Lords of the Land, Lords of the Sea: Conflict and Adaptation in Early Colonial Timor, 1600–1800.* Leiden: KITLV Press, 2012.

Halpern, Joel M. *Laotian Health Problems.* Laos Project Paper 20, Amherst, MA: University of Massachusetts, 1961.

———. *Laotian Health Statistics.* Laos Project Paper 10, Amherst, MA: University of Massachusetts, 1961.

Han Xiaorong. "Spoiled Guests or Dedicated Patriots? The Chinese in North Vietnam, 1954–1978." *International Journal of Asian Studies* 6, 1 (2009): 1–36.

Hangzhoushi renmin weiyuanhui waishi bangongshi [Foreign Affair Office of Hangzhou City People's Commission]. "Dui waibin he huaqiao cheliang tongguo ke mianjian fangxin de yijian" [Instructions on Exempting Quarantine Examination and Clearing Vehicles Carrying Foreign Guests or Overseas Chinese]. Zhejiang Provincial Archives, J166-2-175, 1963.

Harper, Tim. *The End of Empire and the Making of Malaya.* Cambridge: Cambridge University Press, 1999.

———. "The Politics of Disease and Disorder in Post-War Malaya." *Journal of Southeast Asian Studies* 21, 1 (1990): 88–113.

Harrison, Mark. *Contagion: How Commerce Has Spread Disease.* New Haven, CT: Yale University Press, 2012.

Harrison, Mark and Sung Vin Yim. "War on Two Fronts: The Fight against Parasites in Korea and Vietnam." *Medical History* 61, 3 (July 2017): 401–23.

Heggenhougan, H. "Bomohs, Doctors and Sinsehs: Medical Pluralism in Malaysia." *Social Science and Medicine* 14B (1980): 235–44.

Heo, Na Sil. "Rearing Autonomous Children in Cold War Korea: Transnational Formations of a Liberal Order, 1950s–1960s." PhD dissertation, University of Toronto 2020.

Hickey, Gerald. *Free in the Forest: Ethnohistory of the Vietnamese Central Highlands, 1954–1976.* New Haven, CT: Yale University Press, 1982.

Hicks, David. *Tetum Ghosts and Kin: Fieldwork in an Indonesian Community.* Palo Alto, CA: Mayfield Publishing Company, 1976.

Higgins, Benjamin. "Indonesia's Development Plans and Problems." *Pacific Affairs* 29, 2 (1956): 107–25.

Hin, Poey Seng. "Defisiensi Protein Kalori (Kwashiorkor) dan Penjakit Defisiensi Vitamin A" [Kwashiorkor and Deficiency of Vitamin A], in *Research di Indonesia*, ed. M. Makagiansar and Poorwo Soedarmo. Jakarta: Departemen Urusan Research Nasional Republik Indonesia, 1965.

Hing, Lee Kam. "A Neglected Story: Christian Missionaries, Chinese New Villagers, and Communists in the Battle for the 'Hearts and Minds' in Malaya, 1948–1960." *Modern Asian Studies* 47, 6 (2013): 1977–2006.

Hoang, Bao Chau. "The Revival and Development of Vietnamese Traditional Medicine: Towards Keeping the Nation in Good Health," in *Southern Medicine for Southern People: Vietnamese Medicine in the Making*, ed. Laurence Monnais, C. Michele Thompson and Ayo Wahlberg. Newcastle upon Tyne: Cambridge Scholars, 2012, pp. 113–52.

Hoang, Bao Chau, Pho Duc Thuc and Huu Ngoc (ed.). *Vietnamese Traditional Medicine*. Second edition. Hanoi: The Gioi Publishers, 1999.

Homei, Aya and John P. DiMoia. "Integrating Parasite Eradication with Family Planning: The Colonial Legacy in Post-war Medical Cooperation in East Asia." *Social History of Medicine* 34, 4 (2021): 1094–115.

Hong, Young-Sun. *Cold War Germany, the Third World, and the Global Humanitarian Regime*. Cambridge: Cambridge University Press, 2017.

Hu Dalong and Bin Liu et al. "Origins of the Current Seventh Cholera Pandemic." *Proceedings of the National Academy of Sciences of the United States of America* 113, 48 (2016): E7730–E7739.

Huang Shuze and Lin Shixiao (ed.). *Dangdai zhongguo de weisheng shiye* [Health Development in Contemporary China]. Beijing: Dangdai zhongguo chubanshe, Xianggang zuguo chubanshe, 2009.

Huber, Valeska. "The Unification of the Globe by Disease? The International Sanitary Conferences on Cholera, 1851–1894." *The Historical Journal* 49, 2 (June 2006): 453–76.

Hull, Terence and Valerie Hull. "From Family Planning to Reproductive Health in Indonesia," in *People, Population and Policy in Indonesia*, ed. Terence Hull and Valerie Hull. Jakarta: Equinox, 2005, pp. 1–69.

Ileto, Reynaldo C. "Cholera and the Origins of the American Sanitary Order in the Philippines," in *Discrepant Histories: Translocal Essays on Filipino Cultures*, ed. Vincente L. Rafael. Manchester and New York: Manchester University Press, 1988, pp. 125–48.

Institute for Medical Research. *Annual Report of Institute for Medical Research (ARIMR)*. Kuala Lumpur: Institute for Medical Research, 1949.

———. *Annual Report of Institute for Medical Research (ARIMR)*. Kuala Lumpur: Institute for Medical Research, 1950.

———. *Annual Report of Institute for Medical Research (ARIMR)*. Kuala Lumpur: Institute for Medical Research, 1951.

————. *Annual Report of Institute for Medical Research (ARIMR)*. Kuala Lumpur: Institute for Medical Research, 1952.

————. *Annual Report of Institute for Medical Research (ARIMR)*. Kuala Lumpur: Institute for Medical Research, 1953.

————. *Annual Report of Institute for Medical Research (ARIMR)*. Kuala Lumpur: Institute for Medical Research, 1954.

————. *Annual Report of Institute for Medical Research (ARIMR)*. Kuala Lumpur: Institute for Medical Research, 1955.

————. *Annual Report of Institute for Medical Research (ARIMR)*. Kuala Lumpur: Institute for Medical Research, 1956.

————. *Annual Report of Institute for Medical Research (ARIMR)*. Kuala Lumpur: Institute for Medical Research, 1957.

International Bank for Reconstruction and Development. *The Economic Development of Malaya*. Singapore: International Bank for Reconstruction and Development, 1955.

Itsumi, Shigeo. *Futsuryo-Indoshina-Kenkyu* [Research on French Indochina]. Tokyo: Nihon-Hyoron-sha, 1942.

Jaisvasd (Dr Tiao). Former Royal Lao Government Minister of Health interviewed in Torcy, France, 2 December 2012.

James, G.D. *Missionary Tours in Malaya*. Singapore: Malaya Evangelistic Fellowship, 1962.

Jayesuria, L.W. *A Review of the Rural Health Services in West Malaysia*. Kuala Lumpur: Ministry of Health, 1967.

Jennings, Bruce H. *Foundations of International Agricultural Research: Science and Politics in Mexican Agriculture*. Boulder, CO and London: Westview Press, 1988.

Jones, Alun. "The Orang Asli: An Outline of Their Progress in Modern Malaya." *Journal of Southeast Asian History* 9, 2 (1968): 286–305.

Jung, Junho and Ock-Joo Kim. "'It All Started from Worms': Korea–Japan Parasite Control Cooperation and Asian Network, 1960s–1980s." *Korean Journal of Medical History* 27, 1 (2018): 49–88.

Kamal, A.M. "The Seventh Pandemic of Cholera," in *Cholera*, ed. Dhiman Barua and William B. Greenough. New York: Springer, 1974, pp. 1–14.

Kammen, Douglas. *Three Centuries of Conflict in East Timor*. New Brunswick, NJ and London: Rutgers University Press, 2015.

Kammen, Douglas and Jonathan Chen. *Cina Timor: Baba, Hakka, and Cantonese in the Making of Timor-Leste*. Monograph 67. New Haven, CT: Yale University Southeast Asia Studies, 2020.

Katay Don Sasorith. *Le Laos. Son évolution politique. Sa place dans l'Union française* [Laos. Its Political Evolution. Its Place in the French Union]. Paris: Éditions Berger-Levrault, 1953.

Keo Phimphachanh. Unpublished draft manuscript of memoirs, Vientiane, 2020.

Kerkvliet, Benedict J. Tria and Mark Selden. "Agrarian Transformations in China and Vietnam." *The China Journal* 40 (1998): 37–58.

Khammeung Volachit. *Nang Phet Pativat. Xivit tit-phanh kab hongmoh 101 vilaxon* [Revolutionary Female Nurses: Life and the Heroic Hospital 101]. Vientiane: Manthatoulath Press, 2012.

Khamphaï Abhay (Dr). Former Royal Lao Government Minister of Health, interviewed by email, 10 October 2012.

Khamphao Phonekeo. "Les recherches sur la géographie du Laos" [Research on Lao Geography], in *Les Recherches en Sciences Humaines sur le Laos, Actes de la conférence international organiseé à Vientiane, 7–10 décembre 1993*, ed. Pierre-Bernard Lafont. Paris: Publications du Centre d'Histoire et Civilisations de la Peninsule Indochinoise, 1994, p. 29.

Khamsone Sassady. "Contribution à l'étude de la médecine laotienne" [Contribution to the Study of Lao Medicine]. Dissertation for Doctorat en médecine, University of Paris, 1962.

Kheng, Cheah Boon. *Red Star over Malaya: Resistance and Social Conflict during and after the Japanese Occupation, 1941–1946.* Fourth edition. Singapore: NUS Press, 2012.

Kim, Jeong-ran. "The Borderline of 'Empire': Japanese Maritime Quarantine in Busan c.1876–1910." *Medical History* 57, 2 (April 2013): 226–48.

Kim, Jeong-ran. 김정란, "제국의 흔적 지우기: 패전 후 일본에서의 귀환자 검역", 최해별 편, 『질병 관리의 사회문화사: 일상생활에서 국가정책까지 』, 서울, 이화여자대학 교출판문화원 / "jegugui heunjeok jiugi: paejeon hu iboneseoui gwihwanja geomyeok', choehaebyeol pyeon, jilbyeong gwalliui sahoemunhwasa: ilsang-saenghwareseo gukgajeongchaekkkaji" [Erasing the Traces of Empire: Quarantine of Returnees in Japan after Defeat], in *Social and Cultural History of Disease Management: From Daily Life to National Policy*, ed. Hae-byeol Choi. Seoul: Ewha Womans University Press and Cultural Center, 2021, pp. 291–321.

Kim, Kyuri and Buhm-Soon Park. "Infrastructure-Building for Public Health: The World Health Organization and Tuberculosis Control in South Korea, 1945–1963." *Korean Journal of Medical History* 28, 1 (2019): 89–138.

Kim, Sonja. *Imperatives of Care: Women and Medicine in Colonial Korea.* Honolulu: University of Hawai'i Press, 2019.

Kim, Won. "The Race to Appropriate 'Korean-ness': National Restoration, Internal Development, and Traces of Popular Culture," in *Cultures of Yusin: South Korea in the 1970s*, ed. Youngju Ryu. Ann Arbor: University of Michigan Press, 2018, p. 30.

King, John Kerry. "Malaya's Resettlement Problem." *Far Eastern Survey* 23, 3 (1954): 33–40.

———. "Rice Politics." *Foreign Affairs* 31, 3 (1953): 453–60.

Kompantsev, N.F. "Кампания ликвидации малярии в Северном Вьетнаме и помощь Советского Союза" [Malaria Eradication Campaign in Northern Vietnam, and Assistance Given by the USSR]. *Медицинская паразитология и паразитарные болезни* [Medical Parasitology and Parasitic Diseases] 32, 6 (1963): 752–3.

Kotar S.L. and J.E. Gessler. *Cholera: A Worldwide History.* Jefferson, NC: McFarland, 2014.

KOTRA. 세계를 향한 KOTRA 50: 1962~2012 /KOTRA[편] 서울 [Korea to/towards the World 1962–2012 (50 Years History)]. Seoul: KOTRA Korea Overseas Promotion Corporation, 2012.

Kroef, Justus van der. "The Cult of the Doctor and Its Indonesian Variant." *Journal of Educational Sociology* 32, 8 (1959): 381–91.

Kushner, Barak and Sherzhod Muminov. *The Dismantling of Japan's Empire in East Asia: Deimperialization, Postwar Legitimation and Imperial Afterlife.* New York: Routledge, 2016.

Kwon, Heonik. *Ghosts of War in Vietnam.* Cambridge: Cambridge University Press, 2008.

Laderman, Carol. "The Politics of Healing in Malaysia," in *Women and Politics in Twentieth Century Africa & Asia*, ed. V.H. Sutlive, N. Altshuler and M.D. Zamora. Virginia: College of William and Mary, 1981, pp. 143–58.

Langer, Paul F. and Joseph J. Zasloff. *North Vietnam and the Pathet Lao. Partners in the Struggle for Laos.* Cambridge, MA: Harvard University Press, 1970.

Lê, Trần Đức. *Sơ Thảo Lịch Sử Y Học Cổ Truyền Việt Nam* [Brief History of Vietnamese Traditional Medicine]. Hà Nội: NXB Y Học, 1995.

LeBar, Frank and Adrienne Suddard (ed.). *Laos. Its people, Its Society, Its Culture.* Revised edition. New Haven, CT: HRAF Press, 1967.

Lee, Christopher. "At the Rendezvous of Decolonization." *Interventions: International Journal of Postcolonial Studies* 11, 1 (2009): 81–93.

Lee, Jin-kyung. *Service Economies: Militarism, Sex Work, and Migrant Labor in South Korea.* Minneapolis: University of Minnesota Press, 2018.

Lee, Kam Hing. *A Matter of Risk: Insurance in Malaysia, 1826–1990.* Singapore: NUS Press, 2012.

Lee, Sung. "WHO and the Developing World: The Contest for Ideology," in *Western Medicine as Contested Knowledge*, ed. A. Cunningham and B. Andrews. Manchester: Manchester University Press, 1997, pp. 24–45.

Leung, Angela and Izumi Nakayama (ed.). *Gender, Health, and History in Modern East Asia.* Hong Kong: Hong Kong University Press, 2018.

Leung, Angela Ki-Che. *Leprosy in China: A History.* New York: Columbia University Press, 2009.

Li Tana. "In Search of the History of the Chinese in South Vietnam, 1945–75," in *The Chinese/ Vietnamese Diaspora*, ed. Yuk Wah Chan. New York: Routledge, 2011, pp. 52–61.

―――. *Nguyễn Cochinchina: Southern Vietnam in the Seventeenth and Eighteenth Centuries.* Ithaca, NY: Cornell University Press, 1998.

Li, Tania Murray. "Compromising Power: Development, Culture, and Rule in Indonesia." *Cultural Anthropology* 14, 3 (1999): 295–322.

Li, Yushang. "Heping shiqi de shuyi liuxing yu renkou siwang—yi jindai Guangdong, Fujian weili" [Plague and Death Tolls in Peace Time: An Example from Modern Guangdong and Fujian]. *Shixue yuekan* [Journal of Historical Science] 9 (2003): 82–94.

Liang, Yingming. *Jinxiandai dongnanya 1511–1992* [Modern Southeast Asia, 1511–1992]. Beijing: Beijing daxue chubanshe, 1994.

Lin, James. "Sowing Seeds and Knowledge: Agrarian Development in the US, China, Taiwan, and the World, 1920–1980." PhD dissertation, University of California Berkeley, 2017.

Lindsay, Jennifer. "Introduction," in *Heirs to a World Culture: Being Indonesian, 1950–65*, ed. Jennifer Lindsay and Maya Liem. Leiden: Brill, 2012, pp. 1–30.

Litsios, Socrates. "Malaria Control, the Cold War, and the Reorganization of International Assistance." *Medical Anthropology. Cross-Cultural Studies in Health and Illness* 17, 3 (1997): 255–78.

Litvin, Vlu and E.I. Korenberg. "Природная Очаговость Болезней: развитие Концепции к Исходу Века" [Natural Foci of Diseases: The Development of the Concept at the Close of the Century]. *Parazitologiia* 33, 3 (1999): 179–91.

Lockhart, Bruce. "Education in Laos in Historical Perspective." Unpublished paper, 2001.

Loi, Vu Man. "Le système sanitaire et la protection de la santé" [The Sanitary System and Health Protection], in *Population et développement au Viêt-nam*, ed. Patrick Gubry. Paris: Karthala/CEPED, 2000, pp. 135–63.

Luong, Nhi Ky. "The Chinese in Vietnam: A Study of Vietnamese–Chinese Relations with Special Attention to the Period 1862–1961." PhD dissertation, University of Michigan, 1963.

Lysenko, Andreï Yakolevich, Đặng Văn Ngữ, Hồ Văn Hưu and Đặng Tùng Thố. "Studies in Malaria Epidemiology in North Vietnam. 1. Topographical Malariological Exploration of Thai-Nguyen Province." *Med Parazitol (Moskva)* (1961): 293–8. Available at: https://apps.dtic.mil/sti/pdfs/AD0671272.pdf [accessed 19 May 2023].

Lysenko, Andreï Yakolevich and Nguyễn Tiến Bửu. "Studies in Malaria Epidemiology in North Viet Nam. 2. Topographical Malariological Exploration of the Thái Mèo Autonomous Region." *Med Parazitol (Moskva)* 30 (Nov–Dec) (1961): 643–51. Available at: https://apps.dtic.mil/sti/pdfs/AD0671273.pdf [accessed 19 May 2023].

Lysenko, Andreï Yakolevich and I.N. Semashko. *Geography of Malaria*. Moscow, 1968. Available at: https://endmalaria.org/sites/default/files/lysenko.pdf [accessed 09 October 2023].

Malayan Union Report of the Medical Department (MURMD). Kuala Lumpur: The Government of the Malayan Union, 1946.

Mallory, Walter H. "Chinese Minorities in South East Asia." *Foreign Affairs* 34, 2 (1956): 258–70.

Man, Simeon. *Soldiering through Empire: Race and the Making of the Decolonizing Pacific*. Oakland: University of California Press, 2018.

Manderson, Lenore. *Women, Politics, and Change: The Kaum Ibu UMNO, Malaysia, 1945–1972*. Oxford: Oxford University Press, 1980.

———. *Sickness and the State: Health and Illness in Colonial Malaya, 1870–1940*. Cambridge: Cambridge University Press, 1996.

Manivanh Souphanthong. "Kaneseuksa phetsard thi mahavitthayalay vitthayasat soukhaphapsard vivatthanakane 55 pii pheua pitouphoum khong bouangxon lao" [Medical Education at the University of Health Sciences, 55 Years of Service to the Lao People], in *Peum-botkhatyo botthopthouan vixakane Kongpaxoum vitthayasard saleum salong van-sang-tang honghianphed khob-hob 55 pi* [Abstracts for the Scientific Conference to Celebrate the 55th Anniversary of the Establishment of the Medical School], 30 October 2013.

Mantetsu East Asia Economic Survey（満鉄調査局）*Futsuryo-Indoshina ni okeru Kakyo* [Chinese in French Indochina]. Tokyo: The East Asiatic Economic Investigation Bureau, 1939.

Manturin, L. and R. Fontan. "La médecine au Laos" [Medicine in Laos]. *Médecine tropicale* 33, 6 (1973): 641–50.

Marangé, Céline. *Le communisme Vietnamien* [Vietnamese Communism]. Paris: Presse de Science Po, 2012.

Marr, David. *Vietnamese Tradition on Trial, 1920–1945*. Berkeley: University of California Press, 1981.

———. "Vietnamese Attitudes Regarding Illness and Healing," in *Death and Disease in Southeast Asia*, ed. Norman G. Owen. Oxford: Oxford University Press, 1987, pp. 162–86.

Mashad, Dhurudin. *Tahun Penuh Tantangan: Soedjono Djoened Poesponegoro, Menteri Riset Pertama di Indonesia* [A Year Full of Challenges: Soedjono Djoened Poesponegoro: First Indonesian Minister of Research]. Jakarta: LIPI, 2008.

McKeown, Adam. "Conceptualizing Chinese Diasporas, 1842 to 1949." *Journal of Asian Studies* 58, 2 (1999): 306–37.

McMahon, Robert, Harriet Schwar and Louis Smith (ed.). *Foreign Relations of the United States (1955–57), Southeast Asia*, vol. 22 (Washington, DC: US Government Printing Office, 1989.

Means, Gordon. "The Orang Asli: Aboriginal Policies in Malaysia." *Pacific Affairs* 58, 4 (1985): 637–52.

Mekong Circle International. "Those Were the Days." Pamphlet, 2004.

Menyingkap Pemikiran Professor Dr. Sardjito [Thoughts of Professor Dr. Sardjito]. Jogjakarta: UGM Press, 2006.

Metzner, Joachim. "Malaria, Bevölkerungsdruck und Landschaftszerstörung im Östlichen Timor" [Malaria, Population Pressure and Environmental Degradation in East Timor]. *Methoden und Modelle der Biomedizinischen Forschung* [Methods and Models of Biomedical Research]. *Beihefte de Geographische Zeitschrift* 43 (1976): 121–37.

———. *Man and Environment in Eastern Timor: A Geoecological Analysis of the Bacau-Viqueque Area as a Possible Basis for Regional Planning*. Monograph 8. Canberra: Development Studies Centre, Australian National University, 1977.

Meyer, H. *Public Health in Indochina* (prepared for the Health Research Unit of the League of Nations). (Washington, DC, WHO Archives: 8A/43045/21641 (R. 6141), 1944.

Michaels, Paula A. "Medical Propaganda and Cultural Revolution in Soviet Kazakhstan, 1928–41." *The Russian Review* 59, 2 (2000): 159–78.

Miller, Edward. *Misalliance: Ngo Dinh Diem, the United States, and the Fate of South Vietnam.* Cambridge, MA: Harvard University Press, 2013.

Millett, Allen. *The War for Korea: A House on Fire, 1945–1950.* Lawrence, KA: University of Kansas Press, 2015.

Ministério dos Negócios Estrangeiros. "Informação sobre o Oficio no. 15, de 16 de Abril do Ministerio dos Negocios Estrangeiros, sobre o inquérito a realizar pela UNESCO nos territórios ultramarinos" [Information on Official Document No. 15, April 16, of the Ministry of Foreign Affairs, on the Survey Undertaken by UNESCO in the Overseas Territories], 25 April 1951. AHU MU GM mç 1939–1951. Lisbon: Arquivo Histórico Ultramarino.

Ministério do Ultramar, Direcção dos Serviços Hidráulicos. "Recursos Hidroagrícolas da Província de Timor. Elementos para um Programa de Acção" [Hydrological and Agricultural Resources in Timor Province: The Fundamentals of an Action Plan]. MU/T/Cx 82, 6. Lisbon: Arquivo Histórico Ultramarino, 1965.

Mizuno, Hiromi, Aaron S. Moore and John P. DiMoia (ed.). *Engineering Asia: Technology, Colonial Development, and the Cold War Order.* London: Bloomsbury, 2018.

Monnais, Laurence. *The Colonial Life of Pharmaceuticals: Medicines and Modernity in Vietnam.* Cambridge: Cambridge University Press, 2019.

Monnais, Laurence, C.M. Thompson and A. Wahlberg (ed.). *Southern Medicine for Southern People: Vietnamese Medicine in the Making.* Newcastle upon Tyne: Cambridge Scholars, 2012.

Morabia, Alfredo. "'East Side Story': On Being an Epidemiologist in the Former USSR: An Interview with Marcus Klingberg." *Epidemiology* 17, 1 (2006): 115–19.

Moreira, Fausto. "Contribuição para o Conhecimento das Plantas Medicinais do Timor Português" [Contribution to Knowledge on Medicinal Plants of Portuguese Timor]. *Revista Portuguesa de Farmácia* 28 (1968): 13–18.

Mosley, W.H. "Epidemiology of Cholera," in *Principles and Practice of Cholera Control*, ed. World Health Organization. Geneva: World Health Organization, 1970, pp. 23–7.

Mozingo, David. *Chinese Policy toward Indonesia, 1949–1967.* Ithaca, NY: Cornell University Press, 1976.

Mr Choijinsa. "[월남전쟁] 십자성부대 & 비둘기부대 활동" [[Vietnam War] Crusade/Crusaders Unit & Pigeon Unit Activities]. YouTube, 3 July 2018. Available at: https://www.youtube.com/watch?v=4bga2dIm3hY [accessed 09 October 2023].

Neelakantan, Vivek. "No Nation Can Go Forward When It Is Crippled by Disease: Philippine Science and the Cold War, 1950s." *Southeast Asian Studies* 10, 1 (2021): 53–89.

———. *Science, Public Health, and Nation-Building in Soekarno-Era Indonesia.* Newcastle upon Tyne: Cambridge Scholars Publishing, 2017.

———. "The Medical Spur to Postcolonial Science during the Soekarno Era." *IIAS Newsletter* 70 (2015): 14–15.

Nguyen, Duy Lap. *The Unimagined Community: Imperialism and Culture in South Vietnam.* Manchester: Manchester University Press, 2020.

Nguyen, Phuong Thoan. "The Lao Twins Saved and Brought Up by the Truong Son Military Medical Corps—Then and Now," in *History of Vietnam–Laos, Laos–Vietnam Special Relationship 1930–2007*, ed. Vietnamese and Lao Compilatory Steering Committees, Hanoi: National Political Publishing House, 2012, pp. 629–36.

Nguyen, Quang Van and Majorie Pivar. *Fourth Uncle in the Mountain: The Remarkable Legacy of a Buddhist Itinerant Doctor in Vietnam.* New York: St. Martin's Griffin, 2006.

Nguyen, Tien Dinh. "Ten Years of Providing Healthcare for Leaders of the Lao Patriotic Front in the Anti-American Resistance (1966–1975)," in *History of Vietnam–Laos, Laos–Vietnam Special Relationship 1930–2007*, ed. Vietnamese and Lao Compilatory Steering Committees, Hanoi: National Political Publishing House, 2012, pp. 531–8.

Nicolas, Colin and Adela Baer. "Healthcare for the Orang Asli: Consequences of Paternalism and Non-recognition," in *Health Care in Malaysia: The Dynamics of Provision, Financing and Access*, ed. Chee Heng Leng and Simon Barraclough. New York: Palgrave, 2009, pp. 119–36.

Nyce, Ray. *Chinese New Villages in Malaya Community Study.* Kuala Lumpur: Malaysian Sociological Research Institute, 1973.

Oda, Nara. "Betonamu Kingendaishi ni okeru Dento-igaku: Minzoku igaku no tanjo" [Traditional Medicine in the Modern History of Vietnam: Invention of 'National Medicine']. *Tonan Ajia* (Southeast Asia: History and Culture) 40 (2010): 126–44.

———. *Dentou Igakuga Tsukurareru Toki: Betonamu Iryo-seisaku-shi* [The Making of 'Traditional Medicine': A History of Vietnam's Medical Policies]. Kyoto: Kyoto University Press. 2022.

O'Keefe, Brendan G. *Medicine at War: Medical Aspects of Australia's Involvement in Southeast Asia, 1950–1972.* New South Wales: Allen & Unwin, 1994.

Ong, Willie T. "Public Health and the Clash of Cultures: The Philippine Cholera Epidemics," in *Public Health in Asia and the Pacific: Historical and Contemporary Perspectives*, ed. Milton J. Lewis and Kerrie L. MacPherson. Abingdon and New York: Routledge, 2008, pp. 206–21.

Pacific Association (太平洋調査会) (ed.). *Futsuryo-Indhoshina* [French Indochina]. Tokyo: Kawade-shobo, 1940.

Packard, Randall M. "'Roll Back Malaria, Roll in Development'? Reassessing Burden of Malaria." *Population and Development Review* 35, 1 (2009): 53–87.

Panda, S.C. "Medicine: Science or Art?" *Mens Sana Monographs* 4, 1 (2006): 127–38.

Park, Youngsu. "Tempoethics: Envisioning Asian Modernities and Enacting Global Health Projects in Ethiopia." PhD dissertation, Stanford University, 2018.

Pauker, Guy. "Indonesia in 1964: Toward a People's Democracy." *Asian Survey* 5, 2 (1965): 88–97.

Pavlovskyĭ, L.N. "Выдающийся Советский Зоолог и Паразитолог Е. Н. Павловский—Создатель Учения о Природной Очаговости волезней"

[Outstanding Soviet zoologist and parasitologist E.N. Pavlovsky—The Creator of the Theory of Natural Foci of Disease]. *Lik Sprava* 5–6 (2011): 142–9.

Peckham, Robert. *Epidemics in Modern Asia.* Cambridge: Cambridge University Press, 2016.

Pelley, Patricia. "'Barbarians' and 'Younger Brothers': The Remaking of Race in Postcolonial Vietnam." *Journal of Southeast Asian Studies* (1998): 374–91.

Peng Jiali. "Shijiu shiji xifang qinlüezhe dui zhongguo laogong de lulüe" [Plundering and Looting of Western Invaders in China during the Nineteenth Century], in *Huagong chuguo shiliao huibian* [A Compilation of Historical Documents Concerning Chinese Laborers Overseas], ed. Chen Hansheng. Beijing: Zhonghua shuju, 4, 1981, pp. 174–229.

Phan, Vu Thi. *Epidémiologie du paludisme et lutte antipaludique au Vietnam* [Malarial Epidemiology and the Fight against Malaria in Vietnam]. Hanoi: Editions Médicales Vietnam, 1998.

Phee, Tan Teng. *Behind Barbed Wire: Chinese New Villages During the Malayan Emergency, 1948–1960.* Petaling Jaya: Strategic Information and Research Development Center, 2020.

Pholsena, Vatthana. "La production d'hommes et de femmes socialistes nouveaux. Expériences de l'éducation communiste au Laos révolutionnaire" [The Production of New Socialist Men and Women. Experiences of Communist Education in Revolutionary Laos], in *Laos. Sociétés et pouvoirs*, ed. Vanina Bouté and Vatthana Pholsena. Bangkok: IRASEC, 2012, pp. 45–67.

Phua, Kai Hong. "The Development of Health Services in Malaya and Singapore." PhD dissertation, London School of Economics, 1987.

Poesponegoro, Soedjono Djoened. "Address at the Opening Ceremony of the Second Afro-Asian Congress of Paediatrics, August 19, 1964." *Paediatrica Indonesiana* 4 (1964): vii–xii.

———. *Masalah Kesehatan Anak di Indonesia* [Health Problems of Indonesian Children]. Djakarta: Jajasan Pembangunan, 1953.

Pols, Hans. *Nurturing Indonesia: Medicine and Decolonization in the Dutch East Indies.* Cambridge: Cambridge University Press, 2018.

Polunin, Ivan. "The Medical Natural History of Malayan Aborigines." *Medical Journal of Malaya* 8, 1 (1953): 62–171.

Pottier, Richard. *Santé et Société au Laos (1973–1978)* [Health and Society in Laos (1973–1978)]. Paris: Comité pour la Coopération avec le Laos, 2004.

Pravikov, G.A. "The Stalin Prize for the Elaboration and Application of Measures in Malarial Liquidation." *Izvest. Akad. NauklurVmen SSR, Ashkhabad* (1952): 90–1.

Prawirohardjo, Sarwono. "Beberapa Pikiran Tentang Perkembangan Ilmu Pengetahuan dan Penjelidikan di Indonesia" [Several Ideas Regarding the Development of Science and Research in Indonesia], in *Laporan Ilmu Pengetahuan Pertama*, ed. Madjelis Ilmu Pengetahuan Indonesia, Jakarta: MIPI, 1959, n. p.

Purdey, Jemma. *Anti-Chinese Violence in Indonesia 1996–1999*. Singapore: NUS Press, 2005.

Qian Xinzhong. "Fuhuoluan fangzhi gongzuo de qingkuang ji jinhou renwu" [Cholera Prevention and Treatment and Future Work], 12 December 1962, Wenzhou Prefectural Archives, 38-14-7.

―――. "Fuhuoluan fangzhi gongzuo huiyi zongjie" [Summary of the El Tor Cholera Prevention and Treatment Meeting]. Zhejiang Provincial Archives, J166-1-80 1964.

Ramakrishna, Kumar. *Emergency Propaganda: The Winning of Malayan Hearts and Minds, 1948–1958.* London: Curzon Press, 2002.

Ramos, M. Pais de. "Timor: Seus Recursos Hidroagrícolas" [The Hydro-agricultural Resources of Timor]. MU/T/Cx, 82, 5, n.d. Lisbon: Arquivo Histórico Ultramarino.

Raška, Karel. "Surveillance and Control of Cholera," in *Principles and Practice of Cholera Control*, ed. World Health Organization. Geneva: World Health Organization, 1970, pp. 115–25.

Reis, L.M. Moreira da Silva. "Timor-Leste, 1953–1975: O Desenvolvimento Agrícola na Última Fase da Colonização Portuguesa" [Timor-Leste, 1953–1975. Agricultural Development in the Last Phase of Portuguese Colonization]. MA dissertation, Universidade Técnica de Lisboa, Lisbon, 2000.

"Resolutions Adopted at the General Session of the Second Afro-Asian Congress of Paediatrics, Jakarta, August 26, 1964." *Paediatrica Indonesiana* 4 (1964): xxxvi–xxxix.

Rodrigues, Luís Nuno. "Crossroads of the Atlantic: Portugal, the Azores and the Atlantic Community (1943–57)," in *Atlantic Community and Europe 1: European Community, Atlantic Community?* ed. V. Aubourg, G. Bossuat and G. Scott-Smith. Paris: Éditions Soleb, 2008, pp. 456–67.

Rogaski, Ruth. *Hygienic Modernity: Meanings of Health and Disease in Treaty-Port China.* Berkeley: University of California Press, 2014.

Roxborogh, John. *A Short Introduction to Malaysian Church History: A Guide to the Story of Christianity in Malaysia and How to Go About Discovering the History of Your Church.* Kuala Lumpur: Seminari Theoloji Malaysia and the Catholic Research Center, 1989.

Rudner, Martin. "The Draft Development Plan of the Federation of Malaya 1950–55." *Journal of Southeast Asian Studies* 3, 1 (1972): 63–96.

Rusk, Howard. *A World to Care for: The Autobiography of Howard A. Rusk, M.D.* New York: Random House, 1972.

Ryu, Youngju (ed.). *Cultures of Yusin: South Korea in the 1970s.* Ann Arbor: University of Michigan Press, 2018.

Sardjito. *Bangsa Indonesia Seharusnja Dikemudian Hari Mendjadi Bangsa Jang Besar: Tjeramah Diutjapjkan Dimuka Para Mahasiswa Baru Pada Bulan September 1956* [Indonesia Will Become a Great Nation: Lecture Delivered to Incoming Students in September 1956]. Jogjakarta: UGM, 1956.

―――. *Kewadjiban Ilmu Ahli Bakteri dan Ahli Ilmoe Hajat di Djaman Pembangoenan Indonesia Merdeka* [The Role of Indonesian Bacteriologists and Biologists in the Era of National Reconstruction]. Soerakarta: Pergoeroen Tinggi Kedokteran, 1946.

Satrio and Mona Lohanda. "Perjuangan dan Pengabdian: Masuk Kenangan Professor Dokter Satrio, 1916–86" [Struggle and Devotion: Recollections of Professor Doctor Satrio, 1916–86]. *Penerbitan Sejarah Lisan 3.* Jakarta: Arsip Nasional, 1986.

Schrock, Joann L. American University (Washington, DC). Cultural Information Analysis Center. *Minority Groups in the Republic of Vietnam.* Washington, DC: Headquarters, Department of the Army, 1966.

Scott, James. *The Art of Not Being Governed: An Anarchist History of Upland Southeast Asia.* New Haven, CT: Yale University Press, 2009.

———. *Weapons of the Weak: Everyday Forms of Peasant Resistance.* New Haven, CT: Yale University Press, 1985.

Shepherd, Christopher. "Imperial Science: The Rockefeller Foundation and Agricultural Science in Peru, 1940–1960." *Science as Culture, Special Issue: Postcolonial Technoscience* 13, 14 (2005): 113–37.

———. *Development and Environmental Politics Unmasked: Authority, Participation and Equity in East Timor.* London: Routledge, 2014.

———. *Haunted Houses and Ghostly Encounters: Animism and Ethnography in East Timor, 1860–1975.* Singapore: NUS Press, 2019.

Shepherd, Christopher and Andrew McWilliam. "Cultivating Plantations and Subjects in East Timor: A Genealogy." *Bijdragen tot de Taal-, Land- en Volkenkunde* [Journal of the Humanities and Social Sciences of Southeast Asia and Oceania] 169 (2013): 326–61.

———. "Divide and Cultivate: Plantations, Militarism and Environment in Portuguese Timor, 1860–1975," in *Comparing Apples, Oranges, and Cotton: Environmental Histories of the Global Plantation*, ed. Frank Uekotter. Chicago: University of Chicago Press, 2014, pp. 139–66.

Shepherd, Christopher and Lisa Palmer. "The Modern Origins of Traditional Agriculture: Colonial Policy, Swidden Development, and Environmental Degradation in Eastern Timor." *Bijdragen tot de Taal-, Land- en Volkenkunde (Journal of the Humanities and Social Sciences of Southeast Asia and Oceania)* 171, 2–3 (2015): 281–311.

Shin Dong-won. "Hygiene, Medicine, and Modernity in Korea, 1876–1910." *East Asian Science, Technology and Society* 3, 1 (2009): 5–26.

Short, Anthony. *In Pursuit of Mountain Rats: The Communist Insurrection in Malaya.* Singapore: Cultured Lotus, 1975.

Silva, Hélder Lains e. *Timor e a Cultura do Café* [Timor and the Cultivation of Coffee]. Lisbon: Ministério do Ultramar, 1956.

———. "Programa de Desenvolvimento Agrícola 1965–1975" [Agricultural Development Program 1965–1975]. *Comunicação* 47. Lisbon: MEAU, 1964.

Simpson, Bradley R. *Economists with Guns: Authoritarian Development and U.S.-Indonesian Relations, 1960–1968.* Stanford, CA: Stanford University Press, 2010.

Smith, Elta. "Imaginaries of Development: the Rockefeller Foundation and Rice Research." *Science as Culture* 18, 4 (2009): 461–82.

Soekarno. *Soal Hidup atau Mati* [Want to Live or Want to Die Situation]. Djakarta: Kementerian Penerangan, 1952.

———. "Opening Address Given by President Soekarno on 18 April 1955, Bandung." *Asia Africa Speak from Bandung*. Djakarta: Department of Foreign Affairs Republic of Indonesia, 1955.

———. "Applied Sciences and Nation-Building." *Speech Delivered by President Soekarno at the Closing Reception of the Indonesian National Science Conference in Malang, 8 August 1958.* Jakarta: Ministry of Information Republic of Indonesia, 1958.

———. "Lecture by President Soekarno to Students of the Padjadjaran University in Bandung on 17 November 1958." *Presidential Lecture Series*. Djakarta: Ministry of Information Republic of Indonesia, 1959.

———. *Persambahan Hidupmu Kepada Tanah dan Bangsa: Tjeramah Presiden Soekarno didepan pada Para Mahasiswa Universitas Gadjah Mada di Sitinghinggil Jogjakarta, 22 Oktober 1962* [Sacrificing Your Life for the Nation: Lecture Delivered by President Soekarno to Universitas Gadjah Mada Students at Sitinghinggil Jogjakarta, 22 October 1962]. Djakarta: Kementerian Penerangan, 1962.

———. "Mobilizazi Dokter" [Mobilization of Doctors]. *Berita Ketabiban* 1–4 (2604 [1944]): 28.

Somasundaram, Sujit. "Science and the Global: On Methods, Questions, and Theory." *ISIS* 101, 1 (2010): 146–58.

Sreenivasan, B.R. "The Role of Physicians in Developing Countries." *Proceedings of the Conference on Medical Education*. Kuala Lumpur: Faculty of Medicine, University of Malaya, 1965, pp. 22–5.

Stieglitz, Perry. *In a Little Kingdom*. Armonk, NY: M.E. Sharpe, 1990.

Stuart-Fox, Martin. *A History of Laos*. Cambridge: Cambridge University Press, 1997.

Stubbs, Richard. *Counter-Insurgency and the Economic Factor: The Impact of the Korean War Prices Boom on the Malayan Emergency*. Singapore: Institute of Southeast Asian Studies, 1974.

Sweet, Kathryn Dawn. "Limited Doses: Health and Development in Laos, 1893–2000." PhD dissertation, National University of Singapore, 2015.

Syphanom Viravong. Former Operation Brotherhood nurse, interviewed in Sydney, Australia, 25 July 2012.

Tagliacozzo, Eric. "Pilgrim Ships and the Frontiers of Contagion: Quarantine Regimes from Southeast Asia to the Red Sea," in *Histories of Health in Southeast Asia: Perspectives on the Long Twentieth Century*, ed. Tim Harper and Sunil S. Amrith. Bloomington, IN: Indiana University Press, 2014, pp. 47–60.

Tappe, Oliver. "National Lieu de Mémoire vs. Multivocal Memories: The Case of Viengxay, Lao PDR," in *Interactions with a Violent Past: Reading Post-Conflict Landscapes in Cambodia, Laos and Vietnam*, ed. Vatthana Pholsena and Oliver Tappe. Singapore: NUS Press, 2013, pp. 46–77.

Thompson, C. Michele. "Medicine, Nationalism, and Revolution in Vietnam: The Roots of a Medical Collaboration to 1945." *East Asian Science, Technology & Medicine* 21 (2003): 114–48.

———. "Tuệ Tĩnh Vietnamese Monk-Physician at the Ming Court," in *The Illustrated History of Chinese Medicine and Healing*, ed. T.J. Heinrichs and Linda L. Barnes. Cambridge, MA: Harvard University Press, 2013, pp. 134–5.

———. *Vietnamese Traditional Medicine: A Social History.* Singapore: NUS Press, 2015.

Tilman, Robert O. *Bureaucratic Transition in Malaya.* Durham, NC: Duke University Press, 1964.

Toer, Pramoedya Ananta. "Footsteps" [Jejak Langkah]. *Buru Quartet*, 3. Trans. Max Lane. New York: Penguin, 1990.

"Tongnae Rehabilitation Center." Box 344, File 16. United Nations ARMS, New York.

Tran, Khanh. *The Ethnic Chinese and Economic Development in Vietnam.* Singapore: Institute of Southeast Asian Studies, 1993.

Trung Ương Hội Đông Y Việt Nam. *65 Năm Hội Đông Y Việt Nam Trưởng Thành và Phát Triển* [65 Years of the Maturity and Development of the Eastern Medicine Association of Vietnam]. Hà Nội: Nhà Xuất Bản Y Học, 2011.

UNKRA (United Nations Korea Reconstruction Agency). *UNKRA in Action.* New York: United Nations, 1956.

Untuk Perdamaian dan Kesedjahteraan Rakjat [For Peace and Public Welfare]. Djakarta: Bagian Penerangan Besar URSS, 1960.

USAID. "American Aid to Laos." Vientiane: USAID, 1964.

———. "Foreign Assistance to Laos." Vientiane: USAID, 1969.

———. "US Economic Assistance to the Royal Lao Government, 1962–1972." Vientiane: USAID, 1972.

———. "Termination Report. USAID Laos." Washington, DC: USAID, 1976.

Vargha, Dora. *Polio across the Iron Curtain: Hungary's Cold War with an Epidemic.* Cambridge: Cambridge University Press, 2018.

Venediktov, D.D. and V.I. Petrov. *Untuk Taraf Jang Tinggi* [For Better Living Standards]. Djakarta: Soviet Embassy, 1960.

Viện sốt rét ký sinh trùng và côn trùng xuất bản. *Bệnh sốt rét. Phòng chống và tiêu diệt sốt rét ở Việt Nam 1958–1975* [Malaria Prevention and Eradication in Vietnam, 1958–1975]. Hà Nội, 1976.

"Vietnam War 'We've Been There.'" Available at: http://www.vietvet.co.kr/ [accessed 13 June 2020].

Wah, Loh Kok. *Beyond the Tin Mines: Coolies, Squatters and New Villagers in the Kinta Valley, Malaysia, c.1880–1980.* London: Oxford University Press, 1988.

Wahlberg, Ayo. "Revolutionary Movement to Bring Traditional Medicine Back to the Grassroots Level: On the Biopolitization of Herbal Medicine in Vietnam," in *Global Movements, Local Concerns: Medicine and Health in Southeast Asia*, ed. Laurence Monnais and Harold J. Cook. Singapore: NUS Press, 2012, pp. 207–25.

Warman, Adam Aswi. *Sarwono Prawirohardjo: Pembangunan Institusi Ilmu Penge-tahuan di Indonesia* [Sarwono Prawirohardjo: The Development of Institutions of Science in Indonesia]. Jakarta: LIPI, 2009.

Warren, James Francis. *Ah Ku and Karayuki-San: Prostitution in Singapore, 1870–1940.* Singapore: Oxford University Press, 1993.

Watson, Laura. "Lao Malaria Review." Unpublished paper, 1999.

Webster, David. *Fire and the Full Moon: Canada and Indonesia in a Decolonizing World.* Vancouver: University of British Columbia Press, 2010.

Weishengbu gongzuozu [Work Team of the Ministry of Health]. "Jin 25 nianlai shijie fuhuoluan de liuxing he fangzhi gaikuang (1937.9–1962.9)" [Survey of El Tor Cholera Transmission, Prevention and Treatment in the Last 25 Years]. Zhejiang Provincial Archives, J166-2-160, 1962.

Weldon, Charles. *Tragedy in Paradise: A Country Doctor at War in Laos.* Bangkok: Asia Books, 1999.

Wen Xiongfei. *Nanyang huaqiao tongshi* [General History of Nanyang Overseas Chinese]. Shanghai: Dongfang yinshuguan, 1929.

Westermeyer, Joe (Dr). Former USAID doctor, interviewed by email, 13 June 2013.

Whitaker, Donald P. et al. *Laos. A Country Study*, Washington, DC: Foreign Areas Studies, The American University, 1985 [1971].

Woo, Susie. *Framed by War: Korean Children and Women at the Crossroads of US Empire.* New York: New York University Press, 2019.

Woodside, Alexander. "Decolonization and Agricultural Reform in Northern Vietnam." *Asian Survey* 10, 8 (1970): 705–23.

World Health Organization. *Guidelines for Cholera Control.* Geneva: World Health Organization, 1993.

———. "Report on Meeting for the Exchange of Information on El Tor Vibrio Para-cholera, Manila, Philippines, 16–19 April 1962." World Health Organization Western Pacific Regional Office (WPRO) Archives.

———. *50 Years Working for Health in the Lao People's Democratic Republic, 1962–2012.* Manila: World Health Organization, 2013.

Xiaoyuan, Jiang. "The Pasteur Institutes in Vietnam: A Long History." *History of Science in the Multiculture: Proceedings of the Tenth International Conference on the History of Science in East Asia.* Shanghai: Jiao Tong University Press, 2005, pp. 161–72.

Xinhuashe [Xinhua News Agency]. "Jiangfeibang mobuguanxin fangzhi gongzuo, Taiwan fuhuoluan yiqu xunshu kuoda" [Chiang Kai Shek Bandit Clique Did Not Care about Epidemic Prevention and Treatment Work. Cholera Is Spreading Rampantly], *The People's Daily* [RMRB], 1962.

———. "Taiwan nanbu fasheng fuhuoluan" [Cholera Broke Out in Taiwan], *The People's Daily* [RMRB], 1962.

———. "Wo juanzeng de huoluan yimiao yundi feilüebin" [Cholera Vaccines Do-nated by Our Country Have Reached the Philippines], *The People's Daily* [RMRB], 1962.

———. "Xiezhu feiluebin pumie fuhuoluan, Wo hongshizihui jueding zengsong yipi huoluan yimiao" [To Assist the Philippines in Eradicating Cholera, Our China Red Cross Society Decided to Donate a Batch of Cholera Vaccines], *The People's Daily* [RMRB], 1962.

Young, Benjamin. *Guns, Guerillas, and the Great Leader: North Korea and the Third World.* Stanford, CA: Stanford University Press, 2021.

Zalutskaya, L.I. "Comparative Data on the Biology of *Anopheles minimus* and *A. vagus* at Tay-Nguyen (Democratic Republic of Vietnam)." *Meditsinskaya Parazitologiya i Parazitarnyye Bolezni* 28 (1959): 548–53.

Zhonghua renmin gongheguo shanghai weisheng jianyisuo [Shanghai Institute of Health and Quarantine of the People's Republic of China]. "Shijie huoluan yiqing de zhangwo, fenxi yu yingyong" [Collection, Analysis, and Application of the Global Cholera Pandemic]. October 1963, Zhejiang Provincial Archives, J166-2-199.

Zhejiangsheng renmin weiyuanhui bangongting [The General Office of Zhejiang Provincial People's Commission]. "Guanyu huaqiao he gang'ao tongbao yi waihui zhifu lüefei, qi jiaotong zhusu feiyong shixing bazhe youdai de tongzhi" [Circular on Offering 20% Discount to Overseas Chinese and Visitors from Hong Kong and Macau Paying Transport and Accommodation Fees in Foreign Currency]. Pingyang County Archives, Zhejiang Province, 10-16-40, 1964.

Zhejiangsheng weishengting [Zhejiang Provincial Health Department]. "Guanyu dui huaji chuanyuan, guiguo huaqiao, gang'ao tongbao he shuqi fanxiao shisheng kaizhan yiyuan jiansuo de tongzhi" [Circular on Launching the Search for Epidemic Sources among Overseas Chinese Boatmen, Returned Overseas Chinese, Hong Kong and Macau Residents, and Students on Summer Vacation]. Zhejiang Provincial Archives, J166-2-206, 1964.

List of Contributors

Michitake Aso is a global environmental historian at the University at Albany, SUNY, USA. His research has focused on Vietnamese and French agriculture, medicine, and health in the 19th and 20th centuries.

John P. DiMoia is Professor of Korean history at Seoul National University (SNU), where he is also affiliated with the Science and Technology Studies group. He is the author of *Reconstructing Bodies* (Stanford University Press, 2013/WEAI), and one of the co-editors of *Engineering Asia* (Bloomsbury, 2019/WEAI). From June 2022, he has served as the editor of *SJKS* (*Seoul Journal of Korean Studies*).

Xiaoping Fang is an Associate Professor of Chinese Studies at Monash University. He received his PhD in history from the National University of Singapore (NUS), where he majored in Modern China and the history of science, technology and medicine. His research interests focus on the history of medicine, health and epidemics in 20th-century China and the sociopolitical history of Mao's China after 1949. He is the author of *Barefoot Doctors and Western Medicine in China* (University of Rochester Press, 2012) and *China and the Cholera Pandemic: Restructuring Society under Mao* (University of Pittsburgh Press, 2021), and he has published articles in journals such as *Modern China*, *The China Quarterly*, *Modern Asian Studies* and *Medical History*.

Annick Guénel is senior researcher at CNRS, Centre Asie du Sud-Est, France. After a Master's in Microbiology, she turned to the history of biomedical sciences and to their development in the context of the French colonial empire. She has written several articles on the history of the Pasteur Institutes in Vietnam. Her interest in the medical history of this country goes beyond the mid-20th century and she deals with topics such as health systems and nationalism, traditional medicine and globalization.

Por Heong Hong is a lecturer at the School of Social Sciences, Universiti Sains Malaysia. She uses a wide range of conceptual tools across various disciplines of social sciences to interrogate issues pertaining to medicine, health and diseases, bodies, modernity and nationalism. Recently, she has also developed interest in the politics of culture and politics of memory. Her geographical focus is mainly Malaysia, Southeast Asia and East Asia.

Vivek Neelakantan is a 2023 Brocher Fellow. His current research project investigates the evolution of primary healthcare in Southeast Asia whilst his earlier research investigated Indonesia's relation with the WHO during the Cold War and the appropriation of social medicine by local physicians. His monograph *Science, Public Health and Nation-Building in Soekarno-Era Indonesia* (2017) was translated into Bahasa Indonesia. Vivek's forthcoming edited volume with Routledge, entitled *The Geopolitics of Health in South and Southeast Asia: Perspectives from the Cold War to COVID-19*, examines the strengths and weaknesses of a regional approach to global health. In May 2023, Vivek will be co-organizing a one-day interdisciplinary workshop entitled "Cholera in the Indian Ocean World since the Nineteenth Century," with Eva-Maria Knoll, Senior Researcher at the Institute for Social Anthropology, Austrian Academy of Sciences. Since 2015, his research has attracted external funding from the Wellcome Trust, the Rockefeller Foundation, the Truman and Eisenhower Presidential Libraries, the Consortium for the History of Science, Technology and Medicine, and the Brocher Foundation.

Nara Oda is a lecturer at the World Language and Society Education Centre, Tokyo University of Foreign Studies, Japan. She received her PhD in Area Studies from the Graduate School of Asian and African Area Studies at Kyoto University. Her recent research focuses on the modern history of Vietnam in the context of traditional medicine, healthcare and issues related to sexual minorities.

Christopher Shepherd is an independent researcher affiliated with the Department of Anthropology at the Australian National University. He does research on rural development processes, indigenous politics, the history of science, the history of anthropology, extraction industries and human trafficking. Shepherd has two books on East Timor: *Development and Environmental Politics Unmasked: Authority, Participation and Equity in East Timor* (Routledge, 2014) and *Haunted Houses and Ghostly Encounters: Animism and Ethnography in East Timor, 1860–1975* (NUS Press, 2019).

Kathryn Sweet is a social development consultant and social historian of Laos based in Canberra, Australia. She has a PhD in Lao history from the National University of Singapore, and has published on Lao medical and development history.

C. Michele Thompson holds an MA in East Asian History and a PhD in Southeast Asian History. Her research and publications focus on the History of Medicine and the Environment of Southeast Asia. She is Professor of Southeast Asian History at Southern Connecticut State University.

Index

Ho Chi Minh City, 130, 141, 159
Hoà Bình, 154, 162, 163
Hong Kong, 1, 130–2, 200–23, 205,
    212, 221, 224, 234, 247, 259, 265
House of Representatives, Indonesian,
    Dewan Perwakilan Rakjat, 184
Hue, 124, 136, 137, 140, 142, 143, 248
hydroelectric projects, 177

ICA (United States International
    Cooperation Agency), 147, 174
Idris, Mohamed, 69
Ika Dai Gaku (Medical Academy at
    Jakarta), 179
Ikatan Dokter Indonesia (IDI or the
    Indonesian Medical Association),
    180
imperial structures/colonialism/empire,
    4, 7, 15, 18, 21, 22, 25, 26, 28–32,
    37, 38, 48, 78–83, 168–71, 176,
    182, 187, 188, 192, 215, 218, 220,
    230, 233–41, 244, 247, 249, 250,
    253–5, 264, 267
Incheon, 215, 224
indentured laborers, 195
India, 22, 71, 76, 77, 79, 91, 187, 189,
    190, 198, 216, 244
Indian Ocean, 197, 268
indigenous herbal remedies (djamu),
    178
Indochina War, 4, 5, 17, 85, 108, 123,
    124, 153
Indonesia, v, vii, 3, 5, 9, 10, 15, 16–18,
    20, 22–4, 26, 29, 35, 452, 46–8,
    50, 51, 82, 167–94, 197–200,
    202, 205, 207, 209, 211, 212,
    238, 240, 244, 245, 249–51,
    254–62, 264, 268
    Partai Komunis Indonesia (PKI),
        173, 176, 193
Indonesian Chinese, 194, 197–200, 202,
    209, 211, 212

Indonesian Council of Sciences
    (Madjelis Ilmu Pengetahuan
    Indonesia, or MIPI), vii, 180–3,
    186, 192, 259
    First Indonesian Science
        Conference, 167
Indonesian Revolution, 167, 171, 183,
    192
Industrialization, 170, 201, 237, 249
Influenza Institute of Malariology,
    Parasitology and Entomology
    (IMPE), 153, 157, 159, 161, 245
Institute for Medical Research (IMR),
    71, 72, 73, 82, 251, 252
International Agricultural Research
    Centers (IARCs), 41
International Bank for Reconstruction
    and Development (IBRD), 76, 77,
    83, 173, 252
International Labour Organization
    (ILO), 31, 93
    Forced Labor Convention, 31
International Rice Research Institute
    (IRRI), 41, 42, 49, 243
IR5, IR8, IR22 and IR24 varieties of
    rice, 42, 44
Islam, 171, 172, 176
Izi Hoko Kai (Association of Indonesian
    Physicians), 178

Jakarta, ix, 12, 43, 172, 178, 179, 185,
    188–93, 199, 211, 244, 246, 251,
    256, 259–64
Japan, 3, 7, 11, 20, 26, 28, 36, 37, 44,
    55, 71, 74, 78, 79, 88, 89, 91, 123,
    135, 139, 140, 149, 160, 168, 178,
    179, 205, 215, 217–21, 224, 228,
    230, 233, 234–7, 247, 252–4, 268
Japanese imperialism/colonialism/
    empire, 7, 215, 218, 230
Japanese occupation, 26, 36, 37, 49, 55,
    74, 78, 79, 168, 178, 179, 253